MANUAL OF
ORTHOPEDIC ANESTHESIA
and
RELATED PAIN SYNDROMES

MANUAL OF
ORTHOPEDIC ANESTHESIA
and
RELATED PAIN SYNDROMES

Ralph L. Bernstein, M.D.
Chairman
Department of Anesthesiology
Hospital for Joint Diseases Orthopaedic Institute
New York, New York

Andrew D. Rosenberg, M.D.
Vice Chairman
Department of Anesthesiology
Hospital for Joint Diseases Orthopaedic Institute
Instructor
Department of Anesthesiology
New York University School of Medicine
New York, New York

With illustrations by Stan Waine

Churchill Livingstone
New York, Edinburgh, London, Madrid, Melbourne, Tokyo

Library of Congress Cataloging-in-Publication Data

Bernstein, Ralph L.
   Manual of orthopedic anesthesia and related pain syndromes / Ralph
  L. Bernstein, Andrew D. Rosenberg ; with illustrations by Stan
  Waine.
      p. cm.
  Includes bibliographical references and index.
  ISBN 0-443-08843-8
  1. Anesthesia in orthopedics.   I. Rosenberg, Andrew D.
  II. Title.
   [DNLM: 1. Anesthesia—methods. 2. Orthopedics—methods. WO 200
  B531m 1993]
  RD751.B47 1993
  617.9 ' 673—dc20
  DNLM/DLC
  for Library of Congress   93-26437
                                                 CIP

Distributed in the United Kingdom by Churchill Livingstone, Robert Stevenson House, 1–3 Baxter's Place, Leith Walk, Edinburgh EH1 3AF, and by associated companies, branches, and representatives throughout the world.

Accurate indications, adverse reactions, and dosage schedules for drugs are provided in this book, but it is possible that they may change. The reader is urged to review the package information data of the manufacturers of the medications mentioned.

The Publishers have made every effort to trace the copyright holders for borrowed material. If they have inadvertently overlooked any, they will be pleased to make the necessary arrangements at the first opportunity.

Acquisitions Editor: *Nancy Mullins*
Copy Editor: *Lorene K. Johnson*
Production Supervisor: *Patricia McFadden*
Cover Design: *Regina Dahir*

Printed in the United States of America

First published in 1993   7 6 5 4 3 2 1

To my wife, Trudy
and my children, Susan, Ken, Thomas,
Marcy, Paul, Patty, and David.

R.L.B.

To my wife, Maris,
my children, Gabe, Shira, and Alexa,
and my parents.

To my teacher,
Dr. Herman Turndorf.

A.D.R.

Preface

We decided to write the *Manual of Orthopedic Anesthesia and Related Pain Syndromes* after a number of anesthesiologists approached us at national meetings to tell us how our lectures on scoliosis and rheumatoid arthritis, our scientific exhibits, and our nerve block course have helped them pass their boards and enhanced their practice of anesthesiology. Our goal in writing this manual is to provide our readers with a how-to approach based not only on scientific principles but also on our clinical experience gained from the care of patients at the Hospital for Joint Diseases Orthopaedic Institute. While to us some situations such as atlantoaxial subluxation or an infraclavicular block for hand surgery are common, they may be less frequently encountered by other practitioners. We have emphasized this how-to approach by describing anesthetic management techniques and by including specific case studies when appropriate. Since most anesthesiologists deal with patients requiring orthopedic surgery this book has a universal appeal.

The chapter Regional Anesthesia is almost a book in itself. It is complete with detailed drawings and descriptions of all the nerve blocks used in orthopedic surgery. Step-by-step instructions are presented to help facilitate the performance of nerve blocks with the use of the nerve stimulator.

A separate chapter is devoted to the care of the patient with a fractured hip since most anesthesiologists have to contend with this problem.

Problems related to total joint replacement with the various intraoperative changes relating to the use of cement and thromboembolism are addressed.

Since many orthopedic procedures are performed with tourniquets, the proper use of these devices as well as the physiological alterations that occur when they are used are presented. The intraoperative and postoperative complications seen with tourniquets are outlined.

In the chapters Scoliosis and Spinal Surgery the latest techniques in spinal cord monitoring are presented. In addition, positioning, methods of decreasing blood loss, and complications are also addressed.

Pediatric Orthopedics will help guide the practitioner through the difficulties of managing these complex surgical procedures in small children.

Ambulatory Surgery is written with an eye on how to do the surgery and how to get the patient home.

In the chapter Trauma we bring the anesthesiologist into the trauma slot of the emergency room where he is confronted with the patient with cervical spine injuries requiring airway management. Techniques to avoid the well-known pitfalls are discussed. We also tell you how to manage the patient in the operating room after initial care in the emergency room.

Postoperative pain management with patient controlled analgesia, epidural narcotics, and epidural infusions are explained and the protocols for the institution of these techniques are detailed.

We have included the chapter Rheumatological Disorders and Other Medical Conditions so that the anesthesiologist can understand the pathophysiology of some of the diseases that are associated with orthopedic problems.

The chapter Common Pain Syndromes is presented in order for the anesthesiologist to be able to diagnose and treat conditions such as back pain, reflex sympathetic dystrophy, and meralgia paresthetica among others.

In this book we have attempted to fill a need expressed to us by many individuals as illustrated in the following letter:

"During a discussion in a recent morbidity and mortality conference, your name was brought up by several staff members, myself included, as we discussed the management of the patient with severe rheumatoid arthritis. Those of us who have been lucky enough to hear your lecture on this subject have remembered your teaching ever since. I would like to extend an invitation to you to speak to our department."

Through this manual we hope to speak to everyone.

Ralph L. Bernstein, M.D.
Andrew D. Rosenberg, M.D.

Acknowledgments

We wish to thank our editor Nancy Mullins, Eleanor DeSoto for her tireless work in preparing the manuscript, copyeditors Bridgett Dickinson and Lorene Johnson, Stan Waine of the Medical Multimedia Corporation for his beautiful illustrations, and the anesthesiologists in our department who gave us encouragement and advice.

Contents

1. **Rheumatologic Disorders and Other Medical Conditions**   1

2. **Trauma**   43

3. **The Fractured Hip**   91

4. **Total Joint Replacement**   115

5. **Thromboembolism**   151

6. **Regional Anesthesia**   161

7. **Tourniquets**   243

8. **Special Considerations in Surgery of the Extremities**   257

9. **Ambulatory Surgery**   269

10. **Pediatric Orthopedics**   293

11. **Scoliosis**   339

12. **Spinal Surgery**   379

13. **Orthopedic Oncology**   405

14. **Postoperative Pain**   421

15. **Common Pain Syndromes**   447

Index   505

1

Rheumatologic Disorders and Other Medical Conditions

RHEUMATOID ARTHRITIS

Rheumatoid arthritis is a generalized disease in which there are inflammatory changes in the connective tissues of the body.[1] The arthritic changes characteristic of the disease show a symmetric distribution involving the joints, with a chronic proliferative inflammation of the synovial membrane that produces irreversible damage to the joint capsule and articular cartilage. Changes in synovial tissue occur that lead to swelling, hypertrophy, and pannus formation. Granulation tissue develops, which is converted into fibrous scar tissue. This layer of granulation tissue is derived from the synovial membrane and extends over the surface of the cartilage with erosion and destruction of the cartilage. As the granulation tissue is converted into scar tissue, fibrous ankylosis, subluxation, and distortion of the joint causes the deformities characteristic of the disease.[2]

Characteristics

Rheumatoid arthritis is not just a disease of joints (Fig. 1-1).

Bones, Muscles, and Skin

Besides destructive changes in joints, atrophy occurs in bones, muscles, and skin adjacent to the joints. The muscles become atrophic, and the skin over the affected parts is thin, tight, and glossy.

Subcutaneous Nodules

Subcutaneous nodules occur in 20 to 30 percent of patients at some time during the disease[1] and are considered the most characteristic lesion of rheumatoid arthritis. They are often located over bony prominences but can arise in any connective tissue in the body.

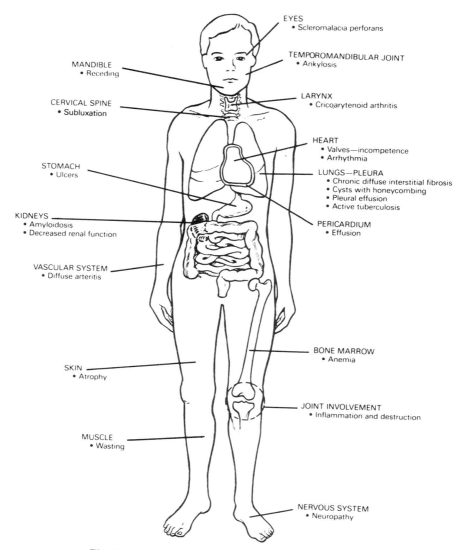

Fig. 1-1. Systemic effects of rheumatoid arthritis.

Cardiac Involvement

Granulomatous involvement of the heart valves and cardiac muscle can produce valvular incompetence and arrhythmias.

Pericarditis and pericardial effusion may be present.

Amyloidosis and focal vasculitis may cause myocardial damage.[2]

Pulmonary Disease

Patients with rheumatoid arthritis suffer from specific pulmonary lesions.[2]

The lesions are rheumatoid nodules, chronic diffuse interstitial pulmonary fibrosis, and cysts with honeycombing of the lungs.

A condition in coal miners known as Caplan syndrome is a lesion seen with pneumoconiosis in rheumatoid lung disease.

Active tuberculosis associated with rheumatoid arthritis may be seen in rheumatoid patients treated with steroids.

Pleural effusion may also be present.

Thoracic Wall Involvement

Chest wall expansion may be limited because of costochondral involvement as well as flexion deformity of the thoracic vertebrae. This condition in association with the pulmonary changes may lead to decreased compliance, diminished diffusing capacity, and diminished arterial oxygen saturation.

Hematologic Disease

These patients frequently suffer from a hypochromic microcytic anemia. This anemia may be due to bleeding from an ulcer secondary to steroid and acetylsalicylic acid therapy. Iron therapy is not successful in improving the hematocrit value, and transfusion is required to raise it.[3]

Because of alterations in immunoglobulins, a hyperviscosity syndrome may occur due to macromolecular polymers.[1] A bleeding diathesis associated with the syndrome may be present leading to epistaxis, petechiae, and purpura. Retinopathy and neurologic deficits may be associated with the hyperviscosity syndrome.

Immunologic Alterations

Rheumatoid disease is associated with an increased frequency of infection and possibly neoplasia. Patients display defects in both the humoral and the cellular components of the immune response.[2] Many different antibodies may be detected in these patients, including immunoglobulins, autologous and heterologous IgG, nuclear antigens, extracellular matrix protein, and B-cell antigens induced by the Epstein-Barr virus. These findings are nonspecific but indicate the potential scope of the humoral derangements.

Increased Risk for Infection

All cell types of the immune system have been demonstrated to function abnormally in association with rheumatoid disease. There is a marked increase in the number of T lymphocytes, and functional T-cell abnormalities have been reported. Neutrophile chemotaxis is diminished, and complement metabolism may be altered. This combination of factors puts patients with rheumatoid arthritis at an increased risk of opportunistic infection. Infection is more apt to occur in those patients with Felty syndrome, which is arthritis associated with splenomegaly and leukopenia.[2]

Renal Problems

Renal function is impaired. The reduction in function is directly proportional to the duration of the disease and may be related to amyloidosis. Creatinine clearance is altered by the impairment.[4]

Arteritis

Vascular lesions may occur with a diffuse arteritis that may be indistinguishable from polyarteritis nodosa.

Scleromalacia Perforans

The eye may be involved with a condition known as scleromalacia perforans, which is a complication of rheumatoid nodules developing in the sclera.[2]

Treatment

Treatment of rheumatoid arthritis includes rest, relief of pain with analgesics, physical measures, and orthopedic surgical procedures. Of particular importance are the side effects of the specific medications used in the treatment of rheumatoid arthritis (Table 1-1).

The Airway

Considerations in securing and maintaining the airway include

Ankylosis of the temporomandibular joint may be present leading to decreased mouth opening.

The distance between the upper and lower teeth should be measured with the mouth fully open. The mouth should be able to be opened to at least 5 cm (i.e., about three fingers).

A receding chin with a hypoplastic mandible (caused by early closure of the mandibular ossification centers usually seen in juvenile rheumatoid arthritis) can be detected by examining the patient in the lateral profile.[2] The upper teeth are seen to extend farther than the lower ones.

Table 1-1. Commonly Used Medications and Potential Side Effects

Medication	Side Effects
Gold	Rash, dermatitis, stomatitis Proteinuria, renal damage, bone marrow depression
Penicillamine	Fever, rash Hematuria, proteinuria Pemphigus, myasthenia gravis Goodpasture syndrome Lupus, jaundice
Plaquenil	Eye problems Central nervous system problems Bone marrow depression
Salicylates	Gastrointestinal bleeding, tinnitus Hepatitis, renal damage
Nonsteroidal anti-inflammatory drugs (NSAIDs)	Gastrointestinal ulceration and bleeding Platelet dysfunction Decrease in renal blood flow Renal failure Hepatic dysfunction
Methotrexate	Hepatic toxicity Interstitial pneumonitis Bone marrow suppression Gastrointestinal ulceration and bleeding Avoid in renal insufficiency Aspirin and NSAIDs increase toxicity by slowing rate of excretion
Azathioprine	Nausea, vomiting Abdominal pain Hepatitis Reversible bone marrow depression
Cyclophosphamide (used in patients with severe vasculitis)	Alopecia Hemorrhagic cystitis Bone marrow depression Sterility Bladder cancer, other malignancies
Azulfidine	Methemoglobinemia

(Data from Bernstein and Rosenberg[1] and Rodman and Schumacher.[2])

Cricoarytenoid arthritis as a result of involvement of the joints in the larynx leads to pain on palpation of larynx and a history of snoring.[5]

The difficulty in visualizing the vocal cords, which results from the above-mentioned changes, is compounded by the destructive changes in the cervical spine, which can result in an unstable neck.

A controlled approach to securing the airway with the aid of a fiberoptic bronchoscope and adequate topical anesthesia has significantly decreased the trauma and the risk to patients with rheumatoid arthritis who have significant airway problems.

Cricoarytenoid Arthritis

Rheumatoid arthritis of the cricoarytenoid joint is fairly common. It is a true diarthroidal joint consisting of two cartilages moving freely on each other, a joint capsule, and a joint cavity lined with synovial membrane.[5-7]

Acute Stage

The signs of cricoarytenoid arthritis during the acute stage are

Acute inflammation

Feeling of fullness in the throat

Foreign body feeling

Pain on swallowing or speaking

Radiation of pain to the ears as a sign of vagal irritation

Hoarseness and stridor, which may be present because of swelling and fixation of the cords

Examination reveals

Bright red swelling of the arytenoid region

Tense mucosal surface

Swollen and red dorsal parts of the aryepiglottic fold and of the false and true cords

Decreased mobility of the cords

Pain elicited by pressure on the larynx and hyoid bone

Acute exacerbation of cricoarytenoid arthritis may even occur during cortisone treatment.

Stage of Remission

After the acute state, periods of symptom-free remission may occur.

Ankylotic Stage

The severity of the final ankylotic stage depends on the position in which the cords become fixed.

Fixation may present as occasional hoarseness or mild respiratory disturbance.

Stridor may occur and is usually noted during sleep. It is probably due to a loss of compensation that occurs when relaxation is present.

Cricoarytenoid arthritis may not become obvious because the general condition of the patient leads to decreased activity with a decrease in the demands on vocal and respiratory resources.

A history of snoring during sleep may be a result of cricoarytenoid arthritis.

Preoperative Evaluation

A history of refractory "asthma," dysphagia, laryngeal tenderness, hoarseness, inspiratory stridor, or dyspnea should lead one to suspect the possibility of cricoarytenoid arthritis in a patient with rheumatoid arthritis. If the diagnosis of cricoarytenoid arthritis is suspected, examination before elective general anesthesia by indirect laryngoscopy is important. The possibility of tracheotomy may have to be considered.

The presence of cricoarytenoid arthritis may be manifest after the patient is anesthetized and airway obstruction occurs. Problems may occur in the postoperative period because intubation may cause trauma to an already injured cricoarytenoid joint.[6] Patients may develop a problem 4 to 6 days after surgery when the danger of complications is normally considered diminished. They develop stridor, dyspnea, and cyanosis as well as hoarseness. In one case, the "attack" was misdiagnosed as asthma, although apparently successfully treated with theophylline only to recur later with cyanosis and loss of consciousness. This patient required emergency tracheotomy.

Cervical Spine Involvement

Instability of the cervical spine is caused by destruction of supporting ligamentous structures that are in close proximity to the synovium-containing joints of the cervical spine.

Involvement of the cervical vertebrae may lead to fixation and ankylosis of these structures, making movement difficult. Airway maintenance may become a serious problem and can make direct and indirect laryngoscopy impossible. This condition alone or in combination with cricoarytenoid arthritis, temporomandibular joint fixation, and a hypoplastic mandible increases the problems of general anesthesia and airway maintenance.

Changes in the Cervical Spine

Major changes in the cervical spine include atlantoaxial subluxation, subaxial subluxation, and superior migration of the odontoid (Fig. 1-2).

Atlantoaxial Subluxation

The *dens* or *odontoid process* of the axis is held in place against the anterior arch of the first cervical vertebrae by the *transverse axial ligament*[8] (Fig. 1-3A). In addition to the transverse axial ligament, other ligaments secure the

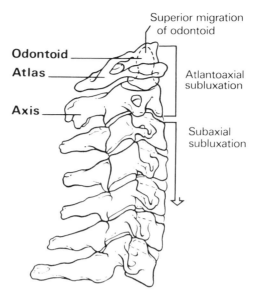

Fig. 1-2. Potential sites of cervical involvement of rheumatoid arthritis.

atlas and the axis to the skull. Apical ligaments attach the peak of the odontoid to the anterior edge of the foramen magnum, while superior and inferior longitudinal bands attach the atlas to the occiput above and the axis below. These ligaments together with the transverse ligaments form the cruciform ligament of the axis.

Laxity or disruption of this ligament by disease process leads to mobility of the odontoid within the spinal canal[9] (Fig. 1-3B).

In extension, the odontoid (dens) is held in position by the anterior arch of C1. In flexion, the odontoid may retain in its position while the arch of C1 and the spinal cord move anteriorly. This can endanger the spinal cord and is why flexion of the neck is an undesirable position (Fig. 1-4).

Steel's rule of thirds states that the odontoid, the spinal cord, and an empty or free space each occupy one-third of the space within the ring of the first cervical vertebrae.[8] This allows for some displacement without compromise to the spinal cord. When the transverse axial ligament is disrupted, the odontoid may move freely and impinge on the spinal cord (Fig. 1-3).

As the neck is moved, the atlas dens interval (ADI) will change. In extension, the dens remains fixed against the arch of C1 and the ADI is small. In flexion, the ADI increases and the safe area for the cord decreases. This may result in

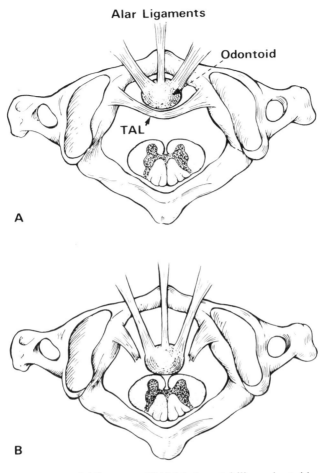

Fig. 1-3. (A) Transverse axial ligament (TAL) helps stabilize odontoid process against arch of C1, **(B)** Disruption of TAL allows free motion of odontoid and compression against cord.

a significant neurologic impairment (Fig. 1-4). Therefore, the neck should be kept in extension.

Evaluation of the Cervical Spine

Radiographs of the cervical spine in flexion and extension should be obtained in all patients with rheumatoid arthritis to determine the ADI. If it is greater than 3 to 4 mm in flexion, there may be neurologic problems.[1,2,10] *The head and neck in such a patient should be kept in extension during surgery.*

Radiographic examination may reveal a large degree of movement from flexion

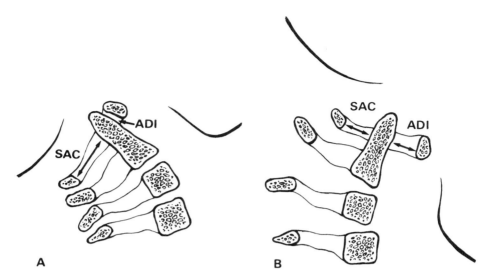

Fig. 1-4. (A) Extension view of cervical spine. In normal patients and many patients with rheumatoid arthritis, the arch of C1 is against odontoid process in extension. Atlas dens interval (ADI) is small, and the safe area of the cord (SAC) is adequate. **(B)** Flexion view of cervical spine. In patients with rheumatoid arthritis, odontoid process moves freely in spinal canal, and SAC decreases as ADI increases.

to extension, even though the patient is asymptomatic. Extreme caution must be used in caring for these patients.

Pathologic changes may result in compression of the second cervical nerve root, causing pain radiating into the neck and the occiput.

Neurologic changes may occur with radiating pain or paresthesias, long tract signs, posterior column dysfunction, and sphincter dysfunction, which indicate involvement of the spinal cord. These changes may progress to quadriparesis or quadriplegia.

Subaxial Subluxation

Subaxial subluxation is a condition in which there is subluxation occurring in two or more cervical vertebrae below the level of C2. Significant subaxial subluxation is considered present if the displacement of the superior on the inferior vertebrae measures 15 percent or more. Subaxial subluxation can cause significant impingement on the spinal cord[10] (Fig. 1-5).

Superior Migration of the Odontoid Process

Severe degrees of bone erosion in the cervical spine allow the odontoid process to migrate superiorly into the foramen magnum.[10] This may occur in conjunc-

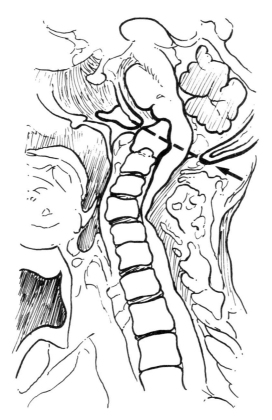

Fig. 1-5. Reconstruction of MRI demonstrating subaxial subluxation as well as superior migration of odontoid process. Note superior migration of odontoid into foramen magnum (designated as dotted line), which has resulted in impingement on medulla and pons. Also note spinal cord and narrowing in the subaxial region as a result of subluxation. (MRI courtesy of Malcolm Dobrow, M.D.)

tion with bone erosion itself or with some form of subaxial subluxation. Lateral magnetic resonance images (MRIs) are useful for noting the presence of the odontoid above the level of the foramen magnum (Fig. 1-5).

Changes in the cervical spine in rheumatoid arthritis may have an effect on the architecture of the larynx and trachea.[10] The semirigid trachea and larynx may become twisted as the result of shortening of the cervical spine, which occurs as alterations in the cervical vertebrae occur. When shortening of the cervical spine occurs, the trachea and larynx rotate because of the tethering effect of the arch of the aorta as it passes posteriorly over the left mainstem bronchus.[10]

Surgical Preparation

Patients undergo surgery for correction of deformities of joints that occur as a result of the arthritis and also for conditions that occur in the general population.

Medication History

Patients who are receiving acetylsalicylic acid therapy, which may interfere with platelet function, may bleed during surgery.

Those patients on steroid medication should have steroids administered before, during, and after surgery to maintain an adequate stress response.

Patients on immunosuppressive agents such as azathioprine may present with leukopenia or thrombocytopenia, macrocytic anemia, and bone marrow depression. Serious infections caused by fungal, viral, and bacterial, as well as protozoal, organisms can occur in patients who are immunosuppressed (Table 1-1).

Airway Evaluation

An evaluation of the airway should be made with an attempt to determine whether endotracheal intubation is possible or fiberoptic intubation is necessary. Upper airway evaluation includes examination of the temporomandibular joint and the mandible to determine the extent of mouth opening. It should be at least three fingers.

Cervical Spine Radiographs

Cervical spine radiographs with lateral views in flexion and extension to determine presence of atlantoaxial instability, subaxial subluxation, and measurements for superior migration of the odontoid process should be obtained.

Adequate History

Records of previous surgical procedures should be secured to determine the anesthetic management, the problems, if any, with intubation, and the postanesthetic course.

Neurologic Evaluation

A careful neurologic examination should be performed before anesthesia and surgery to determine whether any neurologic problems such as long tract signs exist as a result of cervical spine abnormalities.

Vertebral Artery Involvement

Some patients with cervical spine abnormalities may also have vertebral artery compression because these vessels ascend in the foramina transversaria of the cervical vertebrae.[2] Occasionally, a patient will complain of fainting on upward gaze secondary to vertebrobasilar artery insufficiency. Thrombosis of the vertebral artery may occur during surgery.

Other Preoperative Considerations

Pulmonary
> Radiographic findings (fibrosis, cysts with honeycombing, pleural effusion)
> Pulmonary function tests
> Blood gases

Cardiovascular
> Electrocardiogram
> Echocardiogram if valvular lesion or pericardial effusion suspected

Renal
> Urinalysis
> Creatinine clearance
> Blood urea nitrogen

Skin and subcutaneous tissues
> Fragile
> Problematic intravenous access
> Skin damaged by tape removal

Status of joints
> Ankylosis (interferes with positioning)

Hematologic
> Anemia (complete blood count)
> Evaluation of platelet function (bleeding time)

Bones
> Osteoporosis (possibility of fractures during positioning)

Steroids
> Possible steroid preparation

Medications
> Review and consideration of side effects

Endotracheal Intubation: Use of Fiberoptic Laryngoscope

Assessment of the airway and plans for securing endotracheal intubation should be made in advance. If fiberoptic intubation is contemplated, topicalization of the nose with cocaine 4 percent provides anesthesia and vasoconstriction, or if cocaine is not desirable, an anesthetic agent with neosynephrine may be used.

Anesthesia of the mouth and oral pharynx can then be performed with a topical anesthetic. The superior laryngeal nerves should be blocked as they pass near the cornua of the hyoid bone.

Transtracheal injections of local anesthetic provide anesthesia and decrease the hemodynamic responses associated with awake intubation.

A small amount of sedation with midazolam can be given during fiberoptic intubation. Oversedation should be avoided because control of the airway is not guaranteed. Supplemental oxygen should be administered, and a pulse oximeter should be connected to the patient.

We have found that most patients with rheumatoid arthritis are very cooperative when undergoing fiberoptic intubation. Once the airway is secured, the patient can receive general anesthesia.

If general anesthesia is planned with normal oral endotracheal intubation, the neck should be stabilized in extension while laryngoscopy and intubation are performed. This should only be performed if the anesthesiologist is certain the intubation is not difficult and if gross movements of the neck are not necessary.

Before extubation, the patient must be awake enough to maintain the airway. Extubation should be avoided in a patient who will subsequently require a "jaw thrust" or head manipulation to maintain or open the airway.

At the completion of surgery, the patient is observed for postoperative laryngeal problems.

Surgical Procedures

Upper Extremity Surgery

Reconstructive surgery of the hand and wrist is now common.

Regional anesthesia techniques can be used in surgery of the upper extremity, but they must be tailored to the patient's condition.

  Axillary block, which requires abduction of the shoulder to approximately 90 degrees, may not be possible in a patient with a severe shoulder deformity.

  Intravenous regional anesthesia may not be accepted by some surgeons who believe that swelling in the postoperative period will not be tolerated by the poor skin and soft tissue of the rheumatoid patient.

  Interscalene block is a technique that can be used for surgical procedures on the shoulder, hand, wrist, and elbow. This block can be performed in patients with problems in shoulder mobility because it does not require movement of the upper extremity.

Infraclavicular brachial plexus block is useful for surgical procedures on the hand and elbow (see Ch. 6).

Surgery of the Foot

Corrections of deformities of the forefoot lend themselves to ankle block. This block is performed by injecting at the level of the malleoli in the area of the dorsalis pedis pulse between the extensor hallucis longus and the tibialis anterior. Block of the posterior tibial nerve is performed at the level of the medial malleolus, between it and the Achilles tendon. The sural nerve can be blocked at the base of the fifth metatarsal (see Ch. 6).

Total Knee Replacement

Surgery is performed for pain, deformity, and instability of the knee as a result of joint destruction. Spinal or epidural anesthesia can be administered for this procedure. Appropriate padding should be provided because these patients may be quite uncomfortable lying on their backs for the duration of the surgical procedure.

Total Hip Replacement

Patients may develop aseptic necrosis of the femoral head, which may be secondary to corticosteroid therapy. Some patients may not stop acetylsalicylic acid therapy before surgery because they require it for pain relief. Acetylsalicylic acid given within a few days of surgery can lead to excessive bleeding because of its effect on platelets.

If regional anesthesia is chosen, these patients must be made as comfortable as possible during the procedure. Many surgeons perform total hip replacements with patients in the lateral decubitus position. Regional anesthesia techniques have the added advantage of allowing for the administration of spinal or epidural narcotics for postoperative pain relief.

Isobaric bupivicaine administered in the lateral decubitus position with the affected side up is an excellent technique because it does not require further positioning of the patient.

Hip replacement in patients with rheumatoid arthritis can be performed under general anesthesia as well.

General anesthesia with mild hypotension has been used in these patients with a decrease in blood loss and a diminished need for blood transfusions. The Cell Saver and postoperative reinfusion devices can diminish the need for homologous blood requirements (see Ch. 4).

Cervical Spine Surgery

Patients with abnormalities of the cervical spine may require surgical intervention. The decision to operate on patients with cervical spine pathology in rheumatoid arthritis is based on the presence of pain, radiographic deterioration, and neurologic changes.

Stabilization of the cervical spine by means of a properly fitting collar or the placement of the patient in a halo vest or halo traction may be necessary before surgery.

ANKYLOSING SPONDYLITIS

Ankylosing spondylitis (AS) is one of the seronegative spondyloarthropathies, and it is frequently associated with the HLA B-27 antigen.[2] Although there is a strong relationship with patients who have AS being HLA-positive (80 to 95 percent), only 2 percent of HLA B-27-positive patients develop AS.[11–13] There is a strong relationship between the development of AS in HLA B-27-positive first-degree relatives of HLA B-27-positive people who have AS (11 to 29 percent).[13]

AS is present in both men and women (4:1 ratio).[14]
The incidence is one to three per 1,000 people.[12]

Theories that exist concerning the relationship between HLA B-27 antigen and AS include

1. It is a genetic marker.
2. A specific bacterial infection may result in antibody formation that cross-reacts with the HLA B-27 molecule.
3. After an infection, cytotoxic T cells react with a peptide from articular tissue that has bound to HLA B-27 molecule (arthritogenic peptide model).[11]

Pathology

AS is mainly a disease of the sacroiliac joints and the spine with the appearance on radiograph of a "bamboo spine." The spinal involvement ascends from the lumbar area to the cervical spine. There is low back pain and early loss of spinal mobility. The progression of spinal changes leads to fixation of the spine in the lumbar, thoracic, and cervical areas. The degree of limitation of motion of the neck can range from a small degree to complete ankylosis.

Patients with complete ankylosis are at increased risk of sustaining a cervical fracture. These fractures may be difficult to diagnose or visualize on radiographs and should be suspected if the patient has a sudden increase in neck movement, with or without pain. These fractures commonly occur and result from a trivial or unrecognized injury, usually caused by hyperextension, and have most commonly been described in the lower cervical region. Recently, fractures of the dens have been reported in two patients with long-standing AS and pre-existing atlanto-occipital fusion.[15]

ANESTHETIC CONSIDERATIONS

Opening of the mouth may be restricted by temporomandibular joint arthritis.

Cricoarytenoid arthritis may be present, with pain on swallowing, hoarseness, stridor, and snoring at night.

Cervical Spine Involvement

The extent of cervical spine involvement and mobility must be evaluated. The cervical spine may be fixed in flexion or in neutral. Fixation in flexion is probably a result of multiple small fractures with healing in a flexed position. The cervical spine may show several types of fixation, from rigid fixation in a straight upright position to complete flexion of the neck with the mandible touching the sternum. A neck fixed in the "neutral" position may be extremely rigid and present a problem in intubation. Do not be fooled.

Cardiovascular Involvement

Valvular involvement[2]
   Aortic insufficiency and mitral regurgitation may occur.
   Echocardiography may help delineate the extent of involvement.

Conduction defects and *heart block* may require use of a pacemaker.

Cardiomegaly may be present.

Respiratory System Involvement

Limited chest wall expansion occurs because of ankylosis of thoracic vertebrae and costovertebral, costochondral, and sternomanubrial joint involvement. This produces a restrictive respiratory pattern.[2,14,16,17]

Ventilation may ultimately become dependent on diaphragmatic breathing, which may be manifested by slight hyperventilation with rapid, shallow breathing patterns.[14,16,17]

Apical fibrosis of the lungs may be noted in a few patients.[16]

Pulmonary function tests should be performed to evaluate the extent of pulmonary involvement. The presence of cough and sputum production must be determined and treated accordingly.

Neurologic Changes

Vertebrobasilar insufficiency has been noted.

Spinal stenosis may be present and lead to a cauda equina syndrome.

Anemia

A hypochromic microcytic anemia may be present secondary to the disease or as a result of occult gastrointestinal bleeding from anti-inflammatory agents.

Renal Function

Renal involvement from the use of anti-inflammatory agents may be present.

Conduct of Anesthesia

If any question exists concerning the status of the airway, general anesthesia should not be induced until endotracheal intubation has been accomplished. Caution must be exercised in moving the neck because extension may lead to fracture.[18]

Fiberoptic intubation is the most logical choice to secure and maintain the airway.

In one case, anesthesia for total hip replacement was performed using a mask and oral airway 2 weeks apart for replacement of each hip. Another case is reported in which all the front teeth were knocked out during attempted intubation after the administration of succinylcholine. The patient underwent hip replacements using a mask and oral airway.

Warning: Do not attempt this even though it is in the literature. Secure a proper airway first.

Position

After intubation, the head and neck should be moved and positioned carefully. Any undue stresses should be avoided. The neck may have to be kept in its original position and appropriately supported.

Warning: Do not let neck hang free.

Ventilation during Anesthesia

Because of the thoracic involvement and decreased chest excursion, there may be alterations in compliance, which may necessitate the use of high airway pressure to ensure adequate oxygenation and ventilation. Be on the alert for barotrauma.

Regional Anesthesia

Regional anesthesia for surgical procedures such as total hip replacement may be difficult because of the bony ankylosis and calcification of the spine.

Caudal anesthesia may be possible if the sacral hiatus is open.

Surgical Procedures

Total Hip Replacement

This procedure is performed to provide mobility in patients who have fixation of the hip joints. The flexion deformities of the hips are corrected before correction of spinal deformities.

If the procedure is to be performed in the lateral decubitus position, care must be taken to position the head and neck to avoid abnormal stresses that may result in fractures. The cervical spine must be kept in line with the thoracic spine, avoiding flexion or extension.

Intraoperative Problems during Joint Surgery

Extensive ankylosis of joints in flexion may lead to difficulties during the surgical procedure. Some of these difficulties involve the problem of traction on blood vessels after release of the flexed ankylosed joint. The blood vessels cannot be stretched to accommodate the new position. In some instances, shortening of the bones to accommodate this problem is performed.

Ankle Surgery

Some patients develop equinus deformities in the ankles and are treated by Achilles tendon lengthening with capsular releases.

Surgical Correction of Severe Flexion Deformity of the Cervical Spine

Osteotomies of the spine are performed to correct the severe flexion deformities.[19]

In the 1970s, some patients underwent cervical spine surgery under local anesthesia supplemented with nitrous oxide or narcotic analgesia with the patient awake so that intraoperative evaluation of neurologic function could be carried out.[19]

With the advent of fiberoptic endotracheal intubation and somatosensory evoked potential monitoring, awake osteotomies are not necessary because securing and maintaining the airway can be carried out and monitoring of spinal cord function can be evaluated intraoperatively as the surgical procedure progresses (see Ch. 12).

SYSTEMIC LUPUS ERYTHEMATOSUS

Systemic lupus erythematosus (SLE)[2,7] is characterized by inflammatory changes in blood vessels and connective tissues of many organs of the body. These vascular reactions lead to destructive changes in different organs.

Females are affected more often than males by a ratio of 8:1.

Many of these cases present in childhood.

SLE is characterized by an altered immune response, possibly determined by genetic factors.

The disease may be exacerbated by infections, pregnancy, and sunlight.

Manifestations

Skin Involvement

A butterfly rash over the nose and cheeks is frequently seen. The rash may extend over other parts of the body.[2]

Joint Involvement

Arthritis may involve the hands, wrists, elbows, shoulders, knees, and ankles. Avascular necrosis of the femoral head can occur.

Cardiac Involvement

Myocarditis with cardiomegaly, congestive heart failure, arrhythmias, pericarditis, and endocarditis of the mitral valve may occur.[2,7]

Pulmonary Involvement

Pleural effusions, pneumonia, pulmonary infiltrates, and fibrosis may be seen in SLE.[2,7]

Central Nervous System Involvement

Cerebral vascular accidents, psychiatric manifestations, and peripheral neuropathies may be seen.[2,7]

Neurologic Changes

Psychosis may be manifested as a schizophrenic type of reaction.

Organic brain syndrome with inability to perform simple tasks, loss of orientation of time and place, and seizures may occur.

Cranial nerve palsies, major motor weakness, and peripheral neuropathy occur frequently.

Chorea, transverse myelopathy, and aseptic meningitis may be seen.

Migraine headache may be a symptom of active lupus.[2,7]

Gastrointestinal Involvement

Vasculitis involving the gastrointestinal tract can lead to abdominal pain, vomiting, diarrhea, and possibly infarction of the bowel. Hepatosplenomegaly may be present.[2,7]

Hematology

Anemia, leukopenia, thrombocytopenia, and coagulation disorders may occur.[2,7]

Renal Involvement

Significant renal pathology can develop.[2,7]

Anesthetic Considerations

Airway

Changes in the mucosa of the nose or mouth may lead to problems with airway insertion and endotracheal intubation.

Pulmonary System

The extent of the disease must be determined by means of a chest radiograph and arterial blood gases.

Cardiac System

If patients have evidence of endocarditis, antibotic prophylaxis should be administered. If patients have carditis, agents that cause myocardial depression must be avoided. The anesthesiologists should confer with the rheumatologist and surgeon before the operative procedure and develop a plan of management.[2,7]

Renal System

Patients may exhibit significant degrees of renal insufficiency.[7] Agents that rely on kidney function for excretion should be avoided.

Cross-Matching

Antibodies to red blood cells may make cross-matching of blood a problem.

Drug-Related Lupus-like Syndromes

Drugs such as hydralazine, procainamide, and antiepileptic medication have been implicated in their ability to induce a lupus-like syndrome.[2,7]

ACROMEGALY

Pathophysiology

Secretion of growth hormone after puberty results in general overgrowth of skeletal, soft tissue, and connective tissues.[2,20]

Manifestations

There is an increase in the size of the mandible.

The tongue and epiglottis may become enlarged and lead to upper airway obstruction and difficulty in intubation.

Arthropathy or widespread arthralgias, or both, may be present.

Carpal tunnel syndrome may be present.

Problems with the feet are seen because of the abnormal growth of bones.

Back pain is a feature because of the changes in the axial skeleton.[2,20]

Cardiovascular Involvement

Hypertension, arrhythmias, and conduction defects as a result of the effects of the alterations of lipid and carbohydrate metabolism on the cardiac system

Atherosclerosis and heart failure

Left ventricular hypertrophy, ST segment depression, and T-wave abnormalities

Cardiomegaly

Echocardiography revealing increased size of all chambers of the heart with cardiomyopathy[2,20]

Other Systemic Disorders

Diabetes

Hypertension

Anesthetic Considerations

Securing and maintaining an airway may be difficult because of the enlarged mandible, enlarged tongue, and alterations in the oropharynx. Endotracheal intubation should be secured before administration of anesthetics and muscle relaxants.

Fiberoptic intubation may be necessary.[2,20]

Cardiovascular System

Attention must be paid to changes in the cardiovascular system. Anesthetic agents that cause myocardial depression because of the cardiomyopathy should be avoided.[2,20]

General Anesthesia

General anesthesia may be used when indicated.

Spinal or Epidural Anesthesia

Needles of appropriate length should be available if spinal or epidural anesthesia is to be used in patients with large body habitus.

OSTEITIS DEFORMANS: PAGET'S DISEASE OF BONE

Osteitis deformans is a disorder characterized by excessive resorption and formation of bone with extensive local vascularity and increased fibrous tissue in the adjacent marrow.[1,2,21]

This disease occurs in persons older than 45 years of age.[2,22]

Men tend to predominate (3:2 ratio).[22]

The disease may be familial, with 15 percent of patients in the United States having a family history.[22]

A viral etiology may be important in Paget's disease.

Pathology

The pathology involves an intense resorption of bone followed by the deposition of new abnormal bone. The marrow is replaced by loose fibrous connective tissues that appear hypervascular. The bone is poor in structural integrity, is often deformed, and is prone to pathologic fractures.

Sarcoma may develop at the site of pagetic involvement (0.9 to 20 percent).[22]

Sites of Involvement

Common sites of involvement are the spine, pelvis, skull, femur, and tibia.[2]

Manifestations

Osseous Structures

Pain in involved areas

Gross deformities

Pathologic fractures

High-Output Cardiac Failure

The increased vascularity, if extensive, may contribute to the development of high-output cardiac failure. This is due to the many vascular channels in the multiple areas of bone resorption and bone replacement. These areas become extensive arteriovenous fistulas with increased perfusion and a high cardiac output. The heart rate should not be slowed with β-blockers because the tachycardia is a result of the high-output state.

Aortic Valve Calcification

Aortic valve calcification was found on autopsy specimens to be more prevalent than in the general population. More significant calcification and decreased mobility of the aortic valve was noted in patients with more severe Paget's disease. Conduction abnormalities may be present.

Calcification of interventricular septum was also noted at autopsy.[23]

Auditory

Deafness may result from involvement of the small bones of the ear or by compression of the nerves.[2]

Neurologic Changes

Spinal involvement may lead to neural compression with radicular pain.

Joint Involvement

The hip joint may be involved with extensive degenerative changes secondary to the involvement of the subchondral bone.

The knees may become involved in a similar manner. The tibia may develop the classical "saber sword" appearance.

Anesthetic Considerations

Regional anesthesia can be considered.

Note: Involvement of spinal and peripheral nerves by compression can occur.

SCLERODERMA

Scleroderma (progressive systemic sclerosis [PSS])[2,7] is a connective tissue disease involving skin, joints, internal organs, and muscle. Skin thickening and induration are classic signs of the disease.[24]

Incidence

More frequent in women aged 40 to 50 years[2,24]

Female/male ratio of 3:1

Possible genetic predisposition[24]

Manifestations

Skin Involvement

The skin of the hands and feet initially appears puffy and swollen.[2,7,24]

Over time, the skin becomes tight and shiny and loses its normal contours, lines, and wrinkles.

Changes in the skin of the face lead to a mask-like appearance.[7]

Raynaud's Phenomenon

Raynaud's phenomenon may be the initial presentation of PSS and may be present for many years before other symptoms occur. Raynaud's disease is characterized by intermittent decreased blood flow to the fingers. After long-term disease, the fingers may become markedly ischemic with ulceration and gangrene.[2,7,24]

Problems with the Mouth

Mouth opening may be limited because of skin changes.

Esophageal Problems

Marked abnormality in structure and function occur in the esophagus. Esophageal strictures can occur, as can reflux and esophagitis.

Decreased motility and peristalsis can result in inability to swallow food, which may remain lodged in the esophagus.[2,7,24]

Warning: Watch out for regurgitation under anesthesia.

Pulmonary Problems

Many patients complain of shortness of breath on exertion. Pulmonary fibrosis and pulmonary hypertension occur. Pulmonary function testing demonstrates decreased vital capacity, decreased lung volume, and decreased diffusing capacity. Pulmonary hypertension is a major contributing factor to morbidity.[2,7,25,26]

Cardiac Involvement

Cardiac manifestations include

1. Myocardial fibrosis
2. Left ventricular hypertrophy
3. Arrhythmias and conduction abnormalities[7,27]

Renal Disease

Involvement of the kidney can lead to renal insufficiency and marked hypertension with associated systemic side effects.[2,7]

Anesthetic Management

Mouth opening may be limited, making fiberoptic intubation necessary. The patient should not be anesthetized until an airway has been secured.[7]

Airway

Endotracheal intubation by means of fiberoptic broncoscopy in the awake patient placed in the head-up position may be the technique of choice in securing an adequate airway before surgery.

Esophageal Problems

Regurgitation of gastric and esophageal contents may lead to aspiration. These patients should be pretreated with H2 blockers (e.g., ranitidine). The airway must be secured before induction so that the patient does not aspirate.

If there is marked dilatation of the esophagus with retained fluid or possibly food, these drugs may not be successful in preventing aspiration or its complications. Only an awake intubation can prevent the problem.

Hypertension

Hypertension may be present as a result of renal disease.

Pulmonary Considerations

Pulmonary function should be evaluated preoperatively with pulmonary function tests and arterial blood gases.

Circulatory Hemodynamics

These patients may have a low intravascular volume secondary to their vascular disorder.

Arterial Punctures

Note: Arterial punctures for intraoperative blood pressure monitoring or blood gas analysis should be avoided because this procedure may lead to arterial insufficiency.

Case Study

A zealous anesthesiologist *finally* performed arterial cannulation after many attempts only to find that the hand remained poorly perfused for several days after the procedure. Blood flow to the hand finally was re-established, but there were a few sleepless nights in the interim.

Noninvasive blood pressure monitors should be used in this condition. Undue pressure or relatively increased heat may cause injury to skin. Pay attention when a pulse oximeter is used. *Change fingers frequently.*

Regional Anesthesia

Eisele[7] suggested avoiding epinephrine in peripheral nerve blocks because its use may cause problems in circulation to the extremity.

Avoid oversedation because patients

1. Are at risk to aspirate
2. May require being fully awake to ventilate adequately

Postoperative Care in the Postanesthesia Care Unit

The patient should be kept warm. Warming of the skin by direct contact with hot objects should be avoided because this may increase the metabolism of the skin in the areas of poor perfusion.

Ventilatory Support

Ventilatory support in the recovery room may be necessary because of the poor lung and chest wall compliance.

Extubation should be performed when the patient is completely awake and able to breathe adequately. Excessive narcotics and sedatives should be avoided.

ALCOHOLISM

Alcoholism is a major cause of avascular necrosis of the head or the femur.

Hypotension should be avoided to protect the liver.

It should be determined whether patients are in an acute alcoholic state when admitted to the hospital.

The possibility of delerium tremens should be considered.

MARFAN SYNDROME

Marfan syndrome (arachnodactyly) is a congenital defect that affects both sexes equally. The basic defect is the inability to manufacture normal elastin fibers of collagen.

Clinical Features

Tall patients, with long and thin limbs

Pectus excavatum or pectus carinatum

High arched palate

Prognathism

Kyphoscoliosis (increases rapidly during years of rapid vertebral growth)

Diaphragmatic, femoral, and inguinal hernias caused by decreased muscle tone

Dislocation of the lens

Joint dislocation[20,28]

Cardiovascular System

Aortic or mitral insufficiency, or both (echocardiogram determines valvular status)

Dilatation of the ascending aorta

Septal defects

Dissecting aortic aneurysm as a result of weakness of aortic wall (β-blocking agents decrease force of ejection)

Mitral valve prolapse (antibiotic prophylaxis should be considered)

Pulmonary System

Decrease in elastic tissue

Early airway closure

Bronchogenic cysts

Emphysema

Pneumothorax (be careful during positive pressure ventilation)[20,28]

Anesthetic Considerations

The high arched palate may cause difficulties in endotracheal intubation. The patient should be examined before anesthesia to determine if fiberoptic intubation is necessary.

Excess traction with laryngoscope that could result in temporomandibular dislocation should be avoided.

Patients should be kept on β-blocking agents to control heart rate and to decrease force of ejection.

Care should be taken in positioning to avoid joint dislocation.[28]

Inhalation agents should be used alone or in conjunction with narcotics to reduce the velocity of left ventricular contraction to avoid high ejection pressures on the wall of the ascending aorta.

Vasodilators alone must not be administered to control blood pressure. Left ventricular ejection velocity may be increased. These agents must be combined with β-blockers.

The patient should be kept adequately anesthetized to avoid sudden increases in myocardial contractility.[20,29]

NEUROFIBROMATOSIS

Neurofibromatosis (Von Recklinghausen's disease) results from abnormal growths of neural tissue throughout the body.

Diagnosis

Presence of café au lait spots, cutaneous hyperpigmentation, and cutaneous neurofibromas indicates the diagnosis.

Clinical Findings

Café au lait spots

Elephantiasis, cutaneous, and subcutaneous neurofibromas

Kyphoscoliosis of thoracic area[30]

Central nervous system tumors

Neurofibromas in airway resulting in possible obstruction (evaluate carefully before administering anesthesia)[31-35]

Interstitial fibrosis

Cervical spine involvement with atlantoaxial dislocation

Hypertension (neurofibromatosis may be associated with pheochromocytoma)[31-35]

Paraplegia

Patients may develop paraplegia because of destruction of vertebral bodies by neurofibromatous tissue. Traction may result in reversal of paraplegia and should be used only in patients with flexible kyphosis.

Anesthetic Considerations

Hypertension should be controlled before surgery.

Cervical spine involvement may require special attention before intubation.

Airway must be evaluated for presence of lesions.

Kyphosis may lead to pulmonary dysfunction.[32-35]

SICKLE CELL DISEASE

In sickle cell disease, there is a substitution of valine for glutamate at position 6 in the β chain. When a red blood cell (RBC) containing sickle cell hemoglobin becomes desaturated, it alters from the usual oval shape of RBCs to resemble a sickle. The sickle cell (1) may not revert back to its normal shape, (2) being more rigid than normal RBCs, it may get blocked in capillaries, and (3) large clumps or aggregates of sickle cells may obstruct blood flow and result in end-organ damage to the kidneys, spleen, liver, lungs, brain, bones, and heart.[36–38]

Hemoglobin S (HbS) in the presence of other abnormal hemoglobins such as hemoglobin C (HbC) and the β-thalassemia type may show sickling tendencies under appropriate clinical conditions.[36–38]

Manifestations

Children with sickle cell anemia have bone infarcts and osteomyelitis.

Bone development is significantly retarded.

Avascular necrosis of bone affects growing ends of long bones.

Destruction of the femoral head occurs.

Infections

Patients are susceptible to infection. Pneumococcal septicemia and meningitis have been major causes of death.

Prophylactic penicillin has been found to prevent severe pneumoccocal infections.[37]

Neurologic Considerations

Cerebral thrombosis may occur as early as 3 years of age.

Transcranial Doppler ultrasonography is useful in detecting patients who may benefit from transfusion therapy in an attempt to avert cerebral thrombosis.[39]

Osteomyelitis

Salmonella is frequently the causative organism in sickle cell osteomyelitis.

Cardiac Involvement

Severe anemia may lead to abnormal stress on the cardiovascular system, with a rise in cardiac output during exercise.

Pulmonary Involvement

Patients may have frequent respiratory infections or pulmonary infarction.[36–38,40]

Renal Disease

Polyuria, hematuria, or glomerulonephritis may be present. End-stage renal disease may occur, necessitating dialysis or renal transplantation.[36–38,40]

Surgical Preparation

Transfusion Therapy

Different methods exist in how to transfuse patients, if it is necessary, before surgery.[36–38,40,41]

It is desirable to lower HbS levels to less than 45 percent before surgery. Some suggest that levels of 30 percent of HbS or lower be obtained. This can be achieved by transfusion of normal blood.

Direct Transfusion

Transfusion of packed cells to lower the percentage of HbS to less than 45 percent is recommended preoperatively. Transfusion should be carried out over a period of days, not the night before surgery.

Patients are usually anemic and need transfusions to raise the hemoglobin and hematocrit values.

Exchange Transfusion

Exchange transfusion may be helpful to achieve a better rheologic fluid by removing the easily deformed HbS erythrocytes.

Problems of antibodies may exist. It may be difficult to obtain blood with low titers of antigens.

The Montreal Childrens Hospital follows an algorithm for preoperative preparation for surgery for children[41] (Table 1-2).

Table 1-2. Transfusion Algorithm for Patients with Sickle Cell Disease

Condition	Hb Type	Hb Level	Type of Procedure	Transfuse	Aim (%)
Sickle cell trait	HbAs	Normal	All types	No	
Sickle cell anemia	HbSS	Low	Minor surgery	Transfuse	Hct 30–36
Sickle cell anemia	HbSS	Low	Major	Exchange transfuse	Hct 30–36
Sickle cell anemia	HbSC	Low	All types	Exchange transfuse	HbS ≤30
	S-β thalassemia	Low	All	Transfuse	

Abbreviations: Hb, hemoglobin; Hct, hematocrit.
(Modified from Esseltine et al.[41] with permission.)

Transfusion Recommendation

Consultation with a hematologist should be carried out. The preoperative treatment should be determined by the needs of the patient.

Patients with sickle cell trait with normal hemoglobin values are usually not given blood transfusions.

In patients with sickle cell disease (HbSS) with significant anemia, a simple transfusion may be required to elevate the hemoglobin for patients undergoing even minor surgery.

For major procedures, a partial exchange transfusion to a hematocrit value of 30 to 36 percent with a HbS level at 30 percent or less is desirable.

In sickle cell-hemoglobin C disease or hemoglobin S-β-thalassemia, a partial exchange transfusion to a hematocrit value of 30 to 36 percent and a HbS level to 30 percent or less is performed.[36–38,40,41]

Adequate Hydration

Adequate hydration is necessary to decrease the viscosity of the blood and to prevent sludging.

Infection

Adequate evaluation and treatment should be carried out to have the patient free of infection.

Folic Acid

Patients with sickle cell disease usually develop folate deficiencies and should receive folic acid therapy routinely.

Preoperative Visit

The use of sedatives and narcotics should be avoided to prevent hypoventilation and hypoxia.

Anesthetic Management

The patient should be positioned so that there are no areas with undue pressure.

Tourniquets should be avoided if at all possible.[42]

Complete exsanguination may not be possible, leaving trapped RBCs that may sickle. On release of the tourniquet, acid products enter the circulation that may possibly cause sickling.

Low flow states and vena cava or lower extremity compression also must be avoided.

Situations that Might Induce Sickling

Hypotension: Maintain blood pressure in normal range.

Hypercarbia: Ventilate adequately—follow $PaCO_2$ with $ETCO_2$ monitor.

Hypoxia: Ensure adequate FIO_2—monitor with pulse oximeter.

Hypothermia: Warm operating room and IV fluids.

Hypovolemia: Avoid vasoconstriction.

Anesthetic Technique

No one anesthetic technique is beneficial over any other in patients with sickle cell disease. Increased oxygen concentration should be administered. Pulse oximetry is used to ensure adequate oxygen saturation. The patient should be kept warm, adequately hydrated, and adequately ventilated to prevent hypoxia and hypercarbia.

Regional Anesthesia

If regional anesthesia is used, hypotension and hypothermia should be avoided.

Adequate hydration is important, so vasoconstriction is avoided in areas not receiving regional anesthesia.[40]

Surgical Procedures

Total Hip Replacement

Avascular necrosis of the femoral head may require total hip replacement. Because this is elective surgery, adequate preparation of the patient should be carried out.

Regional or general anesthesia can be used as long as all precautions are taken. Hypotensive anesthesia is not used.

One hundred percent oxygen is administered during reaming and during cementing to avoid hypoxia.

Adequate intraoperative fluid replacement is ensured so that hypotension does not occur during cement insertion. Blood is replaced as needed to maintain adequate oxygen carrying capacity.

Blood Salvage Devices

Blood salvage devices *should not be used* in patients with sickle cell disease because sickling occurs during the processing of the blood. Postoperative rein-fusion devices should not be used.

Cell Saver Use

In one report by Brajtbord,[43] it was pointed out that there was a massive amount of sickling seen in the processed blood from a patient with sickle cell trait. It was noted that blood drawn from the reservoir immediately after processing was severely affected with sickling, which was attributed to the Cell Saver washing process.[43]

In another report, a patient with homozygous sickle cell disease received intra-operative autotransfusion of processed blood. This patient had a rare blood type because of extensive isoimmunization to donor cells or HLA antigens. Because this patient had HbSS disease, preoperative exchange transfusions removed 1,800 ml of blood and replaced it with 9 units of homologous packed RBCs. The HbS went down to 25 percent and the HbA went up to 71 percent. The preoperative hemoglobin concentration was 11.5 g. Before the administra-tion of the autologous blood obtained from the intraoperative autotransfusion device, the autologous blood was examined, and it was determined that there was no sickling. It is suggested that intraoperative autotransfusion is possible if exchange transfusions are given preoperatively to decrease the concentration of HbS. These authors further stated that if extensive sickling is apparent after processing of blood as determined by microscopic examination, reinfusion should be aborted.[44]

The Cook group[44] recommends

1. Exchange transfusion to attain 60 to 70 percent HbA and hematocrit value of 30 to 36 percent. Use solutions with a physiologic pH for wound lavage and cell washing.
2. Limit negative pressure at tip of large-bore suction cannula in surgical field to less than 100 mmHg.
3. Compare the smears of the venous and processed blood before reinfusion to determine presence of sickling.
4. Monitor pH, PO_2, and hematocrit value of processed blood.
5. Anticoagulate harvested blood with heparin until processing.
6. Wash RBCs with 1 to 2 L of normal saline to remove waste products and filter before reinfusion.

Case Study

We processed blood from a patient with sickle cell disease lost during a surgical procedure after collection with a blood scavenging device. The blood was exam-ined, and a moderate number of sickled cells were noted. We do not use the Cell Saver nor recommend its use in patients with sickle cell anemia.

Extubation

At the termination of a procedure performed under general anesthesia, the endotracheal tube should be kept in place until adequate ventilation is ensured. After extubation, the patient should be given oxygen for a period of 48 hours and should be monitored with a pulse oximeter.

Postoperative Care

Administer oxygen for 48 hours.

Encourage deep breathing and coughing to prevent respiratory complications.

Administer narcotics and sedatives judiciously to avoid hypoventilation, hypoxia, and hypercarbia.

Monitor oxygen saturation with a pulse oximeter.

Maintain adequate hydration.

Avoid hypothermia and shivering.

If the procedure was performed under regional anesthesia with an epidural, we use epidural morphine to help provide analgesia and decrease the chance of pain inducing a sickle crisis.

SICKLE CELL TRAIT

Patients with sickle cell trait have a combination of HbA and HbS and are heterozygous for the sickle cell gene. The HbS concentration is usually less than 50 percent. This lower percentage of HbS found in patients with sickle cell trait is associated with fewer complications than occur in homozygous patients. In general, it requires extreme circumstances, such as a PaO_2 of 20 mmHg or less to induce sickling in patients with sickle cell trait.[36–38,40]

Anesthetic Management

The same antisickling anesthetic management technique is used, such as avoiding hypoxia, hypotension, hypovolemia, hypercarbia, and hypothermia in patients with sickle cell trait. Increased inspired oxygen concentration is administered during anesthesia and in the early postoperative period.

HEMOPHILIA

Classification

Hemophilia A
  Deficiency of factor VIII
  Occurs in males

Hemophilia B (Christmas disease)
  Deficiency of factor IX

Hemophilia C
  Deficiency of factor XI
  Seen in both males and females

Hemophilia A

Factor VIII deficiency leads to prolonged partial thromboplastin time (PTT).

Hemophilic Arthropathy

Bleeding into joints is the most frequent site of hemorrhage in hemophilia, with pain, swelling, and alterations in the joints.[45]

Fractures

Uncontrolled bleeding secondary to a fracture can lead to Volkmann's ischemic contracture in areas such as the forearm or tibia.

Fractures heal normally.

Nerve Palsy

Compression by a hematoma of a nerve can lead to palsy. The femoral nerve is the most frequently involved.[45]

Laboratory Tests

The PTT is greatly prolonged because of a deficiency of factor VIII.

Surgical Management

Consult with hematologist familiar with patient.

Correct the hemostatic defect with factor VIII.

Treat significant anemia by infusion of whole blood or packed RBCs.[37]

Warning:

Use only superficial veins for intravenous access. Do not poke around.

Do not give any intramuscular injections.

Do not attempt femoral or internal jugular vein punctures.

Use of Factor VIII

Factor VIII is administered to achieve a factor VIII level of 100 percent of normal.

The half-life of factor VIII in plasma is about 8 to 12 hours.

Repeat infusions are necessary to maintain the desired level of activity for 2 to 10 days postoperatively.[36,37,46,47]

Dosage to be administered every 8 hours must be calculated:

$$\text{Dosage} = \text{patients weight (kg)} \times \text{desired plasma level of factor VIII} \times 44$$

Example: $\qquad$ Dosage $= 70 \times 1.0 \times 44 = 3{,}000$ units

To achieve 50 percent $= 70 \times 0.5 \times 44 = 1{,}500$ units[47]

Maintenance

Infuse factor VIII every 12 hours to maintain level at or above 50 percent for several days after surgery.

Check factor VIII activity as well as the clinical condition of the patient to determine the need for further factor VIII infusions.[36,37,47,48]

Cryoprecipitate

One bag of cryoprecipitate contains between 75 and 125 units of factor VIII.

One bag of cryoprecipitate per 5 kg body weight will raise the recipient's level to about 50 percent of normal.[36,37,47–49]

Fresh Frozen Plazma

If factor VIII is unavailable, use fresh frozen plasma (FFP). Infuse 10 to 15 ml/kg every 12 hours. This will provide a plasma level of 10 to 25 percent of normal.[36,37]

Danger: The large volume of plasma necessary to correct clotting deficiency can result in fluid overload. Do not give more than 30 ml/kg of plasma in a 24-hour period.[36,37]

Desmopressin Acetate

Levels of factor VIII can be increased by administration of desmopressin acetate. This may be helpful in patients with mild Hemophilia A.[36,37,47]

A dose of 0.3 mg/kg in 50 ml 0.9 percent NaCl over 15 to 30 minutes may raise factor VIII.[36,47]

Epsilon-Aminocaproic Acid

Epsilon-aminocaproic acid (100 mg/kg every 6 hours) may be indicated in addition to replacement therapy for mucous membrane hemorrhage and dental extractions.[37]

Antibody to Factor VIII

Patients should be tested for the presence of antibody to factor VIII. If present, do not undertake elective surgery. Porcine factor VIII can be used in emergencies if there are antibodies to human factor VIII.[47]

Caution: Problems with instrumentation of the airway may occur.

Be careful during airway instrumentation.

Avoid nasotracheal intubation.

Lubricate endotracheal tubes and airways—insert very carefully.

Avoid esophageal temperature probes—measure body temperature by other means.[36]

Hemophilia B

Hemophilia B (Christmas disease) results from a deficiency of factor IX.

It is an X-linked recessive trait.

It is similar to factor VIII deficiency.[36]

Laboratory Tests

The PTT is abnormal.

Treatment of Bleeding

1. Commercial preparations containing factors II, VII, IX, and X have good levels of factor IX and can be administered in doses similar to that outlined for factor VIII. The half-life of factor IX is about 24 hours.[49]
2. If necessary, FFP can be infused 10 to 15 ml/kg every 12 to 24 hours during bleeding episodes.[36]
3. Cryoprecipitate or factor VIII concentrates should not be used.

Factor IX levels are not usually maintained at 100 percent but run from 60 to 90 percent of normal.[47]

Warning:

Some commercial preparations may transmit infectious disease.

Thrombosis may occur after administration of these concentrates because of their content of activated coagulants.

Hemophilia C

Hemophilia C (factor XI deficiency) is a mild bleeding disorder inherited as an autosomal dominant. Cases are seen in both sexes.

Therapy

FFP is administered in a dose of 10 to 15 ml/kg every 12 to 24 hours for significant hemorrhage to bring the level to 20 to 30 percent of normal.[36]

Universal Precautions

Hepatitis

Patients with hemophilia should be tested for hepatitis. Attention should be paid to universal precautions to avoid transmission of disease from patient to health care worker or from patient to patient.

Acquired Immunodeficiency Syndrome

Patients with hemophilia who have received multiple blood transfusions over many years may carry the acquired immunodeficiency syndrome (AIDS) virus. Again, universal precautions are used to avoid transmission of the virus.

REFERENCES

1. Bernstein RL, Rosenberg AD: Anesthesia for orthopedic surgery. Semin Anesth 6:36, 1978
2. Rodman GR, Schumacher R (eds): Primer on Rheumatic Diseases. 8th Ed. Atlanta Arthritis Foundation, Atlanta, GA, 1983
3. Syndas OA: The anemia of rheumatoid arthritis and its treatment with blood transfusions. Acta Rheum Scand 7:95, 1961
4. Sorensen AW: Investigations of the kidney functions in rheumatoid arthritis. Acta Rheum Scand 7:138, 1961
5. Grossman A, Martin JR, Root HS: Rheumatoid arthritis of the cricoarytenoid joint. Laryngoscope 71:530, 1961
6. Phelps LA: Laryngeal obstruction due to cricoarytenoid arthritis. Anesthesiology 27:518, 1966

7. Eisele JH: Connective tissue diseases. In Katz J, Beneumof JL, Kadis LB (eds): Anesthesia and Uncommon Diseases. WB Saunders, Philadelphia, 1990
8. Steel HH: Anatomical and mechanical considerations of the atlantoaxial articulations. J Bone Joint Surg 50A:1481, 1968
9. Martel W, Page JW: Cervical vertebral erosions and subluxation in rheumatoid arthritis and ankylosing spondylitis. Arthritis Rheum 3:546, 1960
10. Keenan MA, Stiles CM, Kaufman RL: Acquired laryngeal deviation associated with cervical spine disease in erosive polyarticular arthritis. Anesthesiology 58:441, 1983
11. Benjamin R, Parham P: HLA B-27 and disease: a consequence of inadvertent antigen presentation? Rheum Dis Clin North Am 18:11, 1992
12. Rigby AS: Review of UK data on rheumatic diseases. Br J Rheumatol 30:50, 1991
13. Kahn MA: An overview of clinical spectrum and heterogeneity of spondyloarthropathies in spondylarthropathies. Rheum Dis Clin North Am 19:1, 1992
14. Pavlin EG: Respiratory diseases. p. 305. In Katz J, Beneumof JL, Kadis LB (eds): Anesthesia and Uncommon Diseases. WB Saunders, Philadelphia, 1990
15. Miller FM, Rogers LF: Fractures of the dens complicating ankylosing spondylitis with atlanto-occipital fusion. J Rheumatol 18:771, 1991
16. Fisher LR, Cawley MID, Holgate ST: Relation between chest expansion, pulmonary function, and exercise tolerance in patients with ankylosing spondylitis. Ann Rheum Dis 49:921, 1990
17. Sinclair JR, Mason RA: Ankylosing spondylitis. The case for awake intubation. Anaesthesia 39:3, 1984
18. Wittmann FW, Ring PA: Anesthesia for hip replacement in ankylosing spondylitis. J R Soc Med 79:457, 1986
19. Simmons EH: The surgical correction of flexion deformity of the cervical spine in ankylosing spondylitis. Clin Orthop 86:132, 1972
20. Donlon JV: Ear, nose and throat diseases. In Katz J, Beneumof JL, Kadis LB (eds): Anesthesia and Uncommon Diseases. 3rd Ed. WB Saunders, Philadelphia, 1990
21. Singer FR, Schiller AL, Pyle EB et al: Paget's disease of bone. p. 490. In Avoli LV, Krane SM (eds): Metabolic Bone Disease. Academic Press, Orlando FL, 1977
22. Greenspan A: A review of Paget's Disease: radiologic imaging, differential diagnosis and treatment. Bull Hosp Joint Dis Orthop Inst 51:22, 1991
23. Strickberger SA, Schulman SP, Hutchins GM: Association of Paget's disease of bone with calcific aortic valve disease. Am J Med 82:953, 1987
24. Steen VD: Systemic sclerosis in rheumatic diseases. Rheum Dis Clin North Am 16:641, 1990
25. Stupi AM, Stein VD, Medsger TA: Pulmonary hypertension (PHT) in the Crest Syndrome variant of progressive systemic sclerosis (PSS). Arthritis Rheum 29:515, 1986
26. Ritchie B: Pulmonary function in scleroderma. Thorax 19:28, 1964
27. Clements PJ, Furst DE: The relationship of arrhythmias and conduction disturbances to other manifestations of cardiopulmonary disease in progressive system sclerosis (PSS). Am J Med 71:38, 1981
28. Millar WL: Other hereditary disorders. p. 144. In Katz J, Beneumof JL, Kadis LB (eds): Anesthesia and Uncommon Diseases. WB Saunders, Philadelphia, 1990
29. Wells DG, Podalakin D: Anaesthesia and Marfan's syndrome. Case report. Can J Anaesth 34:311, 1987
30. Chaglassian JH, Riseborough EJ, Hall JE: Neurofibromatous scoliosis. Natural history and results of treatment of thirty-seven cases. J Bone Joint Surg 58:695, 1976

31. Chang-Lo M: Laryngeal involvement in Von Recklinghausen's disease: a case report and review of the literature. Laryngoscope 87:435, 1977
32. Fisher MM: Anaesthetic difficulties in neurofibromatosis. Anaesthesia 30:648, 1975
33. Partridge BL: Skin and bone disorders. p. 668. In Katz J, Beneumof JL, Kadis LB (eds): Anesthesia and Uncommon Diseases. 3rd Ed. WB Saunders, Philadelphia, 1990
34. Martz DG, Schreibman LD, Matjasko MJ: Neurological disorders. p. 577. In Katz J, Beneuwof JL, Kadis LB (eds): Anesthesia and Uncommon Diseases. 3rd Ed. WB Saunders, Philadelphia, 1990
35. Smith MF: Skin and connective tissue disorders. In Katz J, Steward DJ (eds): Anesthesia and Uncommon Pediatric Diseases. WB Saunders, Philadelphia, 1987
36. Dewhirst WE, Glass DD: Hematological diseases. In Katz J, Beneumof JL, Kadis LB (eds): Anesthesia and Uncommon Diseases. WB Saunders, Philadelphia, 1990
37. Hain WR: Diseases of blood. p. 489. In Katz J, Steward DJ (eds): Anesthesia and Uncommon Pediatric Diseases. WB Saunders, Philadelphia, 1987
38. Roizen MF: Anesthetic implications of concurrent diseases. p. 793. In Miller RD (ed): Anesthesia. 3rd Ed. Churchill Livingstone, New York 1990
39. Adams R, McKie V, Nichols F et al: The use of transcranial ultrasonography to prevent stroke in sickle cell disease. N Engl J Med 326:605, 1992
40. Dierdorf SF: Rare and coexisting diseases. p. 563. In Barash PG, Cullen BF, Stoelting RK (eds): Clinical Anesthesia. 2nd Ed. JB Lippincott, Philadelphia, 1992
41. Esseltine DW, Baxter MRN, Bevan J: Sickle cells states and the anaesthetist. Can J Anaesth 35:4, 1988
42. Stein RE, Urbaniak J: Use of the tourniquet during surgery in patients with sickle cell hemoglobinopathies. Clin Orthop 151:231, 1980
43. Brajtbord D, Johnson B, Ramsay M et al: Use of the Cell Saver in patients with sickle cell trait. Anesthesiology 70:878, 1989
44. Cook A, Hanowell H: Intraoperative autotransfusion for a patient with homozygous sickle cell disease. Anesthesiology 73:177, 1990
45. Tachdjian MO: Joints in Pediatric Orthopedics. Vol. 1. 2nd Ed. WB Saunders, Philadelphia, 1990
46. Pearson HA: Diseases of the blood. p. 1204. In Behrman R, Vaghan VC III, Nelson W (eds): Textbook of Pediatrics. 12th Ed. WB Saunders, Philadelphia, 1983
47. Berkow R (ed): Hematology and Oncology. p. 1135. In: Merck Manual of Diagnosis and Therapy. Merck and Co., Rahway, NJ, 1992
48. Ellison N: Hemostasis and hemotherapy. In Barash PG, Stoelting RK (eds): Clinical Anesthesia. 2nd Ed. JB Lippincott, Philadelphia, 1992
49. Hoag SM, Johnson F, Robinson J: Treatment of hemophilia B with a new clotting factor concentrate. N Engl J Med 280:581, 1969

Trauma*

Trauma patients frequently suffer major orthopedic injuries in addition to injuries of the brain, spinal cord, and thoracoabdominal area. A rapid, organized approach to these patients is essential to decrease the mortality rate associated with trauma because it is the leading cause of death for persons younger than 45 years of age.

Deaths from trauma occur in a pattern consisting of three phases. Half of the deaths caused by trauma are immediate and essentially unpreventable. Fifty percent of these are due to head injury and 25 percent are due to hemorrhage.

Thirty percent of deaths occur in the second phase referred to as "the golden hour" because mortality results from causes that are secondary to conditions such as hemorrhage, pneumothorax, cardiac tamponade, and intracranial bleeding that are correctible if recognized and treated early.

The third phase occurs after several days, at which time the remaining 20 percent of patients die from sepsis or multiple-organ failure.[1,2]

Essential components in care of the severe trauma patient are listed below[3]:

Establish an airway—be alert for cervical spine injury.

Ventilate.

Oxygenate.

Establish large-bore vascular access.

Obtain blood for laboratory studies and type and cross-match.

Infuse fluids through blood warmers.

Insert Foley catheter.

Stabilize blood pressure.

Place an arterial line.

Obtain an arterial blood gas sample.

Obtain history.

---

* Portions of this chapter are from Rosenberg and Bernstein,[63] with permission.

Evaluate the central nervous system.

Check for intrathoracic and intra-abdominal injury.

Perform a complete physical examination.

Verify patient identification and begin blood transfusion if necessary.

Obtain radiograph—cervical spine, chest, abdomen, pelvis, long bones.
  Do not miss a fracture.

Obtain computed tomography/angiography, if needed.

Assess hemodynamic status and urine output.

Insert central line or pulmonary artery catheter, if indicated.

Insert nasogastric tube if necessary (**not in patients with facial fractures or base of skull fractures**).

Obtain consultations as needed.

TRAUMA SCORES

Scoring systems exist to help determine the severity of injury, predict outcome, and determine treatment.

The most useful scoring system for preoperative injury severity assessment is the trauma score developed by Champion[4] et al. (Table 2-1).

The Champion Trauma Score, which assesses cardiovascular and respiratory status, incorporates the Glasgow Coma Scale, which assesses neurologic status on the basis of behavioral responses such as eye opening, best motor response, and best verbal response.

Use of Champion Trauma Score

Scores range from 1 to 16.

The lower the score, the worse the patient's condition.

Patients with a score of 12 or less benefit from the care of trauma centers.

A score of 3 or less may well predict a fatal outcome even in the best centers. Scores should be used only as a guide because many variations of trauma severity index are in use throughout the country and a single acceptable index has not been established.

Continued re-evaluation and scoring can help one follow the progress of patients.[4,5]

Table 2-1. Trauma Scale Developed by Champion for Field Triage and Evaluation of Care of the Trauma Victim

Trauma Score		Value	Points	Score
A.	Respiratory rate (number of respirations in 15 sec, multiply by 4)	10–24 25–35 >35 <10 0	4 3 2 1 0	A. _____

B.	Respiratory effort
	  Shallow—markedly decreased check movement or air exchange
	  Retractive—use of accessory muscles or intercostal retraction
		Normal
		
		Shallow
		or
		retractive
			1
			
			0
				B. _____

C.	Systolic blood pressure
	  Systolic cuff pressure—either arm—auscultate or palpate
	  No carotid pulse
		>90
		70–90
		50–69
		<50
		0
			4
			3
			2
			1
			0
				C. _____

D.	Capillary refill
	  Normal—forehead, lip mucosa, or nail bed color refills in 2 sec
	  Delayed—more than 2 sec of capillary refill
	  None—no capillary refill
		Normal
		
		Delayed
		None
			2
			
			1
			0
				D. _____

E.	Glasgow Coma Scale		Total GCS	
	1. Eye opening		Points	Score
	Spontaneous	_____ 4	14–15	5
	To voice	_____ 3	11–13	4
	To pain	_____ 2	8–10	3
	None	_____ 1	5–7	2
	2. Verbal response		3–4	1 E. _____
	Oriented	_____ 5		
	Confused	_____ 4		
	Inappropriate words	_____ 3		
	Incomprehensible words	_____ 2		
	None	_____ 1		
	3. Motor response			
	Obeys commands	_____ 6		
	Purposeful movement (pain)	_____ 5		
	Withdraw (pain)	_____ 4		
	Flexion (pain)	_____ 3		
	Extension (pain)	_____ 2		
	None	_____ 1		

Total GCS points (1 + 2 + 3) _____

Trauma score _____

(Total points A + B + C + D + E)

(From Champion et al,[4] with permission.)

ROLE OF THE ANESTHESIOLOGIST

The anesthesiologist is a vital member of the trauma team. Securing and maintaining the airway is the anesthesiologist's main responsibility. Once an airway is established, the anesthesiologist can aid in other resuscitative efforts.

The anesthesiologist provides care outside the operating room in areas such as the emergency department and the radiology suite. The anesthesiologist ensures that these areas have the appropriate equipment and supplies necessary for emergency care of the trauma victim.

Securing and Maintaining an Adequate Airway

Primary Considerations

Obtaining an airway in a trauma patient may prove exceedingly difficult. Aspiration is a major problem, and gastric contents or blood may be present in the oral cavity even on initial evaluation.

If the patient is awake, signs and symptoms that may suggest a difficult intubation include

1. Injury to the face, mouth, or teeth
     Limited opening of the mouth caused by mechanical trauma
     Bleeding or swelling of the mouth or oral cavity
     Facial bone fractures
2. Neck injury
     Open wounds
     Expanding hematomas
     Tracheal disruption or deviation
     Subcutaneous emphysema
3. Head trauma
     Considerations about increased intracranial pressure (ICP)
     Cerebrospinal fluid rhinorrhea
4. Cervical spine injuries
     Acute quadraplegia
     Cervical spine instability

Awake Patient

If the patient is awake but complains of neck pain, neck motion should be avoided while obtaining an airway. In the arousable, uncooperative patient who is thrashing around but requires intubation, a rapid sequence induction with cricoid pressure, thiopental, and succinylcholine is performed. Succinylcholine can be used for up to 24 hours after spinal injury.

Unconscious Patient

Assume that both head and spinal cord injuries have occurred. Keep in mind that manipulation of the neck may cause further injury.

Ensure adequate oxygenation by ventilating with a bag and mask before intubation.

Avoid blind nasotracheal intubation if the patient has facial fractures or if a basilar skull fracture is suspected because an airway or endotracheal tube can lodge in the brain.

Techniques to secure an airway include

1. Intubation while a qualified physician stabilizes the head and neck
2. Fiberoptic intubation (we prefer the oral route in trauma patients as opposed to nasal route)
3. Use of a mask to ventilate that permits fiberoptic intubation at the same time (Patil-Syracuse)
4. Transtracheal jet ventilation until an airway can be secured
5. Retrograde intubation
6. Cricothyrotomy or tracheotomy, if needed

Full Stomach

Attempt to decrease stomach volume with metoclopromide and acidity with ranitidine or cimetidine before intubation. Even so, assume the trauma patient has a full stomach and is at high risk for aspiration.

Use of Cricoid Pressure

The use of cricoid pressure is controversial in patients suspected of having sustained a cervical spine injury because pressure on the cricoid cartilage may theoretically damage the cervical spine further. At the R Adams Cowley Shock Trauma Center, trauma patients requiring intubation are managed with a "modified rapid sequence" technique. Patients are ventilated by mask and intubated while cricoid pressure is maintained. The method has been successfully used in more than 3,000 cases. No appreciable neurologic changes were noted with this technique, even though about 1 percent of the patients were diagnosed as having cervical spine fractures. Other centers prefer to avoid the use of cricoid pressure and recommend fiberoptic intubation.[6]

Motion of the Head and Neck

During normal maneuvers to obtain an "airway," significant motion of the head, neck, and cervical spine occurs. In cases of suspected cervical trauma, it is important that cervical immobilization be ensured. This can be accomplished by taping the head to a spine board with sandbags on either side of the neck. Although Majernick et al.[7] noted marked movements of the cervical spine during intubation, manual in-line traction or stabilization was associated with the least amount of motion.[6]

This technique is advocated at some major trauma centers where a qualified person maintains in-line traction and cervical spine stabilization while another qualified person intubates the patient.

Fiberoptic Intubation

Fiberoptic intubation provides the least amount of neck motion and should be used when neck motion could result in further neurologic damage in a patient with an unstable spine. The Patil-Syracuse mask is a useful aid if ventilation is necessary while fiberoptic intubation is being performed.

Note: When using this mask, do not put the endotracheal tube connector in place until after the mask is removed from the endotracheal tube.

Cricothyrotomy

When an airway must be secured and normal methods are not possible, a cricothyrotomy is performed.

Case Study

A 54-year-old man was struck by an automobile and brought to the emergency department. The patient sustained cervical spine injury with a C4 spinal cord transection. Cervical spine radiographs revealed anterior soft tissue swelling. The patient was hemodynamically stable with worsening mental status and respiratory failure. The patient was manually ventilated easily but was combative and unable to follow commands. Direct laryngoscopy was attempted with axial traction after the administration of lidocaine, pentothal, and double-dose vecuronium. Direct laryngoscopy revealed an extremely edematous oropharynx with inability to visualize laryngeal structures. The patient was once again manually ventilated with no difficulty. After the second attempt at intubation, it was no longer possible to manually ventilate. The patient began to undergo oxygen desaturation. It was decided to perform a cricothyrotomy. Execution time was approximately 10 minutes. The patient went into ventricular tachycardia requiring resuscitation.

Comment

The finding of anterior soft tissue swelling on the radiograph was evidence that there would be difficulty in visualizing the structures in the pharynx, leading to difficulty in intubation. In this situation, an immediate emergency cricothyrotomy would have made it possible to secure the airway and provide ventilation. Attempts at securing the airway by means of fiberoptic intubation in this situation would not be successful because of the soft tissue swelling in the pharnyx.

Performance of a Cricothyrotomy

We use a Pertrach Tracheotomy Set, which we have found to be simple to use and effective (Fig. 2-1).

Procedure

1. Do not extend head.
2. Palpate the cricothyroid interval between the superior border of cricoid cartilage and the inferior border of the thyroid cartilage.
3. Place two fingers of left (or nondominant) hand so that the skin is drawn taut in a lateral direction helping to delineate the interval between the thyroid and cricoid cartilage.
4. With the skin pulled taut, make a 1-cm horizontal incision between the cricoid and thyroid cartilage with the scalpel blade.
5. Insert the needle and syringe through the incision into the trachea, aspirating duration insertion.
6. When the needle is in the trachea, air will enter the syringe.
7. Remove the syringe from the needle.
8. Pass the leader of the dilator into the trachea through the needle.
9. Squeeze the two plastic wings to break the needle apart longitudinally.
10. Push the leader into the trachea followed by the wedge-shaped obturator and tracheotomy tube.
11. Remove obturator.
12. Inflate cuff.
13. Attach Ambu bag or Y connector of anesthesia machine and ventilate patient.
14. Secure tracheotomy tube with ties.

Use of Intravenous Catheter and Jet Ventilation

Jet ventilation should be used if the patient is hypoxic and the need for adequate oxygenation is a pressing concern in the face of a difficult airway.

A 14-gauge intravenous catheter is placed into the trachea, the stylet is removed, and jet ventilation is begun. The catheter must not be kinked as it will prevent jet ventilation. This technique can be used only if there is no upper airway obstruction that hinders the egress of air. Barotrauma leading to subcuta-

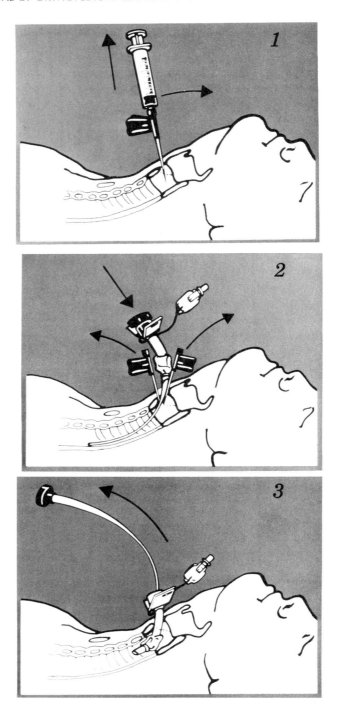

Fig. 2-1. Method of performing a tracheotomy with a Pertrach set (steps 1–3).

neous emphysema and pneumomediastinum are possible problems with this technique if the needle is dislodged from its position in the trachea.

Retrograde Wire Technique

Intubation through a retrograde wire placed through the cricothyroid membrane can be used to help intubate patients whose neck should not be moved.

Procedure
1. Insert a 14-gauge needle through the cricothyroid membrane in a cephalad direction.
2. Pass the guide wire cephalad through the needle.
3. Remove needle and pass the guide wire cephalad until it can be retrieved through the mouth or nose.
4. Pass the guide wire up the suction port and out through the eye piece area of the fiberoptic bronchoscope that already has an endotracheal tube over it.
5. Pass the bronchoscope along the wire and through the vocal cords; when this is accomplished, the wire can be withdrawn.
6. Advance the fiberoptic scope farther into the trachea.
7. Pass the endotracheal tube into the trachea over the fiberoptic scope until it is slightly above the carina. Ascertain final position by direct observation through the fiberoptic bronchoscope. To avoid being in a mainstem bronchus, be sure that the cartilage rings are not completely circumferential right below the tip of the endotracheal tube. In the trachea, the cartilage rings are incomplete and not present posteriorly, whereas in the mainstem bronchi, complete cartilage rings are present.

Ventilation

In a patient *with* head injury, hyperventilation will decrease the possible adverse effects of elevated $PaCO_2$ on ICP. In patients *without* head injury, controlled ventilation is instituted to provide adequate oxygenation as well as maintain the $PaCO_2$ in a normal range.

Airway Pressures

Elevated airway pressures may be noted after intubation. These can be present in patients who

Are "fighting the ventilator"

Have lung contusions, hemothorax, or pneumothorax

Have aspirated

Have developed adult respiratory distress syndrome (ARDS)

Have a misplaced endotracheal tube

May have developed a tension pneumothorax[7]

Circulation

After securing an airway and ensuring adequate ventilation, circulatory volume is restored with blood and fluid. Shock is most commonly caused by hemorrhage and should be treated rapidly. Rapid restoration of intravascular volume during the first hour, "the golden period," is critical in improving patient outcome.

Immediate correction of hypotension and prevention of further episodes will help improve circulation to vital organ systems and possibly prevent permanent damage.[8,9]

Intravenous Access

1. Insert large-bore intravenous catheters with short lengths to maximize infusion rate.
2. Do not use stopcocks or check valves, as they impede flow rate.
3. Secure central venous access if peripheral venous access is not obtainable. Pulmonary artery catheter introducers provide an excellent conduit for fluid infusion.
4. Consider the suspected area of trauma when choosing the site for central venous line insertion. Avoid femoral vein cannulation in a patient suspected of having massive abdominal bleeding or pelvic trauma.
5. If emergency department protocol dictates routine insertion of intravenous lines in all four extremities as soon as major trauma is diagnosed, do not use lower extremity lines if abdominal or pelvic injuries exist.

Rapid Infusion Systems

In addition to placing the largest-bore intravenous catheter with shortest length, use of mechanical infusion pressure devices help improve fluid flow into the patient.

Manually operated pressure cuffs can increase flow rates up to three times that of gravity.

Advanced rapid infusion systems, such as the Level 1, can be valuable when rapid volume infusion is necessary.[10]

Be careful: Large increases in serum potassium levels have been noted after massive blood transfusion in a short period of time.

Autotransfusion Devices

Autotransfusion devices such as the Haemonetics Cell Saver can be used to salvage and reprocess blood to be returned to the patient.

These devices should not be used in

1. Abdominal trauma if there is contamination with bowel contents
2. Patients with sickle cell disease
3. Patients with cold agglutinins

Choice of Fluid

Nonglucose-containing crystalloid solutions in volumes of up to 50 ml/kg should be infused initially to resuscitate hypovolemic patients. This will help establish an adequate blood pressure in many patients with hypovolemic shock and enable time for type-specific blood to be made available.

Giesecke et al[9] suggest infusing crystalloid in a 3:1 ratio of crystalloid infusion to blood volume lost. In addition, Geisecke et al[10] suggest blood transfusions using the following criteria:

When hematocrit value is below 28 percent and significant bleeding continues

When crystalloid infusion exceeds 50 ml/kg and bleeding continues

To increase oxygen-carrying capacity associated with low hematocrit value (In elderly patients or those with known coronary artery disease, higher hematocrit levels may be necessary for optimum oxygen delivery. Optimum blood flow occurs at hematocrit levels in the 30 percent range.)

Fresh whole blood is the first choice

Reconstitute packed cells with normal saline to improve viscosity

In large-volume resuscitations, a combination of blood and crystalloid must be used. Alone, each has been inadequate in survival studies.

Hematocrit levels should be followed and blood administered as needed so that the patient does not become too anemic.[11,12]

Use of Blood

Proper identification procedures should always be carried out before administering blood. Most causes of transfusion reactions are clerical errors.

Cross-Matching

Type and screen patients as rapidly as possible because a full cross-match takes too much time.

Use type-specific blood if possible.

If type-specific blood is not available or not used and the patient has already received 2 or more units of O-negative, continue blood transfusion with O-negative rather than switching back to type-specific blood.[9]

Warm Blood

Blood should be warmed to body temperature to decrease its viscosity. Blood at body temperature flows twice as fast as blood at 10°C.

Caution: Use of excessive pressure during pumping of blood or warming to temperatures above 37°C may cause destruction of red blood cells with release of free hemoglobin and potential kidney damage.

Hemolytic Transfusion Reaction

The most common cause of a hemolytic transfusion reaction is clerical error.

Remember: The usual signs of transfusion reactions—chills, fever, flank pain—are masked by general anesthesia.

The possibility of a transfusion reaction should be considered if

   Urine turns darker or decreases markedly after a transfusion

   Patient develops urticaria and hemodynamic instability

   Bleeding increases in the surgical field or from intravenous sites

Treatment
Steps for treatment of a hemolytic transfusion reaction[13] follow:

1. Stop the transfusion.
2. Maintain urine output at 75 to 100 ml/hr.
      Administer fluids.
      Give mannitol 12.5 to 50.0 g in 10 minutes.
      Administer furosemide 20 mg IV.
      If urine output is still not adequate, repeat furosemide 20 mg IV.
3. Alkalinize urine: administer sodium bicarbonate IV 44.6 mEq/70 kg to raise the urine pH to 8. Administer additional bicarbonate if urine pH does not reach 8.
4. Maintain blood pressure to ensure adequate renal blood flow.
5. Administer blood to maintain adequate hemodynamic state.
6. Obtain platelet count, partial thromboplastin time (PTT), prothrombin time (PT), and fibrinogen level.
7. Check urine and plasma for free hemoglobin levels.
8. Send unused portion of blood and sample of patient's blood for testing.

Dilutional Coagulopathies

Massive bleeding and fluid resuscitation can result in a dilutional coagulopathy. Thrombocytopenia is usually considered to be the cause. Analysis of PT and PTT and platelet count can guide specific therapy.

Urinary Output

Adequate systemic hydration and renal perfusion are critical in preventing renal failure. Urine output should be 0.5 ml/kg/hr.

Adequate hydration should be provided when radiograph studies with radiopaque dyes are performed. The use of mannitol or diuretics such as furosemide does not appear to be beneficial in preventing the development of renal failure secondary to radiopaque days.

Diuretics such as mannitol have a possible role in preventing renal failure when myoglobin is present in the renal tubules, by increasing urinary tubular flow to flush the crystals from the renal tubules.

Position

The patient should not be placed in Trendelenburg's position. This position results in little hemodynamic improvement. It may have deleterious effects on respiratory function and in patients with increased ICP.[14]

Emergency Pain Management in the Injured Patient

Administration of pain medication can unmask hypovolemia and result in hypotension.

Oral or intramuscular medications must not be used in the acute trauma patient even if the patient appears awake, alert, and appropriately oriented.

The administration of pain medication should be considered only after adequate hemodynamic stability is ensured.

Small incremental doses should be used intravenously.

Remember, the patient may be intoxicated or under the influence of drugs, and pain medication may result in respiratory depression.

Central Nervous System

Narcotics and sedatives should be avoided if an altered state of consciousness or intracranial pathology is present or suspected.

Sedatives or narcotics should only be administered if the neurologically impaired patient is first intubated and hyperventilated.

Airway and Respiratory System

Pain medication should not be administered if airway or pulmonary injuries exist.

Gastrointestinal System

Oral analgesics should be avoided. Narcotics can cause vomiting and delay gastric emptying.

Transport to the Operating Room

Do not disconnect vital life support apparatus (oxygen, intravenous lines) and just run to the operating room.

Maintain adequate oxygenation, ventilation, and fluid resuscitation.

Monitor the electrocardiogram (ECG) and blood pressure on the way to the operating room.

Ensure that the oxygen tank is adequately filled and opened to appropriate flow rate if the patient is intubated.

Trauma Operating Room

The designated trauma operating room must be set up and ready for immediate use.

The operating room trauma team should be ready as soon as the patient arrives. In an emergency, it is necessary to mobilize an adequately trained staff, assign specific tasks, and send messengers to obtain blood.

Trauma Operating Room Equipment

Equipment and monitors necessary in the trauma operating room include

Anesthesia machine, checked out and ready for use

Humidified patient breathing circuit

Set up for endotracheal intubation, laryngoscope checked for fresh batteries and good light

Cricothyrotomy set

Tracheotomy set

Fiberoptic bronchoscope

ECG, electrodes ready to be attached to patient (make sure the pads do not get wet)

Inspired oxygen concentration monitor

End-tidal carbon dioxide monitor

Pulse oximeter

Esophageal stethescope, chest stethescope

Pressure monitors with transducers calibrated

Central venous pressure catheter

Arterial blood pressure line

Pulmonary artery catheter

Foley catheter

Body temperature monitor

Peripheral nerve stimulator

Blood pumps

Blood and fluid warmers

Defibrillator

All medications drawn up and labeled

Warning: Be careful. Do not give wrong medication. Do not give wrong blood.

Monitoring

Respiratory Function

Respiratory functions to be monitored include

1. Inspired oxygen concentration
2. Heart and breath sounds
3. End-tidal carbon dioxide
4. Pulse oximetry

One hundred percent oxygen is administered until the patient is stable and a satisfactory blood gas has been obtained. Any subsequent changes of inspired oxygen should be determined by arterial blood gas studies. Heart and breath sounds are auscultated for rhonchi, rales, or secretions.

Pulse oximetry indicates degree of oxygen saturation.

End-tidal carbon dioxide monitors gas exchange and serves as a guide for $PaCO_2$ levels in the head-injured patient.

Arterial Blood Pressure

Direct monitoring of arterial blood pressure is important in trauma patients who are undergoing marked hemodynamic swings in blood pressure. Lower extremity sites should be avoided if aortic cross-clamping may occur intraoperatively. The right radial artery is cannulated in cases of chest trauma as the aorta may be cross-clamped, resulting in a nonfunctional left arterial line.

The arterial pressure wave form often provides an indication of intravascular volume. Cyclic changes of arterial pressure wave form tracings during positive pressure ventilation may suggest hypovolemia and cardiac tamponade.

Central Venous Pressure

The central venous pressure (CVP) reflects right-sided filling pressures, but not volume and pressure relationships on the left side of the heart.

Elevated CVP readings occur with

Pericardial tamponade

Pneumothorax

Hemothorax

Myocardial contusion

Rapid fluid infusion even in hypovolemic patients

CVP line right next to a fluid infusion line[15,16]

Pulmonary Artery Catheter

Pulmonary artery catheters are useful as guides for fluid resuscitation and cardiac output measurements in patients with suspected congestive heart failure, coronary artery disease, valvular disease, or ARDS. In ARDS, fluid status cannot be adequately ascertained unless pulmonary capillary readings are obtained. Patients receiving massive transfusions sometimes benefit from pulmonary artery catheter placement as a guide to left ventricular function and intravascular fluid status.

Temperature

Body temperature decreases rapidly in trauma patients, and it is necessary to perform the following:

Warm operating room.

Humidify inspired gases.

Warm infused fluids.

Cover exposed extremities.

Cover patient with warm airflow devices such as the Bair Hugger.

Use warm irrigating fluids.

Remove cold, wet drapes.

Urine Output

1. Urine output usually reflects renal perfusion. Inadequate urine output probably indicates hypovolemia. Prolonged hypotension before surgery may have already resulted in renal failure; in which case, urine output will not reflect vascular volume status.
2. Frequently, the trauma patient has small amounts of dark urine in the urimeter.
    The differential diagnosis includes
       Markedly concentrated urine
       A transfusion reaction
       Myoglobinuria or hemoglobinuria
    Centrifuging a urine sample is helpful.
    Free hemoglobin will appear pink in color.
    Red blood cells and myoglobin will centrifuge out of the solution.
3. Free hemoglobin can cause renal failure.
4. Massive muscle damage can result in myoglobinuria, which can also lead to renal failure.
5. If hemoglobinuria or myoglobinuria is noted, attempts should be made to increase urine output.[16]

McGoldrick and Capan[17] suggest that alkalinization of the urine with sodium bicarbonate to a pH level above 5.6 may be helpful in patients with myoglobinuria.

Maneuvers to maintain and improve urine output such as diuretics and mannitol may initially be successful, but close observation of urine output is important as the diuretics may provide adequate urine at the expense of intravascular volume.

Renal Failure

Renal failure can result from

1. Hypotensive shock
2. Direct trauma to the kidneys
3. Nephrotoxic agents such as radiopaque dye, free hemoglobin or myoglobin, or antibiotics[17]

An adequate intravascular volume is crucial in avoiding hypotensive shock that will lead to renal failure. All attempts should be made to ensure that intravascular volume and urine output remain optimal.

The use of renal dose dopamine (1 to 2 μg/kg/min) to help maintain adequate urine output should be considered if intravascular fluid volume is adequate.

Pneumothorax

A pneumothorax resulting from injuries may not be readily apparent on physical examination and may possibly be overlooked early in the treatment of a patient. It may manifest itself as hypotension, hypoxia, or even just wheezing. Insertion of chest tubes and proper drainage will usually relieve the problem.

Pneumothorax Developing during Surgery

It is possible that a pneumothorax may only become manifest once endotracheal intubation and intermittent positive pressure breathing has been instituted. Be on the alert for any ventilatory or hemodynamic changes at the beginning of surgery and consider a pneumothorax as a possibility.

Pneumothorax during Surgery after Removal of Chest Tubes

Surgery may be being carried out in the patient in whom chest tubes have been removed with a fully expanded lung before a surgical procedure. Endotracheal intubation and intermittent positive pressure breathing may possibly reopen areas of the injured lung that had been sealed off under normal breathing but have now opened under the pressures of intermittent positive pressure breathing.

Case Study

A 27-year-old patient who had sustained injuries requiring bilateral chest tubes was scheduled for spinal surgery in the immediate post-trauma period.

A consultant thoracic surgeon had removed the chest tubes on the morning of surgery because the preoperative chest radiograph appeared to show that the lungs were fully expanded.

After the administration of general anesthesia, endotracheal intubation, and positioning in the prone position, there was a sudden onset of hypotension, bradycardia, and hypoxia. The diagnosis of pneumothorax was immediately made. Emergency insertion of bilateral chest tubes was immediately performed. After this, the vital signs stabilized.

Comment

It is probably wise to leave any chest tubes that have been present to treat a pneumothorax secondary to trauma in during surgery so that the terrible tragedy of a tension pneumothorax does not develop as in the foregoing case.

ANESTHETIC MANAGEMENT

Warning: Do not use nitrous oxide if there is any problem with oxygenation of the patient. It should only be used if adequacy of oxygenation is confirmed by blood gas studies or pulse oximetry. If a pneumothorax is present or suspected, nitrous oxide should be avoided because it can increase the pressure in the chest cavity with the pneumothorax.

Induction

The ideal induction agent for the trauma patient should produce rapid loss of consciousness while maintaining hemodynamic stability. To avoid hypotension, drugs are administered in small doses slowly because hypovolemia reduces anesthetic requirements.

Stability during induction is important; sedation can be added later.

If severe hypovolemia and hypotension exist, which cannot be corrected with fluid resuscitation, the patient should be induced with oxygen and muscle relaxants.

Barbiturates

Short-acting barbiturates are frequently used in low doses for rapid sequence induction. Myocardial depression, peripheral vasodilatation, and decreased sympathetic tone result in lowering of systolic blood pressure during induction. Low doses of thiopental are used and adequate fluid volume is ensured before induction. In patients with contracted blood volumes, thiopental goes to the brain, leading to rapid induction of anesthesia.

In the hypovolemic state, drugs go directly to the brain because the perfusion to this organ is maintained at the expense of other areas of the body.[18]

Ketamine

Ketamine should not be used in cases of suspected head trauma because it increases ICP.

Ketamine is avoided in the patient with significant coronary artery disease or hypertension because it causes sympathomimetic side effects and increased myocardial oxygen requirements.

In doses of 1 to 2 mg/kg, ketamine plays an important role in induction of anesthesia in trauma patients. It provides excellent analgesia with increase in heart rate, blood pressure, cardiac index, and pulmonary pressures. Cardiac sympathomimetic effects and not direct effects on the myocardium are responsible for the hemodynamic stability noted during induction of patients with *mild* degrees of hypovolemia.

Patients whose catecholamine output has been maximized as a result of injury will not respond appropriately. In the presence of severe hypovolemia (more than 30 percent of blood volume), ketamine has the same cardiovascular depressant effects as thiopental.[19,20]

Midazolam

Midazolam should not be used for rapid sequence induction. Midazolam has a slower onset of action than that of thiopental, and its effect lasts longer. Cardiovascular depression and hypotension may be associated with its use. If midazolam is used, it must be titrated carefully and given in modest doses.[21]

Narcotics

Carefully titrated small doses of narcotics may be used for induction. Fentanyl 2.5 to 5 μg/kg or sufentanil 0.5 to 1 μg/kg administered slowly will be sufficient to induce anesthesia for a patient with adequate vascular volume. The dose is decreased for hypovolemic patients. Rigidity and apnea may occur during administration.

Muscle Relaxants

Succinylcholine

Succinylcholine 1 to 1.5 mg/kg is the most frequently used agent for intubation using rapid sequence induction. This medication should be used only when ease of intubation has been ascertained.

Succinylcholine can be used within the first 24 hours after trauma, but because it causes hyperkalemia after skeletal muscle injury and spinal cord injury, it should be avoided after the first 24 hours.

Alternatives to succinylcholine include

Pancuronium 0.20 mg/kg (pancuronium in doses of 0.2 mg/kg is associated with tachycardia and a long period of muscle relaxation)

Atracurium 0.6 mg/kg (histamine release may be noted with high doses of atracurium)

Vecuronium 0.25 mg/kg

Regional Anesthesia

Regional anesthesia may be useful for an isolated limb injury where a nerve block of that extremity can be performed.

In the face of hypovolemia, spinal or epidural anesthesia should be avoided because of the severe hypotension that may result.

Spinal or epidural anesthesia does not always protect the patient with a full stomach from the possibility of aspiration of gastric contents.

Upper Limb

An interscalene brachial plexus block may be used in patients who have injury to the upper extremity requiring surgery. It must be remembered that Horner's syndrome may develop with this block, which may interfere with neurologic assessment. The axillary approach may be used for patients with head injury requiring surgery of the upper extremity if the site of surgery can be anesthetized by this block.

Brachial plexus blocks can be performed by the axillary, infraclavicular, subclavian perivascular, and interscalene approaches. For operations lasting a long period of time, long-acting anesthetic agents are used. Continuous brachial plexus block techniques are used to provide prolonged anesthesia for surgical procedures as well as prolonged postoperative analgesia[22] (see Ch. 6).

The type of brachial plexus block is determined by the needs of the surgery as well as the ability to move the extremity. Injuries of the upper arm, as well as dislocations of the shoulder, require analgesia extending to the C5 dermatome, which is achieved with an interscalene block.

Lower Limb

In patients with femoral shaft fractures, almost immediate pain relief can be obtained with a femoral nerve block by injecting lateral to the femoral artery below Poupart's ligament. With the nerve stimulator, a low current is used because a violent contraction of the muscles will cause severe pain if the fracture fragments move.

If a sciatic nerve block is needed in the patient with trauma and the position cannot be changed from the supine, an anterior approach to the sciatic nerve can be used[23] (see Ch. 6).

Combined femoral-sciatic nerve block can provide excellent analgesia below the knee and can be used for operations in that area.

MANAGEMENT OF ACUTE SPINAL CORD INJURY

Common causes of spinal cord injury are motor vehicle accidents, falls, and sports-related injuries.

Eighty-two percent of those patients involved are young males in the 15- to 35-year age group. Initial mortality rates after spinal cord injury can be as high as 50 percent.[24]

Be Alert: Five to ten percent of patients with facial trauma have an associated spine injury. If trauma occurs that in any way may be associated with a spinal cord injury, the neck should be stabilized with sandbags until the situation is clarified.[25]

Distribution of Spinal Cord Injuries

Cervical cord	65%
Thoracolumbar T11–L2	19%
Midthoracic T1–T11	16%

Trauma to the spinal cord results in direct cord damage as well as vascular injury. Vascular injury, in turn, can cause further neurologic damage.[26]

Spinal shock with marked physiologic alterations may occur after spinal cord injury.

Hypotension, bradycardia, hemodynamic instability, and inappropriate responses to medications and fluid infusions are noted to occur during spinal shock.

The denervation of the heart and loss of sympathetic tone result in unstable hemodynamics.

Close observation, careful monitoring, and anticipation of hemodynamic instability and respiratory decompensation are all critical to proper management.

Besides spinal shock, pulmonary edema, either neurogenic pulmonary edema or from cardiac dysfunction, has been noted after cervical spine injury.[26,27]

Suspected Cervical Spine Injury

When a patient presents with suspected cervical spine injury, check lateral cervical spine radiographs:

1. All seven cervical vertebrae must be seen. Injury at C7 is the most common site and the most difficult to visualize.
2. Spine should be lordotic. Kyphosis indicates spasm—possible injury.
3. Prevertebral soft tissues should be less than 5 mm at C3 and less than 20 mm at C5, with no nasogastric or endotracheal tube present.
4. Disc spaces are similar at all levels. Narrowing may be due to injury.
5. Alignment should be good along prevertebral, postvertebral, and spinal laminar lines[26,28] (Fig. 2-2).

Early Management

Administer methylprednisolone: 30 mg/kg STAT, 5.4 mg/kg for 23 hours.

Keep blood pressure at 60 to 70 mmHg mean range or higher.

Do not use glucose-containing solution.

Corticosteroid Treatment

Large doses of methylprednisolone administered within 8 hours of spinal cord injury have been demonstrated to improve neurologic recovery. It is believed that steroids suppress the breakdown of cell membranes by inhibiting lipid peroxidation and hydrolysis at the site of injury.

Improvements in motor function and pin-and-touch sensation have been demonstrated at 2 weeks and 6 months in patients treated with high-dose methylprednisolone when compared with those who received placebo. These improvements were seen only in those patients in whom steroids were started within 8 hours of injury. The dosage regimen includes a bolus of 30 mg/kg followed by an infusion of 5.4 mg/kg/hr for 23 hours.[29]

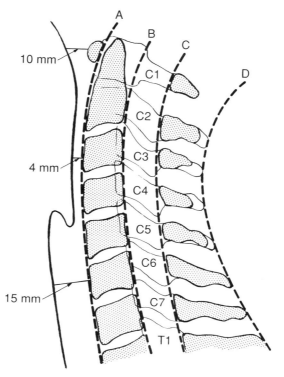

Fig. 2-2. Normal cervical spine alignment and soft tissue measurement. In evaluating lateral radiographs of the neck, the four lines (A, B, C, D) are shown when normal alignment is present. Measurements denote normal width of soft tissues. Changes result from swelling caused by soft tissue injury. A, anterior vertebral line; B, posterior vertebral line; C, spinolaminar line; D, spinous process line.

The mechanism of action of corticosteroids is to enhance the flow of blood in injured spinal cords, preventing the decline in white matter blood flow, extracellular calcium levels, and evoked potentials.[30]

Maintenance of Adequate Perfusion Pressure

Spinal cord perfusion pressure after spinal cord injury is best maintained in the 60 to 70 mmHg mean range.[31]

Glucose Solutions

Increased plasma glucose levels may be associated with a worsened neurologic outcome after spinal cord ischemia; therefore, glucose administration should be avoided.[32]

Injuries and Associated Cord Syndromes

Anterior Cord Syndrome

Anterior cord syndrome results from flexion injury damaging the anterior cord (motor component of cord).

There may be "painful paralysis" because motor function is lost while proproception and deep-pressure sensation remain.[24,26]

Central Cord Syndrome

Central cord syndrome is seen in extension injuries, especially in the geriatric patients with arthritic cervical spines.

Upper extremities are affected to a greater degree than lower extremities.

Abnormalities of bladder function are noted.

Brown-Sequard Syndrome

Brown-Sequard syndrome is a destruction or severing (e.g., knife wound) of one side of the cord, resulting in a loss of motor function on the injured side and loss of pain and temperature sensation on the opposite side. Because pain and temperature fibers cross the spinal cord, the level of loss of these sensations is noted on physical examination to be one or two levels below the level of injury.[26]

Associated Injuries and Problems

Associated injuries occurring in trauma victims who sustain spinal cord injury include

Cervical spine
    Closed head injury
    Facial injury
    Tracheal injury
    Esophageal perforation

Thoracic spine
    Rib fracture
    Flail chest
    Tear of the aorta
    Myocardial contusion
    Cardiac tamponade
    Pneumothorax

Lumbar spine
    Pelvic fractures
    Retroperitoneal hemorrhage
    Rupture of bladder

Associated respiratory problems with spinal cord damage include

C3–C5
    Variable phrenic nerve dysfunction
    Paralysis of intercostal and abdominal muscles
    Paradoxical respiration
    May need ventilatory support

C5–C8
    Intercostal and abdominal muscle paralysis
    Inability to cough

T1–T8
    Poor intercostal muscle function
    Cough weak

T8–T12
    Variable abdominal muscle strength

Management Considerations

Manage the airway (see p. 46).

Decrease neck motion by fixing the patient in a neutral position.

Support the neck with sandbags and a hard collar.

Maintain position with traction—manual in-line traction or Gardner Wells tongs.[26]

Maintain traction when moving patient. Pay attention to the weights—do not let them swing about leading to abnormal stresses on the cervical spine. The weights can also "hang-up" on the edge of the patient's bed, so make certain the weights are free.

Caution: If the patient is brought to the operating room for cervical fusion and stabilization, watch for

Flexion or extension of the neck (may exacerbate any injury)

Excess traction on the head and neck (may extend neurologic damage)

Lifting of the epiglottis or applying pressure to the valleculae during direct laryngoscopy (may result in damage)[7]

Indications for tracheal intubation of patients with cervical spine injury are

1. Relief of airway obstruction
2. Treatment of ventilatory failure
3. As an aid for pulmonary toilet
4. Prevention of aspiration of gastric contents
5. Hyperventilation to reduce or prevent elevated ICP
6. Establishment of an airway for surgery

Cardiac Considerations during Intubation

Note: Administer atropine 0.4 to 0.8 mg before airway manipulation to avoid sinus arrest.[33]

In the patient with a spinal cord injury above the level of T1, the effects of cardioaccelerator fibers are lost, leading to marked vagal tone.

Respiration

The level of injury to the spinal cord will determine the extent of respiratory impairment and whether the patient will require intubation.

The patient should be monitored with pulse oximeter and arterial blood gases and administered oxygen as needed.

Respiratory problems may exist in specific neurologic injuries.

Above C4, voluntary diaphragmatic respiration is impossible.

Patients with lesions at C5, C6, and lower are usually able to ventilate adequately.

Loss of intercostal and abdominal muscle function may result in decreased ability to cough and clear secretions.

Hemodynamic Responses to Injury

Initial injury results in massive catecholamine discharge with increased systemic and pulmonary vascular pressures, increased extravascular lung water, and increased ICP.

This is then followed by hypotension.

Table 2-2. Cardiac Effects of Atropine in Quadriplegics with Spinal Shock

	Before	After	P
Pulse	60 ± 12.2	85 ± 10.3	
Cardiac index	3.0 ± 0.76	4.2 ± 1.40	<.05
Pulmonary capillary wedge pressure	13 ± 8.2	14 ± 6.7	NS
Pulmonary artery	85 ± 18.8	109 ± 24.5	<.05

(From MacKenzie and Shin,[33] with permission.)

Pulmonary Edema

Pulmonary edema has been reported to develop in up to 50 percent of patients with cervical cord injury because of alterations in autonomic activity and catecholamine discharge.

By the time a pulmonary artery catheter is placed, the pulmonary hypertension may have resolved, but the pulmonary edema may still be present.[26]

Role of Fluid Overload

Early postinjury patients tend to be hypotensive. To maintain blood pressure and urinary output, these patients may receive large quantities of fluid. When spinal shock resolves and vascular tone returns, congestive heart failure may occur.

MacKenzie and colleagues[34] observed left ventricular function in a group of young patients with spinal shock. They demonstrated the difficulty in predicting changes in pulmonary artery pressure during fluid infusion. The use of a pulmonary artery catheter is very helpful in directing therapy to optimize cardiac output in patients with spinal shock.[34]

Bradycardia

Bradycardia is due to vagal activity in the absence of high thoracic sympathetic output. Bradycardia and sinus arrest have been noted with airway manipulation. Use of atropine 0.4 to 0.8 mg IV will increase heart rate, cardiac index, and arterial blood pressure (Table 2-2).

Spinal Shock

Etiology

Hypotension may be due to hemorrhagic shock, but patients with spinal cord injuries above T5 may experience spinal shock with hypotension, bradycardia, and vasodilatation.

If the lesion is T1 or higher, cardioaccelerator reflexes are lost with a decrease in ability to increase heart rate and cardiac output. Atropine is used to prevent bradycardia during endotracheal intubation and suctioning.[24,26]

Duration

Spinal shock lasts for 3 to 8 weeks after injury. Patients are sensitive to IV fluids, drugs, and anesthetics. The patient is monitored with arterial and pulmonary artery catheters, and urinary output is followed to determine the hemodynamic state.

Autonomic Hyperreflexia

Autonomic hyperreflexia is the result of uninhibited catecholamine discharge at spinal levels above the level of spinal injury. This is characterized by hypertension, flushing, and bradycardia.

If anesthesia is not used in patients with complete cord lesions undergoing surgery in an area without sensation, there is a high incidence of autonomic hyperreflexia. Anesthesia is needed in patients with complete lesions at T7 or above.

Symptoms of autonomic hyperreflexia include

  Facial tingling

  Nasal obstruction

  Severe headache

  Shortness of breath

  Nausea

  Blurred vision

Signs of autonomic hyperreflexia include

  Hypertension

  Bradycardia

  Arrhythmias

  Sweating

  Goose flesh

  Seizures[26]

How to Avoid Autonomic Hyperreflexia

Autonomic hyperreflexia can be avoided by administering anesthesia to the patient. In lower extremity and genitourinary surgery, regional anesthesia may be preferable.[35,36]

Surgical Approach

1. In neurologically intact patients, the neck must be stabilized to prevent injury.
2. In patients with incomplete injury, traction or surgical intervention may be necessary to decompress the spinal cord. These patients may demonstrate recovery after spinal realignment.
3. In patients with complete neurologic lesions, early stabilization is performed to reduce edema and prevent extension of the injury.[26,27]

Considerations in Surgery

If somatosensory evoked potential (SSEP) monitoring is used, a narcotic, nitrous oxide, oxygen-relaxant technique is used to avoid the effect of inhalation agents on SSEPs.

When stabilization of the spine is carried out or when bone fragments are removed from the spinal cord, it may be possible to note improvements in spinal cord function as evidenced by increase in the amplitude or decrease in the latency of the SSEPs.

Perioperative considerations include

1. Stabilize the neck.
2. Administer methylprednisolone.
3. Give atropine 0.4 to 0.8 mg to prevent bradycardia during intubation.
4. Secure and maintain the airway.
5. Use monitoring equipment (ECG, blood pressure, end-tidal carbon dioxide, pulse oximeter).
6. Insert arterial line.
7. Insert pulmonary artery catheter.
8. Insert Foley catheter.
9. Use SSEP monitoring.

Thoracic Spinal Cord Injuries

A burst fracture of the thoracic spine requiring early surgery may be present. Chest radiograph, ECG, and echocardiogram should be obtained.

Look for

Respiratory complications

Rupture of the aorta

Intrathoracic bleeding

Contusions of the lung

Myocardial contusion

Cardiac tamponade

Attention should be directed to intrathoracic injuries before attempts at surgical stabilization of the spinal column injury.

Injuries to the Lumbar Spinal Cord

Look for

- Retroperitoneal hematomas
- Bowel injury
- Bladder injury

After stabilization and treatment of associated injuries, surgical procedures in the lumbar spinal area can be performed.

MUSCULOSKELETAL INJURIES

Historically, the multiply injured patient with fractures underwent surgery directed to the head, abdomen, and thoracic areas. Orthopedic injuries, such as open fractures or long bone fractures, were not immediately repaired definitively.

The recent approach to treatment of musculoskeletal injuries is to repair all fractures on the day of admission. LaDuca et al[38] showed that immediate repair of open fractures did not result in any major complications and episodes of fatal, post-traumatic pulmonary failure or fat embolism did not occur.

The benefits of early surgery include

1. Eliminating casts, thus allowing improved local wound care
2. Decreasing wound complications
3. Allowing early mobilization, thus avoiding cardiopulmonary complications[38,39]

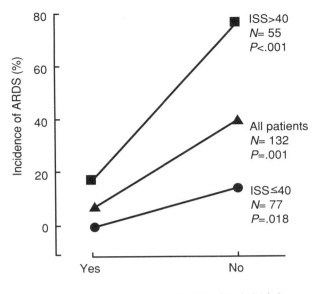

Fig. 2-3. Incidence of ARDS as related to early and late operative stabilization and injury severity score (ISS). (From Johnson et al,[40] with permission.)

In 1985, Johnson et al[40] were able to demonstrate that the incidence of ARDS resulting from trauma increased as time to fracture fixation increased. ARDS was more common in those patients not stabilized within the first 24 hours (Fig. 2-3).

The overall incidence of ARDS was 7 percent in those who had early fracture fixation. Those with less-severe injury severity scores (ISS less than 40) had a 0 percent incidence of ARDS when early fixation occurred. Delay resulted in an 8 percent incidence of ARDS. Patients with high ISS had ARDS 17 percent of the time with early fixation and 75 percent of the time with delayed fixation.

Seibel et al[41] demonstrated that the incidence of pulmonary and septic complications increased if stabilization was delayed for 10 to 30 days. The number of days on a ventilator, days in the intensive care unit, febrile days, and positive blood cultures, were all increased if immediate fixation was not performed.[39,41]

The studies of LaDuca, Johnson, and Seibel support the concept of early fracture repair to

1. Decrease motion and decrease the incidence of fat embolism
2. Allow the patient to sit in an upright position to improve pulmonary function

3. Decrease pain
4. Remove hematoma and necrotic tissue and decrease septic complications
5. Decrease incidence of ARDS[38-41]

Warning: Although early fixation improves outcome, it does not allow repair of all fractures on patients regardless of the severity of associated injuries.

An inflated limb tourniquet on a head-injured patient can result in an increase in ICP when the tourniquet is inflated and deflated. Blood pressure and heart rate tend to increase during tourniquet inflation. On deflation, released acidotic products result in an increase in $PaCO_2$, which may result in elevation of the cerebral blood flow and ICP[4] (see Ch. 7).

MANAGEMENT OF FRACTURES AND DISLOCATIONS
Fracture of Long Bones
Open Fractures

An open fracture is an acute emergency.

Immediate operation is required within a "golden period" of 6 hours or less to prevent infection in open fractures. Intravenous antibiotics should be administered, and débridement of the area carried out.

If a tourniquet is to be used, antibiotics must be infused before tourniquet inflation.

External fixation devices may be applied to stabilize bony fragments to prevent pain and decrease the possibility of fat embolization.

Closed Fractures

Treatment may include open reduction and internal fixation with plates and screws, application of external fixators, or intramedullary rodding. Intramedullary rodding provides good stabilization with the ability for early ambulation, causing compression of the fracture site with better healing.

Dislocations

A dislocation is an acute emergency.

In any dislocation, neurovascular status must be evaluated. Closed or open reduction should be carried out almost immediately to prevent long-term damage. Adequate anesthesia and muscle relaxation is provided to allow closed reduction.

Warning: Do not miss a fracture.

In unconscious or obtunded patients, musculoskeletal injury may be missed easily during initial evaluation. In one study, injuries of the spine, pelvis, femur, or tibiofibula complex occurred in 31 percent of obtunded head trauma victims. This underscores the importance of routine radiologic evaluation of these patients.[42,53,54]

Pelvic Fractures

Pelvic fractures are associated with high mortality rates, significant blood loss, and major hemodynamic swings. The high mortality is usually due to exsanguination.[39,43-46]

Management

Warning: Lower extremity intravenous lines must be avoided.

Associated Hemorrhage
Application of pneumatic antishock garment (PASG) or military antishock trousers (MAST) may help achieve hemodynamic stability once applied.

Inflation of the PASG may actually reduce fracture fragments.

During evaluation in the hospital, PASGs may be placed, although they may not be inflated. Some centers avoid PASGs unless necessary, as they may interfere with intravenous line placement and patient evaluation (C. Grande, personal communication).

Inflation pressures of 30 to 40 mmHg are acceptable. These inflation pressure levels can be kept up to 48 hours.[44] Elevated pressures or prolonged inflation may lead to tissue necrosis.

Deflation should be performed by sections.

Hypovolemia in the face of an inflated PASG may be the result of intra-abdominal or intrathoracic bleeding. Diagnostic peritoneal lavage via a supraumbilical tap may help delineate whether intra-abdominal bleeding is occurring and whether an exploratory laparotomy is necessary.

Case Study

A 27-year-old man involved in a motor vehicle accident was transferred to our institution for repair of a pelvic fracture. While he was being treated with PASGs, he was not able to maintain an adequate blood pressure, although he was receiving blood and fluid. We suspected that the patient was bleeding from a site other than the pelvis. Abdominal exploration was performed, and a ruptured spleen was removed. After stabilization, treatment of the pelvic fracture was undertaken.

Application of External Pelvic Fixators

External pelvic fixators can be applied in the emergency department to reduce the fracture and help decrease bleeding. Fractures with disruption of the symphysis pubis, known as *open book* fractures, are well suited for this type of fixation.

Arteriography

Arteriography is used to identify and embolize disrupted vessels.

Associated Respiratory Problems

Respiratory problems are frequently noted in association with pelvic trauma. These can be exacerbated if PASGs are applied or if a large retroperitoneal hematoma displaces the diaphragm.

Endotracheal intubation and mechanical ventilation should be instituted immediately on the application and inflation of PASGs if ventilation is hindered.

Anatomic Considerations

A large amount of bleeding can occur with pelvic fractures because many arterial anastomoses are present in the pelvis, and the arteries are anatomically adjacent to the pelvic bone. Also, marked venous bleeding can occur.[39,40]

Hemodynamic stability in massive pelvic trauma may result from the tamponade of blood vessels in the retroperitoneal space. Relief of the tamponade may result in death.[39]

Mucha and Welch,[45] in reporting the Mayo Clinic experience, noted high mortality rates with hemodynamically unstable pelvic fractures (42 percent) compared with stable pelvic fractures (3.4 percent). Also, 15.7 units of blood were required per patient.[45]

Cryer et al,[47] in a review of pelvic fractures, noted that fractures of more than 0.5-cm distraction were associated with greater blood transfusion requirements and increased mortality rate. Fractures involving posterior bony fragments, comminuted and open fractures, are associated with the highest mortality rates.[39,46]

Protocols for Exsanguinating Pelvic Fractures

1. The hemodynamically unstable patient who is exsanguinating is taken directly to the operating room.
2. If the patient is somewhat hypotensive and has associated injuries, diagnostic supraumbilical peritoneal lavage is performed.
3. If the patient is hypotensive without major associated injuries and does respond to fluid, the patient can go to the angiography suite. If the patient has received 4 units of blood within 24 hours or 6 units within 48 hours or if an enlarged expanding hematoma is noted, exploratory laparotomy is performed.[45,47]

Embolization

Embolization is an effective treatment for bleeding in pelvic fractures. Embolization can be performed when the patient is in the operating room.

Embolization success rates can be as high as 85 to 90 percent. Failure of embolization is due to severe arterial disease, cardiopulmonary arrest, or coagulopathy.

Panetta et al[48] performed 27 successful embolizations in 31 patients. The average transfusion requirement was 18.6 units, with only 2 to 4 units required after successful embolization.

The patient should be observed carefully for renal dysfunction after the use of radiopaque dye.

Mechanism of Injury

The mechanism of injury determines associated complications.

1. *Anteroposterior compression* includes the open book fracture, in which the symphysis pubis "pops open." When the symphysis pubis separates by more than 3 cm, the pelvic volume is doubled, enabling large volumes of blood to be lost. External fixation devices can reduce open book fractures. Disruption may occur posteriorly at the posterior sacral iliac joint. Along with posterior fractures, the superior gluteal and lateral sacral arteries are at risk.
2. *Lateral compression fractures* are associated with pubic rami fractures, sacroiliac complex fractures, and straddle fractures.
3. *Vertical shear fractures* may disrupt the sacrum and its arterial supply from the rest of the pelvis. These fractures result when a fall occurs from a height.[34,45,46]

Associated Problems

Problems associated with pelvic fractures include pelvic organ injury, coagulopathy from massive blood loss, and pelvic venous thrombosis.[39]

Acetabular Fractures

If the patient is stable, three-dimensional computerized reconstructions of the pelvis and acetabulum can be obtained. These allow planning of acetabular and pelvic reconstructive surgery.

Anesthetic Technique

General anesthesia with a narcotic, nitrous oxide/oxygen, relaxant technique is used for acetabular repairs.

A central venous line, arterial line, Foley catheter, and a blood salvage device are used.

The procedures may be associated with 3 to 4 L of blood loss.

SSEPs are monitored to ascertain the integrity of the sciatic nerve. Changes in sciatic nerve SSEPs have been noted during acetabular repair and, in particular, during femoral traction. We have specifically noted deterioration and resolution of the SSEP wave forms during manipulation of the femur.

Postoperative Pain Relief

An epidural catheter is placed after the patient is anesthetized to provide postoperative pain relief because these patients are immediately placed on continuous passive motion machines (CPMs).

In the early postoperative period, patients are transported for radiation treatment to prevent the formation of myositis ossificans. Epidural narcotics help provide pain relief during the patient's transport to and from radiation therapy.[39]

Vascular Injuries

Vascular injury may be associated with fracture dislocations.

Prompt recognition and repair of vascular injuries is the most important consideration in preventing loss of limb.[41,49]

Arterial injuries commonly associated with specific fractures include

1. Axillary artery injury from humeral fracture, and anterior dislocation of the shoulder.
2. Subclavian artery injury from high upper extremity trauma
3. Brachial artery injury from posterior dislocation of the elbow
4. Popliteal artery injury from posterior dislocation of the knee or from tibial femoral fracture[50]

Presenting Signs

Consider vascular injury if any of the following are present:

1. *P*ulselessness
2. *P*allor
3. *P*ain
4. *P*aresthesias
5. *P*aralysis

In patients with vascular injury and a fracture, the vascular injury is repaired first to avoid prolonged ischemia time.

Heparinization may be required during vascular repair. This must be taken into consideration in assessing bleeding in other areas of the body.

COMPARTMENT SYNDROME

Compartment syndromes may develop after injuries as a result of the development of increased pressure within a closed space, leading to compromise of neurovascular structures within that space.

Compartment syndromes can result from

1. Fractures
2. Bleeding
3. Soft tissue injuries
4. Postischemic states

The area of potential involvement is at or distal to the area of a fracture. Ischemia to muscles and nerves in areas of elevated compartment pressures can ultimately result in necrosis of these tissues.

Five compartments exist in the lower extremity. The posterior tibial compartment is now considered to be an individual compartment.

Compartment syndrome is suspected when pain is out of proportion to the injury or pain on stretching is noted in the involved compartment.[51]

Diagnosis

Anterior Compartment Syndrome

Anterior compartment syndrome consists of weak toe extension, pain on passive flexion, and decreased sensation in the first web space.[51]

Posterior Compartment Syndrome

Posterior compartment syndrome consists of weakness with toe flexion, pain on passive extension, and decreased sensation in the sole of the foot.[51]

Pressure Measurement

Diagnosis of a compartment syndrome is made by measuring intracompartmental pressures by inserting a wick or slit catheter into the compartment at risk. Digital readouts are available on hand-held monitors (Stryker).

Measurements of 30 to 35 mmHg or higher, in combination with clinical findings in the presence of a normal diastolic blood pressure, are considered diagnostic.[51]

Differential Diagnosis

Differential diagnosis of a compartment syndrome includes

Arterial occlusion

Neuropraxia, which may coexist with a compartment syndrome

Deep vein thrombosis[51]

Treatment

Treatment involves early fasciotomy to decrease intracompartmental pressures and prevent nerve, arterial, and muscle ischemia. If pressures are elevated in all compartments and the entire extremity is involved, all compartments need to undergo fasciotomy.[51]

NERVE INJURIES

Nerve injuries may occur in extremity trauma, and specific injuries may be associated with specific deficits.

Neurologic status of both sensory and motor function should be carefully documented before surgical intervention.

Sciatic nerve injury may occur after posterior dislocation of the hip.

Ulnar nerve injury may occur with elbow fractures.

Radial nerve injury may occur with humeral fractures.[52]

FAT EMBOLISM SYNDROME

Embolization of marrow fat after long bone fractures may result in respiratory failure, significant hypoxia, a petechial rash, central nervous system disturbances, and even death. Fat embolism syndrome (FES) is usually seen after pelvic and long bone fractures but has been noted after vertebral and small bone fractures.

Most frequently, FES is associated with

Long bone and pelvic fractures (tibia, fibula, femur)

Vertebral and small bone fractures occasionally

Movement of fracture fragments

Closed fractures

Reaming of long bones intraoperatively

Increased pressure within a marrow cavity (e.g., pressurization during cementing)[34,55,56]

Pathophysiology

FES is believed to occur in two stages:

1. Initial mechanical obstruction caused by fat present in the lungs (this occurs immediately and is similar in presentation to a pulmonary embolism)
2. Chemical phase during which lipase breaks down fat to free fatty acids and glycerol (it is the free fatty acids that cause destruction of lung tissue; phase occurs after 1 to 2 days)[39,58]

Fat Embolism in the General Circulation

Although most embolized fat goes to the lungs, some fat may gain access to the arterial circulation across a patent foramen ovale, which opens as a result of increases in right atrial and ventricular pressure. This embolized fat can reach the brain, kidney, and myocardium.[58]

Signs and Symptoms

Signs and symptoms of fat embolism as described by Peltier, Lindique, and others may include

Hemodynamic instability

Petechial rash present in 50 percent of patients—usually on upper torso especially in axillary region

Hypoxemia on room air—PaO_2 less than 60 mmHg

A picture similar to ARDS, with pulmonary symptoms of tachypnea, dyspnea, rales, and cyanosis

Tachycardia

Fever

Central nervous system signs with restlessness, anxiety, confusion, and coma

Cerebral edema

Change in hematocrit value

Retinal artery occlusion by fat—evident as fluffy white exudates

Delayed awakening from anesthesia—a sign that may be missed

Laboratory data will demonstrate

Low PaO_2—PaO_2 less than 60 mmHg room air

Elevated $PaCO_2$—$PaCO_2$ greater than 55 mmHg or pH less than 7.3

Thrombocytopenia with platelet counts of less than 150,000 mm^3

Fluffy chest radiograph—"snowstorm appearance"

Lipuria, serum lipase, and fat droplets are nonspecific findings and considered too sensitive a test[39,58,59]

Be Alert: Always suspect fat embolism if

Any change in central nervous system status occurs in the trauma patient

Coma from fat embolism begins several hours after trauma (rule out subdural or epidural hematoma, alcohol intoxication, or drug overdose)

Patient fails to awaken from anesthesia[59]

Treatment

Supportive treatment is the mainstay.

Treat hemodynamic instability by improving intravascular volume status.

Treat hypoxia as necessary with supplemental oxygen, mechanical ventilation, and positive end-expiratory pressure (PEEP).

Prophylactic Treatment and Prevention

Early stabilization of fractures is important in decreasing the incidence of FES.

Steroids have been demonstrated to be efficacious in treating FES only if they are administered prophylactically. Kallenbach et al[60] showed a significantly lower incidence of fat embolism in patients receiving 9 mg/kg of steroids than control patients. Severe hypoxemia occurred significantly less frequently ($p <$ .005).[39,57-60]

Case Study

A 68-year-old man underwent a total hip replacement under general anesthesia. During reaming and cementing of the femur, the oxygen saturation level decreased into the 80 percent range. The patient demonstrated unstable hemodynamics, which were corrected with vasopressors and fluid. Oxygen saturation and PaO_2 remained low despite an FIO_2 of 1.0 and use of PEEP. The patient did not awaken postoperatively. Computed tomography scan performed on the second postoperative day demonstrated cerebral edema. Shortly thereafter, the patient died.

Comment

This appears to be a classic case of massive fat embolism. Right heart strain and increased atrial pressures probably enabled fat to embolize across a patent foramen ovale. That the patient did not awaken made us suspect that paradoxical embolism had occurred.

Case Study

A 45-year-old man fell from a roof and sustained a T12 burst fracture. When the patient was brought to the operating room for stabilization, his oxygen saturation was noted to be 82 percent. Arterial blood gases demonstrated a PaO_2 of 47 mmHg. Chest radiograph did not reveal any obvious pulmonary contusion or other pathology. Consultation with the patient's internist revealed that previous PaO_2 levels on room air were in the 75 mmHg range. The possibility of fat embolism was entertained. Platelet count was slightly below normal. The case was postponed while pulmonary toilet and supplemental oxygen were administered. The patient stabilized and underwent surgery without problem, but oxygen saturation remained in the mid 90s despite FIO_2 of 1.0.

Comment

Vertebral fractures are not frequently associated with FES. However, this diagnosis should be entertained when the evidence is sufficient.

POSTOPERATIVE CONSIDERATIONS

Mental Status

Agitation in the postoperative period may be a sign of hypoxia, fat embolism, distended bladder, elevated ICP, or pain and must be evaluated before treatment is instituted.

If the patient fails to awaken after an appropriate period of time, a full neurologic assessment must be carried out.

Causes to be considered include

Residual anesthesia

Fat embolism

Intracerebral bleeding or contusion

Brain stem herniation

Early computed tomography scan may be valuable.

Neck

Airway obstruction from an acute expanding hematoma may occur.

Chest

Obtain chest radiograph on arrival to postanesthesia care unit.

Look for a pneumothorax, which may appear as a result of chest tube malfunction or rupture of the lung.

Obtain arterial blood gas studies—adjust ventilator settings accordingly.

Be on the alert for
ARDS
Fat embolism
Aspiration

Heart

If tachycardia is present, consider

Hypovolemia

Persistent unrecognized hemorrhage

Pneumothorax

Abdomen

Check for
Distention—may be result of nitrous oxide effect on bowel gases

Bleeding in abdomen

Bladder distention from obstructed urinary catheter

Urine

Decreased urinary output may be caused by

Renal failure

Hypovolemia

Myoglobinuria

Transfusion reaction

Operative Site

Check for swelling, which may be due to bleeding. This can lead to hypovolemia. Swelling can also result in compartment syndrome.

Acute Post-Traumatic Pain Management

Morphine is commonly used to treat acute pain. Analgesia after an IV dose may be delayed. Small 1- to 2-mg IV doses of morphine can be given while observing patient until pain relief is achieved. Careful observation of the patient to detect respiratory depression or excess sedation is mandatory.

Meperidine, in IV doses of 12.5 mg, may be administered every 5 to 10 minutes to reach adequate analgesia. Meperidine is a cardiovascular depressant, and it should be used carefully in the hypovolemic trauma victim.[61,62]

Patient Controlled Analgesia

The requirement for pain management after trauma depends on the degree of injury and the mental status of the patient. Modalities include IV or IM injections, patient controlled analgesia (PCA), nerve blocks, and epidural narcotics or infusions (see Ch. 14). PCA is very effective for postoperative pain management. The patient must be capable of understanding what is required to obtain adequate relief. Mental obtundation or fractured upper extremities may make it difficult to press the PCA button at the appropriate time. The patient must be able to understand what is required to obtain adequate pain relief.

REFERENCES

1. Capan LM, Miller SM, Turndorf H: Trauma overview. p. 3. In Capan LM, Miller SM, Turndorf H (eds): Trauma Anesthesia and Intensive Care. JB Lippincott, Philadelphia 1991
2. Baker CC: Epidemiology of trauma: the civilian practice. Ann Emerg Med 15:1389, 1986
3. MacKenzie RC, Schackford SR, Garfin SR, Hoyt DB: Major skeletal injuries in

the obtunded blunt trauma patient: a case for routine radiologic survey. J Trauma 20:1450, 1988

4. Champion HR, Sacco WJ, Carnazzo AJ et al: The trauma score. Crit Care Med 9:672, 1981

5. Morris JA, Auerbach PS, Marshall GA et al: The trauma score as a triage tool in the pre-hospital setting. JAMA 256:1319, 1986

6. Grande CM, Stene JK, Bernhard WN: Airway management: considerations in the trauma patient. p. 37. In Grande CM (ed): Overview of Trauma Anesthesia and Critical Care. Vol. 6. WB Saunders, Philadelphia, 1990

7. Majernick TG, Bienick R, Houston JB, Hughes HG: Cervical and spine movement during orotracheal intubation. Ann Emerg Med 15:417, 1986

8. Boyd DR: Comprehensive regional trauma/emergency medical service (EMS) delivery systems: The United States Experience. World J Surg 7:149, 1983

9. Giesecke AH, Grande CM, Whitten CW: Fluid therapy and resuscitation of traumatic shock. In Grande CM (ed): Overview of Trauma. Anesthesia and Critical Care. Vol. 6. WB Saunders, Philadelphia, 1990

10. Millikan JS, Cain TL, Hansbrough J: Rapid volume replacement for hypovolemic shock: a comparison of techniques and equipment. J Trauma 24:428, 1984

11. Lucas CE: Renal considerations in the injured patient. Surg Clin North Am 12:133, 1982

12. Lucas CE: Resuscitation of the injured patient: the three phases of treatment. Surg Clin North Am 57:3, 1977

13. Miller RD: Transfusion therapy. p. 1486. In: Anesthesia. 3rd Ed. Vol. 2. Churchill Livingstone, New York, 1990

14. Coonan TJ, Hope CE: Cardiorespiratory effects of change of body position. Can Anaesth Soc J 30:424, 1983

15. Pavlin EG: Anaesthesia for the traumatized patient. Can Anaesth Soc J 30:S27, 1983

16. Capan LM, Gottlieb G, Rosenberg A: General principles of anesthesia for major acute trauma. p. 259. In Capan LM, Miller SM, Turndorf H (eds): Trauma Anesthesia and Intensive Care. JB Lippincott, Philadelphia, 1991

17. McGoldrick MD, Capan LM: Acute renal failure in the injured. p. 755. In Capan LM, Miller SM, Turndorf H (eds): Trauma Anesthesia and Intensive Care. JB Lippincott, Philadelphia, 1991

18. Weiskopf RB, Bogetz MS: Haemorrhage decreases the anaesthetic requirement for ketamine and thiopentone in the pig. Br J Anaesth 57:1022, 1985

19. Weiskopf RB, Bogetz MS, Roizen MF, Reid DA: Cardiovascular and metabolic sequelae of inducing anesethesia with ketamine or thiopental in hypovolemic swine. Anesthesiology 60:214, 1954

20. White PF, Wagner Trevor AJ: Ketamine: its pharmacology and therapeutic uses. Anesthesiology 56:119, 1982

21. Adams P, Gelman S, Reves JG: Midazolam pharmacodynamics and pharmacokinetics during acute hypovolemia. Anesthesiology 63:140, 1985

22. Manriquez RG, Pallares VS: Continuous brachial plexus block for prolonged sympathectomy and control of pain. Anesth Analg 57:128, 1978

23. Beck GP: Anterior approach to sciatic nerve block. Anesthesiology 26:222, 1963

24. Schriebman DL, MacKenzie CF: The trauma victim with an acute spinal cord injury in anesthesia and trauma. p. 459. In Matjasko MJ, Shin B (eds): Problems in Anesthesia. Anesthesia and Trauma. Vol. 4. JB Lippincott, Philadelphia, 1990

25. Stene JK: Management of airway problems in trauma patients. p. 431. In Matjasko MJ, Shin B (eds): Problems in Anesthesia. Anesthesia and Trauma. Vol. 4. JB Lippincott, Philadelphia, 1990

26. Sommer RM, Bauer RD, Errico TJ: Cervical spine injuries. p. 447. In Capan LM, Miller SM, Turndorf H (eds): Trauma Anesthesia and Intensive Care. JB Lippincott, Philadelphia, 1991

27. Poe RH, Reisman JL, Rodenhouse TG: Pulmonary edema in cervical spinal cord injury. J Trauma 18:71, 1978

28. Crosby ET, Lui ACP: Trauma and the adult cervical spine. Implications for airway management. p. 13. In Lui ACP, Crosby ET (eds): Problems in Anesthesia. Anesthesia and Musculoskeletal Disorders. Vol. 5. JB Lippincott, Philadelphia, 1991

29. Bracken M, Shepard MJ, Collins WF et al: A randomized controlled trial of methylprednisolone or naloxone in the treatment of acute spine cord injury. Results of the Second National Acute Spinal Cord Injury Study. N Engl J Med 322:1504, 1990

30. Young W, Flamm ES: Effect of high dose corticosteroid therapy on blood flow, evoked potentials, and extracellular calcium in experimental spine injury. J Neurosurg 57:667, 1982

31. Griffiths IR, Trench JG, Crawford RA: Spinal cord blood flow and conduction during experimental cord compression in normotensive and hypotensive dog. J Neurosurg 50:353, 1979

32. Drummond JC, Moore SS: The influence of dextrose administration on neurologic outcome after temporary spinal cord ischemia in the rabbit. Anesthesiology 70:64, 1989

33. MacKenzie CF, Shin B: Cardiac effects of atropine in bradycardic quadriplegics during spinal shock. Crit Care Med 9:150, 1981

34. MacKenzie CF, Shin B, Krishnaprasad D et al: Asessment of cardiac and respiratory function during surgery on patients with acute quadriplegia. J Neurosurg 62:843, 1985

35. Lambert DH, Deane RS, Mazuzan JE: Anesthesia and the control of blood pressures in patients with spinal cord injury. Anesth Analg 61:344, 1982

36. Guttman L: Spinal Cord Injury. Comprehensive Management and Research. 2nd Ed. Blackwell, London, 1976

37. Brunnette DD Rockswold GL: Neurologic recovery following rapid spinal realignment for complete cervical spinal cord injury. J Trauma 27:445, 1987

38. LaDuca JN, Bone LL, Seibel RW et al: Primary open reduction and internal fixation of open fractures. J Trauma 20:580, 1980

39. Patel KP, Capan LM, Grant GL et al: Musculoskeletal injuries. p. 511. In Capan LM, Miller SM, Turndorf H (eds): Trauma Anesthesia and Intensive Care. JB Lippincott, Philadelphia, 1991

40. Johnson KD, Cadambi A, Seibert GD: Incidence of adult respiratory distress syndrome in patients with multiple musculoskeletal injuries: effects of early operative stabilization of fractures. J Trauma 23:375, 1985

41. Seibel R, LaDuca J, Hassett JM et al: Blunt multiple trauma (ISS 36), femur traction and pulmonary failure—septic state. Ann Surg 202:283, 1985

42. Eldridge PR, Williams S: Effect of limb tourniquet on cerebral perfusion pressure in the head-injured patient. Anaesthesia 44:973, 1989

43. Trunkey DD: Pelvic injuries. p. 147. In Najarian JD, Delaney JP (eds): Trauma and Critical Care Surgery. Year Book Medical Publishers, Chicago, 1987

44. Brotman S, Soderstrom CA, Oster-Granite M et al: Management of severe bleeding in fractures of the pelvis. Surg Gynecol Obstet 153:823, 1981

45. Mucha P Jr, Welch TJ: Hemorrhage in major pelvic fractures. Surg Clin North Am 68:757, 1988
46. Cryer HM, Miller FB, Everes BM et al: Pelvic fractures classification: correlation with hemorrhage. J Trauma 28:973, 1988
47. Flint LM, Brown A, Richardson JD et al: Definitive control of bleeding from severe pelvic fractures. Ann Surg 189:709, 1979
48. Panetta T, Sclafani SJA, Goldstein AS et al: Percutaneous transcatheter embolization for massive bleeding from pelvic fractures. J Trauma 25:1021, 1985
49. Rittman WW, Schibi M, Matter P et al: Open fractures: long term results in 200 consecutive cases. Clin Orthop 138:132, 1979
50. Gustilo RB Mendoza RM, Williams DN: Problems in the management of type III (severe) open fractures: a new classification of type III open fractures. J Trauma 24:742, 1984
51. Bourne RB, Rorabeck CH: Compartment syndromes of the lower leg. Clin Orthop 240:97, 1989
52. Ransom KJ, Shatney CH, Soderstrom CA, Kali RA: Management of arterial injuries and blunt trauma of the extremity. Surg Gynecol Obstet 153:241, 1981
53. MacKenzie RC, Shackford SR, Garfin SR et al: Major skeletal injuries in the obtunded blunt trauma patient: a case for routine radiologic survey. J Trauma 28:1450, 1988
54. Riska E, von Bonsdorff H, Hakkinen S: Primary operative fixation of long bone fractures in patients with multiple injuries. J Trauma 17:111, 1977
55. Karb CA Jr, Hillnaj JW: Fat embolism. p. 122. In American Academy of Orthopaedic Surgery (eds): Instructional Course Lecture. American Academy of Orthopaedic Surgeons, Chicago, 1961
56. Duis HJT, Nijsten MWN, Klasen JH et al: Fat embolism in patients with an isolated fracture of the femoral shaft. J Trauma 28:383, 1988
57. Peltier LF: Fat embolism. A perspective. Clin Orthop 232:263, 1988
58. Peltier LF: Fat embolism. III. The toxic properties of neutral fat and free fatty acids. Surgery 40:665, 1956
59. Lindeque BGP, Schoeman HS, Dommisse GF et al: Fat embolism in the fat embolism syndrome. A double blind therapeutic study. J Bone Joint Surg 69(B):128, 1987
60. Kallenbach J, Lewis M, Zaltzman M: "Low dose" corticosteroid prophylaxis against fat embolism. J Trauma 27:1173, 1987
61. Mather LE, Phillips GD: Opioids and adjuvants. Principles of use. Crit Care Med 8:77, 1986
62. Bond AC, Davies CK: Ketamine and pancuronium for the shocked patients. Anaesthesia 29:59, 1974
63. Rosenberg AD, Bernstein RL: Perioperative anesthetic management of orthopedic trauma. p. 555. In Grande CM (ed): Textbook of Trauma Anesthesia and Critical Care. CV Mosby, St. Louis, 1993

3

The Fractured Hip

Hip fractures tend to occur in the elderly patient. Compared with younger people, the geriatric patients who fracture their hips tend to suffer from comorbidities that have significant impact on their daily lives and may affect the outcome of their surgery.

It has become evident to us that special attention to the medical conditions present in these patients is important in improving their outcome. At the Hospital for Joint Diseases Orthopaedic Institute (HJDOI), a comprehensive approach to the geriatric hip fracture patient has been instituted that addresses all aspects of care and rehabilitation.

In a comparison of 431 program patients with matched controls, there were

Fewer postoperative complications ($P < .001$)

Fewer intensive care unit transfers—10.2 percent versus 20 percent ($P < .05$)

Fewer discharges to nursing homes

Decreased length of stay

Improved ambulatory status ($P < .001$)[1]

PATIENTS AT RISK

Predisposing factors to fractures have been identified. In women, these include

Lower limb dysfunction

Visual impairment

Previous stroke

Parkinson's disease

Use of long-acting barbiturates[2]

Other factors include

Increased age

Sex—ratio of women to men 2:1

Race—higher in white women

Institutionalized patients

History of previous fracture

Psychotropic medications

Dementia

Osteoporosis

Comorbidity

Cold climate[3]

MORTALITY RATES

Mortality associated with hip fractures is highest in the first 6 months after injury, with overall mortality rates after fracture ranging from 14 to 36 percent.[3]

COMORBIDITY

Patients often suffer from several medical conditions at the time of fracture.

Frequent comorbidities observed include

Hypertension

Diabetes

Cardiac problems (previous myocardial infarction, congestive heart failure, angina, abnormal electrocardiogram [ECG])

Chronic obstructive pulmonary disease and pulmonary dysfunction

Neurologic disorders and dementia

Renal or metabolic disorders

Gastrointestinal disorders

Genitourinary disorders

COMORBIDITY AND OUTCOME

The effect of comorbidity has been studied in relation to the outcome of patients with fractured hips. Kenzora et al[4] found that patients with four to six comorbidities had an increased mortality rate when compared with those with fewer comorbidities (zero to three).

AMERICAN SOCIETY OF ANESTHESIOLOGISTS CLASSIFICATION AND OUTCOME

An association can be made between the American Society of Anesthesiologists (ASA) classification and morbidity. White et al[5] noted that patients with hip fractures and ASA classifications of I or II were at no more risk for mortality

Table 3-1. Factors Associated with Increased Mortality in Geriatric Patients with Hip Fractures in Different Studies

Author	High ASA Classification	Concurrent Medical Problems	Increased Age	Male Sex
White, Fisher, and Laurin[5]	X			
Valentin et al[6]	X		X	
Kenzora et al[4]		X	X	
Davis et al[7]		X	X	
Clayer and Brauze[8]		X	X	X

(From Rosenberg and Bernstein,[35] with permission.)

than age- and sex-adjusted controls (8 percent death rate per year). However, those with ASA III or IV status had mortality rates of 49 percent or 6.3 times that of their controls.

Table 3-1 reviews some studies of factors associated with mortality after hip fracture.

DIABETES AND OUTCOME

In our geriatric trauma program at HJDOI, in 70 diabetic patients there was a 26 percent mortality rate compared with an 11 percent mortality rate in nondiabetic controls (JD Zuckerman and R Feldman, personal communication).

COMORBIDITY AND MORTALITY IN SURGICAL PATIENTS

Although not specifically addressing the hip fracture patient, the study of Browner et al,[9] shows that comorbidity may be a predictor of postoperative mortality in the surgical patient undergoing non-cardiac surgery.

The presence of the following risk factors are associated with increased in-house mortality in hospitalized patients undergoing surgery.

1. Decreased renal function (low creatinine clearance)
2. History of hypertension or use of antihypertensive agents
3. "Severely limited activity"

The greater the number of these risk factors a patient had, the greater the chance of death.

A mortality rate of about 20 percent was noted in patients with two or more risk factors, which was about eight times that of patients with zero or one risk factor.

Long-term mortality (within 2 years) increased in patients with pre-existing medical conditions and was associated with cancer, renal dysfunction, congestive heart failure, and obstructive pulmonary disease. Mortality was noted to be higher the greater the number of associated medical conditions present.[9]

ANATOMY FOR THE ANESTHESIOLOGIST

Hip fractures have been divided into two major anatomic subgroups (Fig. 3-1).

1. Intracapsular fractures or fractures of the femoral neck
2. Extracapsular fractures, comprising intertrochanteric and subtrochanteric fractures

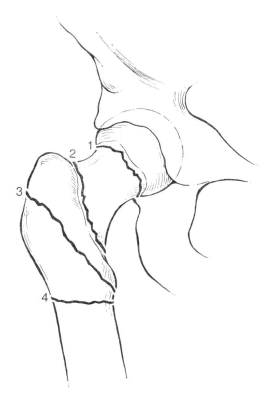

Fig. 3-1. Diagramatic representation of different fractures of the femur. 1, Subcapital fracture of neck of femur; 2, fracture through base of neck; 3, intertrochanteric fracture; 4, transverse subtrochanteric fracture.

Intracapsular Fractures

Intracapsular fractures occur more frequently in younger, healthier patients.[3,10]

They can occur as a result of direct trauma, but the fracture may occur before a fall as the result of a slip or twisting injury. Even if the patient does not fall, tightening and contraction of the muscles around the hip joint may result in fracture of osteoporotic bone.[3,11]

The blood supply to the femoral head arises from a branch of the profunda femoris artery and flows from distal to proximal up the femoral neck. Disruption of this blood supply as a result of femoral neck fractures can lead to aseptic necrosis of the femoral head.[3]

If the fracture of the femoral head can be reduced under fluoroscopy, pins can be placed across the fracture site. If the femoral head appears unsalvageable or closed reduction is unsuccessful, a hemiarthroplasty is performed. Closed reduction and pinning is associated with lower blood loss.

Extracapsular (Intertrochanteric and Subtrochanteric) Fractures

Intertrochanteric fractures tend to occur after a fall or injury. Transient ischemic attacks, stroke, arrhythmia, myocardial infarction, or other cause for falling should be considered.

These fractures are associated with higher blood loss.

In the elderly, intertrochanteric fractures occur more commonly than subtrochanteric fractures, which only account for approximately 5 percent of hip fractures in geriatric patients at HJDOI.[3]

These fractures are repaired with a nail through the femoral neck and into the femoral head, which is attached to a side plate and screws for fixation along the femoral shaft.

ARE ALL FRACTURED HIPS EMERGENCIES?

Although fractured hips are considered urgent cases, data exist to suggest that obtaining an optimal medical state before surgery is advantageous. Merely pushing in 2 units of packed red blood cells and rushing the patient to the operating room is not the best way to approach the patient with a fractured hip. Schultz et al[12] decreased their mortality rate from 29 to 2.9 percent by placing pulmonary artery catheters and correcting the altered physiologic state.

Kenzora et al[4] reported a significantly higher mortality rate (34 percent versus 6.9 percent) in patients operated on within the first 24 hours when compared with those patients undergoing surgery 2 to 5 days after fracture.

At HJDOI, in a study of 315 patients, those with two or fewer comorbidities fared worse if surgery was delayed, whereas delay in patients with three or more comorbidities was associated with decreased mortality.[13]

Our practice is to evaluate the patient's medical status, identify medical conditions that need to be improved, and obtain necessary laboratory work and diagnostic tests. Central venous pressure or pulmonary artery catheters are placed when indicated, and then surgery proceeds. Most patients are operated on within 24 to 48 hours, but surgery will be delayed when indicated by the medical condition.

Case Study

An 89-year-old hypertensive, confused, hyponatremic woman with an anginal history presented for repair of a fractured hip. Current medications were nifedipine, propranolol, and a nitroglycerine patch. The hyponatremia had been treated by fluid restriction. Blood pressure on arrival to operating room was 290/130 mmHg.

The operation was postponed, and the patient was treated with her usual medications plus labetalol. A pulmonary artery catheter was placed because of concern about dehydration in this fluid-restricted hypertensive patient. Because many hypertensive patients tend to become hemodynamically unstable intraoperatively, we were especially concerned with this patient who had been fluid-restricted. Initial pulmonary artery pressure readings were 2 to 3 mmHg. Rehydration with saline solutions in combination with antihypertensive agents improved the patient's physiologic profile. General anesthesia was selected because the patient was too uncooperative and we were concerned about the physiologic response to spinal anesthesia. The patient was induced with etomidate, atracurium, and fentanyl and maintained on nitrous oxide/oxygen, narcotics, and muscle relaxants. The operation proceeded uneventfully, and the patient did well postoperatively.

Comment

In this case, surgery was postponed because of marked hypertension and dehydration. Without specific knowledge as to the state of hydration and adequate control of the blood pressure, the patient would be at risk for severe hypotension on induction.

PREOPERATIVE EVALUATION AND PREPARATION

Proper preoperative evaluation and preparation includes a review of systems geared toward the geriatric patient. Why did the patient sustain a fracture? Is there a history of syncope, palpitation, loss of consciousness, stroke, transient ischemic attack, arrhythmia, myocardial infarction, or just tripping?

Medications

Current medications must be continued because a few days without medications such as antihypertensive agents or β-blockers may lead to hemodynamic instability.

Hypertension

This is a common finding among geriatric patients. Associated damage to the heart, kidney, and brain may be present. These patients may be volume-depleted from hypertension, antihypertensive agents, diuretics, and blood loss into the thigh. Spinal and general anesthesia in the face of volume depletion can result in marked hypotension.

Preoperative Plan

The preoperative evaluation must include a determination of whether end-organ problems exist. Left ventricular hypertrophy, renal disease, and cerebrovascular insufficiency are considered. The patient's antihypertensive medications should be continued.

Diabetes

If diabetes is present, serial glucose determinations should be obtained preoperatively, and a management plan should be outlined.

These patients may suffer from silent myocardial ischemia, renal insufficiency, vascular disease, and decreased gastric motility.

Preoperative Plan

Preoperative evaluation must include a baseline glucose determination and a management plan for glucose control. Patients should be protected from hypoglycemia. Fingersticks, not urine samples, should be relied on to determine dosing.

The insulin-dependent patient should receive insulin only after a glucose-containing infusion is started.

Administration of metoclopramide to avoid gastric regurgitation should be considered.

Pulmonary System

The pulmonary system deserves special attention because it is always argued that "we have to do surgery now or the patient will get pneumonia and die." Immobilization before surgery may lead to pneumonia, and therefore any pulmonary abnormalities should be noted and corrected as soon as possible. Factors that contribute to poor lung function in geriatric patients include decreased muscle power, chest wall compliance, and elastic recoil of the lung, smaller intervertebral spaces, chronic obstructive pulmonary disease, smoking, or history of other pulmonary disorders.[14]

Baseline PaO_2 levels in the low 70-mmHg range are not uncommon in the geriatric patient. Levels may be decreased from this secondary to immobilization, fat emboli, or platelet and fibrin deposition in the lung.[15,16]

Preoperative Plan

Obtain a preoperative arterial blood gas.

Evaluate the chest radiograph.

Obtain baseline pulmonary function tests, if indicated.

Administer medications such as steroids or bronchodilators, when necessary.

Consult with respiratory therapist to administer treatments to correct abnormalities in pulmonary function.

Cardiac Risk

Goldman helped us to evaluate and determine cardiac risk in surgical patients. He determined nine conditions that independently correlate with perioperative cardiac morbidity and assigned point values for each.[17,18]

Point totals are determined by adding the points for each risk factor present. Morbidity and mortality can be estimated based on the point total.

Table 3-2. Factors Related to Perioperative Cardiac Complications[a]

Disease	Points
Preoperative congestive heart failure	11
Myocardial infarction in the previous 6 mo	10
Preoperative electrocardiogram rhythm other than sinus	7
History of >5 premature ventricular contractions	7
Age >70 yr	5
Aortic stenosis	3
Poor general medical status	3
Site of operation	3
Emergency nature of the procedure	4

[a] Note that many of these risk factors are present in patients with fractured hips.
(From Rosenberg and Bernstein,[36] with permission.)

Higher point scores are associated with higher risk[17,18] (Table 3-2). A recent study of predictors of postoperative myocardial ischemia noted preoperative comorbidities associated with postoperative cardiac problems. The five preoperative predictors of postoperative myocardial ischemia were (1) left ventricular hypertrophy by ECG, (2) a history of hypertension, (3) diabetes mellitus, (4) definite coronary artery disease, and (5) use of digoxin. The risk of ischemia increased with the number of predictors present (22 percent with no predictors to 77 percent with four predictors).[19]

Preoperative Plan

Examine the patient to determine whether any cardiac disease is present.

Listen to the heart and lungs for murmurs and rales.

Check for the presence of diabetes.

Obtain a history of cardiac medications.

Evaluate the chest radiograph for heart size and increased vascularity.

Check the ECG for changes; obtain old ECG for comparison. We use our facsimile machine constantly for this.

Postpone surgery on patients in active congestive heart failure, treat the patient with the aid of a pulmonary artery catheter, and then operate when the patient's congestive heart failure (CHF) is under control.

Obtain an echocardiogram in patients with valvular heart disease to determine which valves are involved so an intelligent decision can be made concerning anesthetic technique (e.g., avoid spinal or epidural anesthesia in patients with moderate or severe aortic stenosis).

Recent Myocardial Infarction

Patients with recent myocardial infarctions pose problems in that surgery within the first 6 months is associated with increased risk of reinfarction and death.[20]

Consideration must be given to the extent of myocardial damage as determined by evaluation of left ventricular function, the presence or absence of angina, and the state of the heart as determined by imaging techniques.

We have operated on a few patients in the 3- to 6-month period after a myocardial infarction with the aid of a pulmonary artery catheter and postoperative monitoring in the intensive care unit. These were patients who had minor myocardial damage and good left ventricular function on echocardiogram.

Neurologic Considerations

Many patients with hip fracture suffer from some degree of organic mental syndrome. They should be evaluated preoperatively and the degree of dementia determined and recorded to be compared with the mental status postoperatively.

Parkinson's Disease

Patients with Parkinson's disease need special attention. Studies have demonstrated that these patients have a higher morbidity and mortality after fracture than others.[3,21,22]

These patients may be rigid, have a tremor, suffer from bradykinesia, and have loss of postural reflexes, all caused by dopamine deficiency in the brain. Many patients also suffer from dementia. It is important to continue anti-Parkinson medications in the perioperative period to maintain the patient in a stable condition.[23]

Note: Medications to be avoided in these patients include dopamine antagonists such as butyrophenone derivatives (droperidol and haloperidol) and centrally acting antihypertensives such as methyldopa (Aldomet).[24]

Abnormalities in muscular function and coordination of the airway resulting in abnormal airflow patterns have been noted in these patients.[25]

This airway problem in association with abnormalities of the gastrointestinal tract places the patient at risk for aspiration. In one recent case in our hospital, after induction of anesthesia and endotracheal intubation, more than 500 ml of gastric contents were suctioned from the stomach of a patient with Parkinson's disease who had a fractured hip.

Stroke

Patients who have strokes and sustain fracture of the hip are high-risk surgical candidates. These patients have circulatory instability for several weeks after the stroke. We wait about 3 weeks after a cerebral vascular accident until hemodynamic stability returns before we repair the fracture.

PREOPERATIVE LABORATORY DETERMINATIONS

Hemoglobin and Hematocrit Values

Levels are usually low secondary to age and bleeding into the fracture site. Although there is a tendency to avoid giving blood transfusions, we prefer to have these patients with a hematocrit value of 30 percent or above. Adjustments are made when necessary based on the presence of cardiac and pulmonary disease. The patient with an anginal history may not tolerate a lower hematocrit value than his or her baseline level without the onset of symptoms. One must be careful that the hematocrit level was not obtained in a dehydrated patient because rehydration can result in an hematocrit level in the low 20 percent range.

Warning: Do not start the operation unless you are sure that the blood for the patient has been typed and cross-matched and *is readily* available.

Electrolytes

Hyponatremia may result because of the administration of D5 one-third normal saline to "protect" the patient from an overload of sodium. In the elderly, there may also be an increased secretion of antidiuretic hormone. Low sodium levels may lead to confusion.

Dehydration and abnormal electrolyte levels are avoided by administering proper fluids based on serum electrolyte determinations. Urinary output should be followed and a central venous pressure line placed if necessary. *Hypokalemia* can result from diuretic therapy. Marked hypokalemia needs to be treated. Intracellular potassium will not be corrected by a few boluses of potassium rapidly administered overnight. We accept values above 3.0 mEq.

MONITORING

Blood Pressure

Blood pressure may be measured by noninvasive means. Arterial monitoring is useful because it allows beat-to-beat analysis of the blood pressure. An intra-arterial line provides easy access to obtain samples for blood gas determinations.

Pulse Oximetry

Many elderly patients arrive in the operating room with a low PaO_2 and low oxygen saturation. Pulse oximetry is a valuable tool in the patient who is at risk for fat embolism, decreases in oxygenation during reaming of the femur, and changes caused by methylmethacrylate cement[26] (see Ch. 4).

We have noted oxygen desaturation during both reaming and cementing of the femoral shaft and acetabulum.

Electrocardiogram

We routinely use leads II and V5 to monitor for myocardial ischemia. If we have specific knowledge that one area of the heart tends to become ischemic, we will direct our monitoring to the appropriate lead.

Central Venous Pressure and Pulmonary Artery Pressure Monitoring

The decision to monitor central venous or pulmonary artery pressures is based on anticipated fluid shifts, blood loss, and the presence of significant cardiac disease. A pulmonary artery catheter is especially valuable in the patient with a history of CHF to manage fluid status and avoid overload and dehydration.

We have seen patients with a history of CHF arrive in the operating room very dehydrated because of

1. Blood loss secondary to fractures
2. Continued use of diuretics because these were taken before admission
3. An extra "shot" of furosemide administered just before coming to the operating room by the internist to keep the patient "out of failure"
4. Diuretics used before and after transfusion

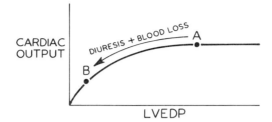

Fig. 3-2. Patient with chronic congestive heart failure and elevated left ventricular end-diastolic pressure (LVEDP) (**A**) may have lowered LVEDP and low intravascular volume after aggressive preoperative diuresis and blood loss into fracture site (**B**). Resulting hypovolemia may cause hypotension after spinal or general anesthesia is induced (see text).

Patients with a history of chronic CHF exist on the flat part of the "Frank-Starling curve" with elevated left ventricular end-diastolic pressures (Fig. 3-2). After aggressive diuresis, these patients may now rest on the ascending steep part of the Frank-Starling curve with low end-diastolic pressures but also decreased stroke volumes and cardiac output (Fig. 3-2). This degree of diuresis leads to hypovolemia, which may result in marked hypotension after a spinal anesthestic is administered. We are very concerned when a patient with a history of CHF arrives in the operating room with a pulmonary capillary wedge pressure of 3 mmHg. Fluid infusion may be necessary before induction of anesthesia if the pulmonary capillary wedge pressure is low. If rehydration is not adequate and blood pressure falls after induction, careful fluid infusion, while observing the pulmonary capillary wedge pressure, not inotropes, may be necessary to treat the low blood pressure and cardiac output.

We use pulmonary artery catheters in patients with significant valvular disease, idiopathic hypertrophic subaortic stenosis, and ischemic heart disease with left ventricular dysfunction.

Urine Output

Foley catheters are inserted in all patients with hip fractures. Adequate urine output on arrival to the operating room is a good indication of adequate hydration. In patients with borderline renal function, pharmacologic and physiologic interventions such as dopamine or fluid challenges are administered.

BEST ANESTHETIC TECHNIQUE

"Patient cleared for repair of hip fracture under spinal anesthesia." Although many of our internist colleagues write clearance notes such as this and believe that patients do better if they receive a regional anesthetic, there are no convincing data to support this concept.

Table 3-3. ASA Classification and Anesthetic Technique

Anesthetic Technique	ASA Classification				
	I	II	III	IV	Nonclassified
General	10	156	86	7	17
Spinal	2	64	97	11	9

ASA I and II patients received general anesthesia more frequently ($P < .001$).

In one study by Valentin et al[6] of 578 patients with a mean patient age of 79.0 years, no significant difference occurred in short- or long-term mortality based on anesthetic technique. In another study conducted by Davis et al[7] of 538 patients with a mean age of 79.5 years, there was also no difference between short- and long-term mortality. Davis et al[7] noted that increased mortality was associated with patients who had dementia.[35]

HJDOI Experience

We reviewed 459 patients with fractures of the hip repaired at HJDOI between 1987 and 1991 to determine the effect of ASA classification on anesthetic technique, the number of comorbidities on anesthetic technique, and the effect of anesthetic technique on mortality[28] (Table 3-3). Of the 459 patients reviewed, 60.1 percent received general anesthesia and 39.9 percent received regional anesthesia. (Data from the Database Geriatric Trauma Program of HJDOI [JD Zuckerman, Director].)

Evaluation of patients classified as ASA III or IV demonstrated that 46.3 percent received general and 53.7 percent received regional anesthesia.

Comorbidity and Anesthetic Technique

Anesthetic technique was not influenced by the number of comorbidities from which the patient suffered. There was no statistically significant difference on anesthestic technique if the patient had zero to two comorbidities or three or more comorbidities. Patients having three or more comorbidities received general anesthesia 48 percent of the time and regional 52 percent of the time.

Relationship of Choice of Anesthesia to
In-Hospital Mortality

There was no statistically significant difference in in-hospital mortality rates for those who received general or regional anesthesia (Table 3-4).

Table 3-4. Mortality

	Number	Percent
General anesthesia	8/279	2.9
Spinal anesthesia	5/183	2.7

Table 3-5. Practical Considerations in Choosing an Anesthetic Technique

Anesthesia	Pros	Cons
Regional	Avoids pulmonary irritation in patients with chronic obstructive pulmonary disease	May require additonal sedation causing respiratory depression
	Decreases stress response	Bad for hypovolemic patient
	Patients with history of congestive heart failure tolerate it well	Bradycardia
	Decreases afterload	Time factor
	Patients more awake postoperatively	Not for patients with moderate to severe aortic stenosis
	May prevent thromboembolism	Not for very confused or disoriented patients
		Not for patients with uncorrected coagulopathy
General	Ease of administration	Myocardial depression
	Patient comfort	Not protective against thromboembolism
	Higher FıO$_2$ if necessary	Airway manipulation necessary
		Prolonged effects of medications (narcotics, muscle relaxants, inhalation agents)

The results in our hospital are similar to those of Valentin and Davis in that anesthetic technique does not affect mortality.[6,7]

Considerations for determining which anesthetic technique should be used for a given patient are presented in Table 3-5.

SPINAL ANESTHESIA

Spinal anesthesia is utilized in many patients with histories of congestive heart failure or pulmonary disease (Table 3-5).

Two examples of how we took care of a complicated problem follow.

Case Study

A 51-year-old woman with a fractured hip and severe chronic obstructive pulmonary disease was scheduled for surgery. On room air, her PaO$_2$ was 50 mmHg and oxygen saturation was 88 percent.

The following technique was used:

1. The patient was placed on the operating table in the lateral decubitus position with the fracture site up. Change of position was not necessary, and there was no need for the patient to lay on the painful fractured hip.
2. Three milliliters of isobaric bupivacaine 0.5 percent with 0.3 mg of epinephrine plus 0.3 mg of preservative-free morphine was administered intrathecally.
3. Onset of anesthesia was rapid, with a stable hemodynamic state.

Patient tolerated the procedure well.

Case Study

A 74-year-old woman presented for repair of a hip fracture. The patient had a history of mild aortic stenosis, aortic insufficiency, cardiomegaly, recent CHF, a pleural effusion, shortness of breath, bladder tumor, and anemia.

On physical examination, the patient was in moderate respiratory distress, with a respiratory rate of 25 breaths/min and the head of the bed was elevated 45 degrees. Jugular veins were prominent. With the bed placed flat, the respiratory rate increased to 35 breaths/min and the patient appeared in obvious respiratory distress. Auscultation revealed diminished breath sounds over the left lung and a murmur heard over the entire precordium. Chest radiograph demonstrated a left pleural effusion. Laboratory data demonstrated a marked anemia.

Because of the condition of the patient, surgery was delayed while a controlled diuresis and a blood transfusion were carried out over a few days. The patient improved and was no longer short of breath.

On arrival to the operating room, the pulmonary artery catheter demonstrated a wedge pressure of 10 mmHg. Intravenous fluids were kept to a minimum. The patient received a spinal anesthetic. Phenylephrine was used to treat decreases in blood pressure. The patient tolerated the procedure well.

In the postanesthesia care unit (PACU), the pulmonary capillary wedge pressure increased to 12 mmHg as the spinal anesthesia level receded. No diuretics or vasopressors were required postoperatively. Had the pulmonary capillary wedge pressure risen too high, small doses of furosemide would have been administered. The patient remained in the intensive care unit for 2 days postoperatively without any problems.[36]

Comment

This patient with complex medical problems and a Goldman score of 27 out of a possible 53 points (Table 3-2) required extensive preoperative preparation and intraoperative attention.

Problems and Solutions

Hypotension

We have noted that fewer instances of hypotension are associated with the use of isobaric bupivacaine.

Infusion of large amounts of fluid for hypotension should be avoided because this may result in fluid overload when the spinal anesthesia wears off.

A small dose of a vasopressor such as neosynephrine or even a neosynephrine drip will counteract the effects of vasodilatation and help maintain a stable blood pressure.

Nausea and Vomiting

Spinal anesthesia can block the sympathetic nervous system, resulting in brady-cardia, nausea, and vomiting. Vagolytic medications such as glycopyrrolate or atropine are helpful in increasing the heart rate and relieving gastrointestinal symptoms.

Valvular Heart Disease

We avoid spinal anesthesia in patients with moderate to severe aortic stenosis because myocardial perfusion may suffer if a decreased afterload occurs as a result of hypotension.

Sedation during Regional Anesthesia

Warning: Be careful in the use of sedation.

Case Study

At another hospital, an elderly woman with a hip fracture received intravenous sedation while in the lateral decubitus position before the administration of a spinal anesthetic. Because the patient was still uncooperative, an intravenous injection of sodium thiopental was given. Attention was directed to performing the spinal injection. Suddenly, it was noted that the patient had suffered respiratory and cardiac arrest. Resuscitation efforts were unsuccessful.

Comment

Any benefits that may be derived from the use of spinal anesthesia will be lost if excess sedation is used to carry the patient through the operation.

GENERAL ANESTHESIA

Medications used for induction should be decreased and sufficient time allowed for physiologic and hemodynamic effects to occur.

Thiopental and lidocaine should be administered slowly in decreased dosages, as they may result in a more significant physiologic effect than observed in younger patients. We have noted substantial decreases in blood pressure when lidocaine was injected to blunt the physiologic response to intubation.

Inhalation agents may lead to vasodilatation and myocardial depression. Nitrous oxide may result in myocardial depression in patients with angina or coronary artery disease.[27]

Most general anesthetics are conducted with a nitrous oxide/oxygen, narcotic, muscle relaxant technique. Specific agents are chosen based on effects desired and resultant hemodynamic side effects. Isoflurane may be added in small concentrations to manage rises in blood pressure.

Vecuronium and atracurium are used for muscle relaxation and to avoid tachycardia.

Epidural, lumbar plexus block and even a combination of femoral nerve and lateral femoral cutaneous nerve blocks are used for repair of fractured hips (see Ch. 6)

Position

Use of Fracture Table

Patients are placed on fracture tables to aid in the reduction of the fractured hip and maintain position during repair. After administration of anesthesia, a post is inserted in the perineal area to stabilize the patient while traction is placed on the fractured hip.[36]

Proper padding of the perineal post and proper positioning are essential to avoid pressure on the genitalia, which can result in skin breakdown, necrosis, and nerve damage. The Foley catheter should not be crimped against the post. You will be giving large fluid challenges and diuretics to "promote urinary output" during the operation to no avail.

The foot of the injured extremity is then carefully padded and placed in the traction boot. Adequate muscle relaxation must be present at this time to ensure ease of manipulation for positioning. Intracapsular fractures are reduced at this time for fixation. If reduction is successful, the fracture is pinned. If reduction is unsuccessful, a hemiarthroplasty may have to be performed, necessitating transfer to an operating table where the patient is repositioned.

Intertrochanteric fractures are opened and repaired once reduction has been obtained.

Conduct of Anesthesia

After induction, the patient is positioned on a fracture table.

Hemodynamic alterations may occur when the patient's position is changed, either when the patient is placed on the fracture table or into the lateral decubitus position.

If invasive arterial monitoring is placed, we prefer to use the down hand of the patient in the lateral decubitus position.

Blood loss is monitored during the procedure and replaced as necessary. Before extubation, neuromuscular status is evaluated with a monitor. The patient should be awake and alert and should have regained airway reflexes. Respiratory parameters are evaluated. In a few elderly patients, we have noted both "renarcotization" and diminished respiratory function after extubation. Small doses of naloxone or reversal of muscle relaxants has been advantageous. We dilute our naloxone into 0.04 mg/dose to avoid a marked increase in blood pressure and heart rate with the return of pain.

USE OF CEMENT

Methylmethacrylate is used when a hemiarthroplasty is cemented. The use of methylmethacrylate has been associated with hypoxia, hypotension, cardiopulmonary complications, cardiac arrest, and death.

Methylmethacrylate monomer, bone marrow elements, bone marrow fat, and thromboplastic elements have all been implicated in causing the side effects noted with the use of methylmethacrylate cement[28-33] (see Ch. 4).

We noticed that patients tend to desaturate during reaming and cementing of the femur as well as the acetabulum even if they are given 100 percent oxygen during this period. Patients arriving in the operating room at lower oxygen saturation tend to desaturate more frequently intraoperatively. We suggest that patients receiving general anesthesia receive 100 percent oxygen during cementing and that patients under regional anesthesia receive supplemental oxygen during the procedure.[26]

INTRAOPERATIVE BLOOD LOSS

Significant blood loss can occur during surgery, especially with intertrochanteric fractures. Drapes, suction bottles, lap pads, and the floor should be checked. Transfusions should be administered based on the patient's medical condition and the degree of blood loss. A necessary transfusion should not be withheld in an octagenarian with a significant anginal history just because you are afraid of blood-borne infections.

MANAGEMENT OF THE UNCOOPERATIVE PATIENT

The uncooperative patient may be suffering from chronic organic mental syndrome. Check with family members as to prefracture mental status because these manifestations can be a result of acute head trauma, toxic effects of medications, hypoxia, or metabolic derangement.

If organic mental syndrome is the underlying cause for uncooperativeness, our approach is to

Administer small amounts of a sedative while the patient is observed.

Protect intravenous lines, arterial lines, and the Foley catheter from being pulled out.

Pad all sharp surfaces on the operating table so that the patient does not hurt himself.

Spinal or general anesthesia may be chosen based on the physiologic profile. Organic mental syndrome is certainly not a contraindication to regional anesthesia.

POSTANESTHESIA CARE UNIT

Regional Anesthesia and the Patient with Congestive Heart Failure

In the patient with a history of CHF who had a pulmonary artery catheter placed to aid in management, PACU nurses should be reminded to keep a close eye on the pulmonary artery measurements as the spinal anesthesia recedes. A small dose of diuretic such as furosemide (2 to 5 mg) may be required to avoid pulmonary edema as pressures rise as the spinal anesthesia recedes.

General Considerations

Besides the routine evaluation and monitoring performed on all patients, major considerations in the geriatric patient in the PACU include

1. Effect of altered metabolic rate
2. Neurovascular status
3. Hypothermia
4. Cardiac, pulmonary, and intravascular volume status
5. Pain management
6. Orientation—mental status

Altered Metabolic Rate

Because metabolic rate is diminished in the elderly, medications used intraoperatively are frequently still exerting a physiologic effect in the PACU. Even careful anesthesiologists have experienced situations in which geriatric patients develop respiratory depression or appear to be renarcotized in the PACU.

Neurovascular Status

On arrival, the neurovascular status should be evaluated and recorded. The presence of peripheral pulses and status of motor and sensory nerves should be checked and compared with preoperative findings. The extremity is observed for swelling because bleeding into the thigh can cause neurovascular compromise.

Hypothermia

Hypothermia is a common problem in the elderly, especially after regional anesthesia. Because the elderly do not regulate their temperature as well as younger people, they will remain colder for longer.

Return of thermoregulatory control may result in shivering, which is associated with increased oxygen consumption. This may be dangerous in the elderly patient with coronary artery disease because it increases oxygen consumption in skeletal muscle at the expense of myocardial oxygen supply.[34]

The following steps may be taken to treat hypothermia and shivering:

1. Apply forced air warming devices such as the Bair Hugger or heat lamps.
2. Administer meperidine—use low doses (e.g., 12.5 mg IV) in the elderly. Observe for respiratory depression.
3. Warm infused fluids.
4. Keep exposed areas covered.
5. Use heat and moisture retainers if the patient remains intubated in the PACU.

Pulmonary Status

Geriatric patients are operated on expeditiously to avoid pulmonary complications. Postoperatively, the chance for pneumonia still exists, and a postoperative respiratory therapy plan should be instituted early.

We suggest the following:

1. Preoperative education in use of incentive spirometry and deep breathing reinstituted early in the PACU
2. Use of supplemental oxygen
3. Avoidance of excess narcotics that will result in respiratory depression, decreased cough, and atalectasis
4. Early mobilization

Cardiac Status

If the patient has a history of cardiac disease, attention should be directed to the following:

Supply supplemental oxygen.

Obtain postoperative ECG if indicated—compare with preoperative ECG for rate, rhythm, and ST segments.

If an arrhythmia is noted, check old ECG to see if it was present preoperatively. Check electrolytes and blood gases for abnormalities.

If patient has a history of CHF, listen for rales—observe for signs of CHF as spinal anesthesia recedes.

If patient has anginal history, evaluate for ischemia.

Treat pain—avoid tachycardia and hypertension.

Restart cardiac medications.

Check hematocrit value to make certain the patient does not become too anemic. Administer blood as needed.

Keep patient warm—avoid shivering.

Intravascular Volume Status

Fluid infusion rates, hourly urine output, hematocrit values, and if present, central venous pressure measurements are followed to help to determine the intravascular status.

Drains are checked for blood loss because bleeding may result in hypotension.

Postoperative Pain Management

Pain medication should be administered judiciously to the elderly patient. Although we are not desirous of allowing patients to be in pain, we are concerned about oversedation in a patient who may still have residual effects of narcotics present.

Doses of medication should be decreased and, if administering intravenous medications, sufficient time allowed for a physiologic effect to occur. If spinal narcotics have been administered, parenteral narcotics are avoided if the patient complains of pain. Acetaminophen or ketorolac are used.

Because of our concern about respiratory depression after spinal or epidural narcotics, we currently monitor these patients in a postoperative unit.

We do not usually provide patient controlled analgesia for elderly patients because it is difficult for the patient to understand the concepts involved in this technique. We are worried about the patient being confused and that an elderly spouse may push the patient controlled analgesia button for the patient.

Orientation—Mental Status

On arrival, the patient's current mental status should be noted as well as the status before anesthesia. Although the residual effects of anesthesia may play a role, return to baseline status should be observed before discharge. It is very common for the geriatric patient to become very confused postoperatively. Frequently, a familiar face is necessary to help calm the patient.

REFERENCES

1. Zuckerman JD, Sakales SR, Fabian DR et al: Hip fractures in geriatric patients. Clin Orthop 274:213, 1992
2. Grisso JA, Kelsey JL, Strom BL et al: Risk factors for falls as a cause of hip fracture in women. N Engl J Med 324:1326, 1991
3. Zuckerman JD, Schon LC: Hip fractures. p. 23. In Zuckerman JD (ed): Comprehensive Care of Orthopaedic Injuries in the Elderly. Urban & Schwarzenberg, Baltimore, 1990
4. Kenzora JE, McCarthy RE, Lowell JD et al: Hip fracture mortality. Relation to age, treatment, preoperative illness, time of surgery and complications. Clin Orthop 186:45, 1984
5. White BL, Fisher WD, Laurin CA: Rate of mortality for elderly patients after fracture of the hip in the 1980s. J Bone Joint Surg 69(A):1335, 1987
6. Valentin N, Lomholt B, Jensen JS et al: Spinal or general anaesthesia for surgery of the fractured hip? A prospective study of mortality in 578 patients. Br J Anaesth 58:284, 1986
7. Davis FM, Woolner DF, Frampton C et al: Prospective, multi-centre trial of mortality following general or spinal anesthesia for hip fracture surgery in the elderly. Br J Anaesth 59:1080, 1987
8. Clayer MT, Brauze RJ: Morbidity and mortality following fractures of the femoral neck and trochanteric region: analyses of risk factors. J Trauma 29:1673, 1989
9. Browner WS, Li J, Mangano DT: The study of perioperative ischemia research group: in-hospital and long-term mortality in male veterans following non-cardiac surgery. JAMA 268:228, 1992
10. Patel KP, Capan LM, Grant GJ et al: Musculoskeletal injuries. p. 511. In Capan LM, Miller SM, Turndorf H (eds): Trauma Anesthesia and Intensive Care. JB Lippincott, Philadelphia, 1991
11. Frankel VH: Biomechanics of the hip joints. AAOS Instructional Course Lectures 35:3, 1986
12. Schultz RJ, Whitfield GF, LaMura JS et al The role of physiologic monitoring in patients with fractures of the hip. J Trauma 25:309, 1985
13. Zuckerman JD, Skovron ML, Kessel K et al: The role of surgical delay in the long-term outcome of hip fractures in geriatric patients. Orthop Trans 16:750, 1992

14. Wahba WM: Influence of aging on lung function: clinical significance of changes from age 20. Anesth Analg 62:764, 1983
15. Kakkar VV, Corrigan TP, Fossard DP: Prevention of fatal pulmonary embolism by low dose heparin. Lancet 2:45, 1975
16. Siegel JH: The aged and high risk surgical patient. In: Seigel JH, Chodoff PD (eds): Medical, Surgical and Anesthetic Management. Grune & Stratton, Orlando, FL 1976
17. Goldman L: Cardiac risks and complications of non-cardiac surgery. Ann Intern Med 98:508, 1983
18. Goldman L, Caldera DC: Risks of general anesthesia and elective operation in the hypertensive patient. Anesthesiology 50:285, 1979
19. Hollenberg M, Mangano DT, Browner WS et al: Predictors of postoperative myocardial ischemia in patients undergoing noncardiac surgery. JAMA 268:205, 1992
20. Tarhan S,Moffitt EA, Taylor WF et al: Myocardial infarction after general anesthesia. JAMA 220:145, 1972
21. Coughlin L, Templeton J: Hip fractures in patients with Parkinson's disease. Clin Orthop 148:192, 1980
22. Eventor I, Moreno M, Geller E et al: Hip fractures in patients with Parkinson's syndrome. J Trauma 23:98, 1983
23. Fahn S: Parkinsonism. p. 2143. In Wyngaarden JB, Smith LH (eds): Cecil Textbook of Medicine. 18th Ed. WB Saunders, Philadelphia, 1988
24. Stehling LC: Anesthetic cnnsiderations for the patient with a fractured hip. In Zauder H (ed): Anesthesia for Orthopedic Surgery. FA Davis, Philadelphia 1980
25. Vincken WG: Involvement of upper airway muscles on extra pyranudal disorders. N Engl J Med 311:438, 1984
26. Rosenberg AD, Bernstein RL, Bernstein DB et al: Oxygen desaturation during cemented hip replacement—who desaturate and when. Anesthesiology 67:A551, 1987
27. Eisele JH, Rectan JA, Mossumi R et al: Myocardial performance and N_2O analgesia in coronary artery disease. Anesthesiology 44:16, 1976
28. Dhamee MK, Ramic R, Asidao CB: Arterial oxygen tension during application of methylmethacrylate for total hip arthroplasty. Anesth Rev 13:17, 1986
29. Heindon JH, Bechtol CO, Crichenberger DP: Fat embolism during total joint hip replacement. J Bone Joint Surg 56(A):1350, 1974
30. Kallos T: Impaired arterial oxygenation associated with the use of bone cement in the femoral shaft. Anesthesiology 42:210, 1975
31. Kepes ER, Underwood PS, Becsey L: Intraoperative death associated with acrylic bone cement. JAMA 222:576, 1972
32. Modig J, Busch C, Olerud S et al: Arterial hypotension an hypoxemia during total hip replacement: the importance of thromboplastic products, fat embolism and acrylic monomers. Acta Anaesthesiol Scand 19:28, 1975
33. Park WY, Balingit P, Kenmore PI et al: Changes in arterial oxygen tension during total hip replacement. Anesthesiology 39:642, 1973
34. Bay J, Nunn JG, Prys-Roberts C: Factors influencing arterial PO_2 during recovery from anaesthesia. Br J Anaesth 40:398, 1986
35. Rosenberg AD, Bernstein RL: Perioperative anesthetic management of orthopedic trauma. p. 551. In Grande CM (ed): Textbook of Trauma Anesthesia and Critical Care. CV Mosby, St. Louis, 1993
36. Rosenberg AD, Bernstein RL: Anesthesia. p. 583. In Zuckerman JD (ed): Comprehensive Care of Orthopedic Injuries in the Elderly. Urban & Schwarzenberg, Baltimore, 1990

Total Joint Replacement

One of the most exciting advances in orthopedic surgery has been the successful replacement of diseased joints. Replacement of the hip joint was accomplished as a result of the work of many investigators, but the major contribution must be given to Sir John Charnley who developed the low friction arthroplasty. The femoral component with a specially designed head is placed into the femoral canal and a prosthetic socket is inserted into the acetabulum.

Charnley's unique contribution to total joint replacement is the use of acrylic cement to fix the components to the bone.

Since the innovative work of Charnley, many advances in design and metallurgy have been developed. Newer techniques in fixation of the components without cement using porous in-growth methods, as well as special coatings on the prostheses such as hydroxyapatite, have been introduced.

Total joint replacement at present most frequently involves hip, knee, and shoulder replacement.

The anesthesiologist is presented with a unique opportunity to take part in advances in orthopedic surgery as well as to assume responsibility for management of patients with several rare and complicated systemic disorders associated with joint destruction.

TOTAL HIP REPLACEMENT

Conditions associated with deterioration of the hip joint (see Ch. 1 for diseases) are

Osteoarthritis

Rheumatoid arthritis

Ankylosing spondylitis

Failed fracture repair

Failed previous surgery

Congenital dislocation of the hip

Metabolic disorders (Charcot joint)

Neuropathic arthropathy

Hemophilia

Acromegaly

Paget's disease

Gout

Hip dysplasias

Neoplasms

Aseptic necrosis of the femoral head

Causes of aseptic necrosis of the femoral head include

Fracture of the femoral neck

Traumatic dislocation of the hip

Trauma to hip without fracture or dislocation

Slipped capital femoral epiphysis

Alcoholism (see Ch. 1)

Chronic liver disease

Systemic steroid administration

Systemic lupus erythematosus (see Ch. 1)

Caisson disease (decompression sickness)

Exposure to high altitudes

Hemoglobinopathies (sickle cell-hemoglobin S disease, sickle cell-hemoglobin C disease, S-β-thalassemia) (see Ch. 1)

Coagulopathies

Pancreatitis

Hyperlipidemias

Burns

Pregnancy

Gout

Gaucher's disease

Fabry's disease

Arteriosclerosis and other vascular occlusive disorders

Radiation

Osteoarthritis

Osteoarthritis, or degenerative joint disease, is the most common disease of peripheral joints. It may arise without any apparent etiologic factor or may result from an injury or mechanical derangement of the joint. Although osteoarthritis increases with advancing age, not all aged cartilage develops this condition. Osteoarthritis results from cartilage destruction followed by bony changes that lead to derangement in joint function and mechanics. This leads to joint pain, stiffness, and limitation of motion.

Osteoarthritis by itself is usually not associated with other medical problems.

Indications for surgery are persistent pain and limitation of motion.

Associated Problems

Age

Because of the increase in average life expectancy, there will be an increasing number of elderly patients in the population.

Because the incidence of different forms of arthritis is increased with aging, older patients will become candidates for surgery.

General Medical Condition

Special consideration exists in caring for elderly patients (see Ch. 3).

As aging occurs, the incidence of associated diseases is increased.

The general medical condition of the patient should be considered in preparation for total joint replacement. The following conditions are noted in elderly patients[1]:

Hypertension

Diabetes

Renal disease

Atherosclerosis

Myocardial infarction

Congestive heart failure

Angina

Cardiomyopathy

Chronic obstructive pulmonary disease

Cerebrovascular accidents

Neurologic dysfunction

Perioperative Problems

Pettine et al.[2] compared perioperative complications in patients older than 80 years of age undergoing total hip arthroplasty with a control group (ages 64 to 67 years).

There were 2.5 times more minor postoperative complications and 3.5 times more major ones in the elderly group than in the controls. Perioperative mortality was not increased in the elderly patients.

This study showed that proper emphasis should be placed on preoperative evaluation of the urinary system, postoperative cardiac monitoring, prophylaxis against deep vein thrombosis, and prevention of postoperative dementia.[2]

For elective total joint replacement, patients must be properly evaluated. Special attention should be directed toward hypertension, diabetes, cardiac status, pulmonary status, renal status, hematologic status, and neurologic status.

Hypertension

Check blood pressure on preoperative rounds yourself. Check present medications and see whether the patient has continued to take them. Some patients discontinue their medication before entering the hospital.

Some internists also give very large doses of medication to try to decrease a high blood pressure quickly so that the patient can go to the operating room. These patients may become hypotensive on induction. Hypertensive patients may also have decreased blood volume.

Make sure patients receive antihypertension medication on schedule preoperatively and in the immediate postoperative period.

Diabetes

Determine whether patient is insulin- or noninsulin-dependent. Formulate a coverage plan for patient. Obtain preoperative fingerstick. If insulin coverage is to be administered, have dextrose-containing intravenous solution started before administering insulin.

Cardiac Status

Evaluate for angina, coronary artery disease, valvular disease, cardiomyopathy, or history of myocardial infarction.

Obtain electrocardiogram (ECG), echocardiogram, or stress test as required by history and physical examination.

Pulmonary Status

Check for emphysema, asthma, or chronic obstructive pulmonary disease.

Obtain preoperative arterial blood gas studies and pulmonary function tests based on history, physical examination, and chest radiograph.

Renal Status

Obtain history and baseline values of blood urea nitrogen and creatinine as well as history of problems with prostatic disease.

Hematologic Status

Hematocrit value may be low secondary to predonation of blood. Patients with rheumatoid arthritis are chronically anemic.

Neurologic Status

Determine history of transient ischemic attacks, carotid artery disease, and neurologic disorders such as Parkinson's disease (see Ch. 3).

Anesthetic Management

Preoperative Evaluation and Preparation

Total joint replacement is elective surgery.

The patient should be in the best possible condition.

History of Analgesic Therapy

A careful history concerning the use of analgesics such as aspirin and nonsteroidal anti-inflammatory drugs, which may interfere with platelet function, must be obtained. These medications should be discontinued for 3 days before the surgical procedure; however, some surgeons do not stop aspirin preoperatively.

Warning: Patients with rheumatoid arthritis may not stop taking aspirin because of the severe pain.

Obtain a coagulation profile if any question exists.

Check for anemia secondary to gastrointestinal bleeding from aspirin or nonsteroidal anti-inflammatory agents. A low hematocrit value may be present secondary to gastrointestinal bleeding.

Preoperative Medication

Premedication is advantageous in that it decreases anxiety and decreases the amount of pain the patient experiences when lying on stretchers or the operating table before surgery. Although patients may be admitted the day of surgery, premedication can be administered once appropriate consents are obtained.

The nothing by mouth after midnight rule should not preclude asthmatic, hypertensive, or cardiac patients from receiving their usual daily medications. Special considerations for the diabetic patient include fingerstick blood glucose measurement, starting a glucose-containing intravenous solution, and dosage modification of insulin as needed.

Total Joint Operating Room

A patient who develops an infected total joint may require removal of the prosthesis and 6 weeks of intravenous antibiotics. The toll is enormous on the patient, the family, the surgeon, and the health care system. Fear of infection has resulted in innovations in infection control. These innovations have decreased the rate of infection as compared with other surgical procedures.[3]

Role of the Anesthesiologist

The anesthesiologist should be aware of the concern of the surgeon and participate in promoting an infection-free environment for the patient. This may require the anesthesiologist to wear special glasses to protect the eyes from ultraviolet rays or to wear more head covering than usual. Extra care should be taken with sterility of the medications, needles, and syringes you are using.[3]

Laminar Flow Operating Rooms

Many orthopedic surgeons use laminar flow systems and wear hooded gowns with air supply and return hoses to isolate the patient from the surgeon and decrease the chance of infection. These systems decrease both the number of airborne particles in the room and particles from the surgical team that can contaminate the surgical wound.[3]

Laminar flow, which is used to decrease turbulent airflow in an operating room, has air flowing in parallel. This airflow pattern keeps floor dust particles near the floor and ceiling air near the ceiling. Objects in the path of the laminar flow disrupt the flow pattern by causing turbulence. Horizontal laminar airflow systems use a panel of laminar units that deliver the air at one end of the operating room and air vents at the other end. The anesthesiologist and other personnel not wearing hooded gowns with air return systems should not walk between the laminar flow panels and the patient. This will demonstrate lack of knowledge about laminar flow and give the surgeon an opportunity to tell you to move.

In vertical laminar flow systems, the panels are above the patient and air flows down.[3]

Complicated vertical flow systems may have a glass enclosure or "greenhouse" in which the surgeon, the patient from the neck down, and the scrub nurse are inside the laminar flow. The anesthesiologist, the anesthesia equipment, the patient's head and neck, and the circulating nurse are outside the enclosure. Necessary surgical equipment is passed into the system through glass doors. The anesthesiologist must have obtained intravenous access before the patient enters the glass enclosure.

Newer systems include helmets that have hoses attached to small canisters that are worn on the surgeon's back.

With laminar flow, airborne particles can be directed toward the anesthesiologist. The anesthesiologist should be aware of this and wear appropriate protection.

Room Noise

The laminar flow systems can be noisy, and if you want to communicate important information to the surgeon, it is necessary to speak loudly and make sure the surgeon acknowledges what was said. Remember, it is even noisier inside the gowns. The noise in the operating room may mask the background ventilator sounds and other noises that the anesthesiologist relies on to help care for patients.[3]

Ultraviolet Light

Some surgeons believe an improved infection-free environment is obtained with the use of ultraviolet light. This may be used during preparation of the patient or even during surgery itself. Satisfactory eye and skin protection must be worn to protect from damaging rays.

Monitoring and Equipment

Electrocardiogram

> In general, leads II and modified V5 are monitored. If specific knowledge of an ischemic area is known, the appropriate lead should be used.

Pulse oximeter

> Besides routine monitoring for hypoxia, the pulse oximeter is very valuable in detecting clinically relevant desaturations during reaming and cementing.

End-tidal carbon dioxide monitor

> Besides routine use, it may help detect episodes of fat and pulmonary emboli that might occur with reaming and cementing.

Nerve stimulator

Arterial line

> An arterial line is placed
>
> In geriatric hypertensive patients
>
> In patients with diabetes or cardiac, renal, or pulmonary disease
>
> If the use of some degree of hypotensive anesthesia is anticipated
>
> **Warning:**
>
>> Placement may be very difficult to obtain in patients with rheumatoid arthritis.
>>
>> An arterial line should be avoided in patients with scleroderma and Raynaud's disease.

Central venous lines

> Central venous lines are used if
>
>> Significant fluid shifts are anticipated
>>
>> Underlying disease process deems central access necessary
>>
>> Central volume status measurements are important
>>
>> Peripheral intravenous access is difficult

Pulmonary artery lines

> Indications are as for central venous lines, but more precise data on pulmonary artery pressure and left-sided filling pressures are required to aid in management (e.g., patients with congestive heart failure or significant valvular disease).

Esophageal stethoscope

Temperature probe

Foley catheters

> Perioperative use of Foley catheters is frequently a "bone" of contention between orthopedic surgeons and anesthesiologists. Concern about bacteremia and seeding of the operative site with subsequent infection has led many surgeons to shun the use of catheters. Anesthesiologists desire knowledge of urine output to help assess renal function and fluid

status and to note such occurrences as blood transfusion reactions. At the Hospital for Joint Diseases Orthopaedic Institute (HJDOI), we do not place catheters for primary total hip replacements unless an underlying pathologic disease state requires its use. Even though patients may not have a catheter inserted in the operating room, it is not uncommon for patients to require catheters in the postanesthesia care unit (PACU). If this is placed in the PACU, antibiotic coverage should be discussed with the surgeons.

Position

The operation is performed in the supine or the lateral decubitus position.

If performed in the supine position, the upper extremity on that side is folded across the chest. The arm should not be taped down so tightly that chest excursion is inhibited on inspiration.

In the lateral decubitus position, concern should be directed toward

1. *Axillary compression on the lower arm*—place an adequate axillary roll so the axillary artery and nerve are not compressed.
2. *Radial pulse in the lower arm*—inability to obtain a pulse by palpation or via a pulse oximeter indicates arterial occlusion.
3. *Head and neck*—position carefully to avoid strain on the brachial plexus. Place a pillow or support under the head so the cervical spine is aligned with the thoracic spine. In patients with cervical spine pathology and in those with ankylosing spondylitis, pay careful attention to support of the neck with adequate pillows and padding.
4. *Nonoperated lower extremity*—make sure it is properly padded.
5. *Lateral positioner on the iliac crest*—check for appropriate placement.

Case Study

A patient with an abdominal renal transplant underwent elective total hip replacement in the lateral decubitus position. Despite adequate fluid administration and minimal reduction in blood pressure from baseline values, no urine output was noticeable in the tubing even when traced back to its origin. Examination of the abdomen underneath the drapes to see whether the bladder was distended revealed that the lateral positioner was malpositioned and was compressing the abdomen and transplanted kidney. Repositioning resulted in an adequate urine output.

Description of the Operation

Exposure of the hip joint

Excision of the capsule of the hip

Excision of the femoral head from the acetabulum

Reaming of the acetabulum (this is where sciatic nerve injury may occur)

Placement of methylmethacrylate bone cement into the acetabulum

Insertion of the acetabular prosthesis or preparation of the acetabulum for screwing in of the noncemented acetabular prosthesis

Preparation of the femoral shaft

Broaching, reaming, and widening of the femoral canal (canal is suctioned and cleaned to remove residual blood, bone, and marrow elements)

Insertion of cement into femoral canal

Insertion of prosthesis into cement in the femoral canal

Hardening of cement (no movement must occur at this time)

Reduction of hip joint

Insertion of drainage systems

Closure

Radiographic examination

Surgeon's acceptance of radiograph (do not wake the patient until the surgeon sees the radiograph)

Induction of Anesthesia to Incision

The time required to prepare and drape a patient for total hip replacement can be 10 to 30 minutes, depending on the surgeon's preparation and draping procedure. During this time, there is no surgical stimulation to a patient who has just received induction doses of medication. The blood pressure should be carefully monitored because lack of stimulation may result in hypotension.

This time can be used to obtain additional intravenous access and to start an arterial line if a noninvasive blood pressure device was used during induction.

Depth of anesthesia is evaluated just before incision to ensure that the patient is adequately anesthetized and does not move with incision.

Choice of Anesthesia

Regional Anesthesia

If regional anesthesia is contemplated, the use of spinal narcotics to provide postoperative pain relief should be considered. Patients are very appreciative of the postoperative pain relief they obtain from epidural and spinal narcotics. The patient should receive supplemental oxygen. Sedation can be administered as allowable by pre-existing medical conditions so that the noise in the operating room does not cause anxiety.

Spinal Anesthesia

After appropriate monitoring devices are placed, the patient is positioned in the lateral decubitus position with the side to be operated uppermost.

Spinal anesthesia can be administered with any acceptable agent that lasts for the length of the procedure.

We favor isobaric bupivacaine dose: 0.5 percent 3 ml with 1:200,000 epinephrine.

Onset of anesthesia is rapid and lasts for up to 3 hours.

Intrathecal morphine up to 0.5 mg can be administered with the bupivacaine.

An appropriate anesthetic level must be obtained so that no pain is present when the surgeon places a draping clamp at the midabdominal level (T8 level). If the patient complains of pain with this maneuver, which occurs before incision, the surgeon will not have much confidence in the anesthetic technique.

Epidural Anesthesia

The patient is placed in the lateral decubitus position. An epidural catheter is placed, and the medication is added to raise the level of anesthesia. Again, an adequate anesthetic level to the mid-upper abdomen should be obtained.

Toward the end of the procedure, preservative-free morphine can be added to provide pain relief after surgery before the effect of the epidural anesthesia wears off.

With spinal and epidural anesthesia, we have noted a drier surgical field and less blood loss, and the patients are more alert in the PACU.

With regional anesthetic techniques, no attempt is made to induce hypotensive anesthesia. We prefer regional anesthesia for its antithrombotic characteristics (see Ch. 5).

General Anesthesia

After appropriate monitoring devices are attached, general anesthesia is induced and the patient is positioned as required. If the patient is elderly, lowering induction and maintenance doses of medications is considered, as well as waiting an appropriate amount of time for the medication to work.

Adequate muscle relaxation should be provided during

1. Dislocation of the hip
2. Testing of the fit of the femoral component before cementing
3. Reduction of the femoral prosthesis into the acetabulum

Special Considerations During Total Hip Replacement

These special considerations include blood pressure control, blood loss, and decreasing homologous transfusions during total joint replacements.

Approach during 1970s and 1980s

During the 1970s and early 1980s, attempts were made to decrease intraoperative blood loss during total hip replacement. Regional anesthetic techniques and general anesthesia with induced hypotension were associated with

1. Less intraoperative blood loss than general anesthesia
2. A dry surgical field
3. A dry cement–bone interface at the time of cementing

When compared with general anesthesia, Sculco and Ranawat[4] showed that spinal anesthesia decreased blood loss by 600 ml.

In a review of 533 procedures performed under general anesthesia at our institution before the use of the Cell Saver and predonation of autologous blood, blood loss during total hip replacement was 1,740 ml with neuroleptanesthesia, 1,483 ml with inhalation anesthesia, and 1,102 ml when a hypotensive technique was combined with an inhalation technique. Transfusions were required in 70 percent of patients receiving general anesthesia compared with 21 percent in the hypotensive group.

Current Concepts of Intraoperative Blood Pressure Control

Although many total joint replacements have been performed under induced hypotension, there is always a concern about significant decreases in mean arterial blood pressure in geriatric patients, as well as in patients with coronary, carotid, or renal disease.

Autologous predonation and the use of blood salvaging devices have obviated the need for induced hypotension.

In our institution, total hip replacements performed under general anesthesia are conducted with slightly reduced blood pressure from the patient's normal pressure, but not fully induced hypotension.

Marked decreases in blood pressure from baseline are avoided.

Healthy patients receiving regional anesthesia are allowed to have their blood pressure decrease somewhat below normal levels but not as low as induced hypotension levels.

Alternatively, increases in blood pressures should be avoided because they will lead to difficulty in surgical exposure and increased requirement for transfusion.

Methods to avoid homologous transfusion include

1. Autologous predonation
2. Use of Cell Saver
3. Postoperative wound drainage reinfusion
4. Acceptance of lower postoperative hematocrit level before transfusing

(For an in-depth discussion of avoiding homologous transfusion see Ch. 11.)

Autologous Predonation

Many patients undergoing elective total hip replacement in HJDOI predonate at least 1 or 2 units of blood and occasionally more if revision surgery is scheduled. Predonation is performed either at our institution or a regional blood center and the blood transported to the hospital. *Make sure this has arrived before the procedure.* During the predonation period, patients are placed on iron therapy to help improve iron stores.

Erythropoietin

There may be a role for erythropoietin in patients who have to donate a large number of units of blood before surgery. In a study of 47 adults scheduled for elective orthopedic surgery in which 31 underwent hip replacement, the use of erythropoietin and iron increased the number of predonated units; only 1 of 23 patients in the erythropoietin-iron group was unable to donate 4 or more units, whereas 7 of 24 in the placebo-iron group were unable to predonate 4 or more units. Also, the red blood cell mass of the units that were predonated was higher in the erythropoietin-treated group.[5]

Danersund et al[6] studied the physiologic response of erythropoietin to predonation in patients scheduled for total hip replacement. The authors noted that while the normal physiologic response of erythropoietin production to anemia did occur with predonation it was not as significant as the response usually seen with severe anemia. If prephlebotomy hematocrit levels are considered important, the authors suggest the use of erythropoietin in combination with predonation.[6]

Predonation and the Elderly

Because patients who undergo total hip replacement are usually elderly, the question is often raised, "Can the elderly patient be allowed to predonate?"

The elderly are not at increased risk for complications by predonating blood, and therefore, age is not a contraindication to predonation.[7-11]

In general, it is the first-time donor, the patient of low body weight, women, and anyone who has had a prior donation reaction who is at increased risk for complications with predonation.[8,11]

Because patients undergoing cardiac surgery are allowed to predonate, cardiac disease itself is not a contraindication to predonation. However, these patients should be observed very carefully. Patients with unstable angina or severe aortic stenosis are not candidates for predonation, but they are also probably not candidates for elective total hip replacement.[11] Other underlying conditions such as pulmonary and renal disease must be considered when allowing patients to predonate.

The initial hematocrit and hemoglobin levels of patients who have predonated should be evaluated. It may be very low and decrease quickly after surgery starts and initial blood loss is accompanied by infusion of crystalloid.

Cell Saver

The Cell Saver has gained widespread use in salvaging blood during total hip replacement. Blood is salvaged and washed; the heparin, bone, fat, and debris from the surgical site is removed; and the washed blood is reinfused into the patient. We very frequently return between 125 and 375 ml of processed shed blood to patients during total hip replacements. Usually, enough blood has been salvaged so that approximately 85 percent of patients undergoing primary total hip replacement and close to 100 percent of those undergoing revision hip surgery have benefited from the use of the Cell Saver.

Problems with the use of the Cell Saver include

Coagulopathy
     Infusion of large volumes of Cell Saver blood
     Inadequate removal of heparin during washing

Disseminated intravascular coagulation[12]
     Results from high suction pressure during collection of shed blood
     Insufficient washing of blood

Postoperative Wound Drainage Devices

Blood that is lost into wound drains, which previously had been discarded, is now salvaged in postoperative reinfusion devices and returned to patients after being washed or filtered. These devices are routinely used after total hip replacement at HJDOI. The hematocrit level of blood returned by this method is usually less than the patient's own hematocrit level.

Concern about reinfusion of wound drainage blood includes

1. Dilutional coagulopathy
2. Reinfusion of anticoagulants
3. Disseminated intravascular coagulation
4. Complement activation
5. Renal insufficiency caused by hemolyzed cells
6. Acute respiratory distress syndrome (ARDS)

Controversy exists as to whether the reinfused blood should be washed or unwashed. We currently do not wash our drainage blood and have noted only a minimal number of reactions for the large number of reinfusions. Occasionally, red urine has been noted. When this occurs, a diuresis is promoted so that free hemoglobin does not cause renal damage.

Acute Respiratory Distress Syndrome

Another concern is the development of ARDS after reinfusion of blood. A few patients have had an ARDS pattern on chest radiograph after receiving this type of blood, but it has not been clear that reinfusion caused the ARDS.

Use of Anticoagulant

We do not use anticoagulant in the drainage devices because the prothrombin time and partial thromboplastin time of the blood we collect has been demonstrated to be markedly elevated. Thus, we avoid the possible complications associated with infusion of anticoagulant.

However, some studies suggest that blood lost in the postoperative period be washed before return. Clements et al[13] published a report of four complications in 16 patients receiving unwashed blood and zero in 19 patients receiving washed blood. Two patients had immediate hypotension probably caused by anticoagulant, one had a fever, and one had a myocardial infarction postoperatively.[13]

Complement Activation

A systemic anaphylactic reaction from complement activation is also a concern. Bengston et al[14] demonstrated complement activation in shed blood canisters but was not able to demonstrate it in patients after they received the shed blood.

In another study, a patient developed upper airway edema after reinfusion of shed blood. This was believed to be the result of complement activation, specifically C3a and C5a fragments.[15]

Best Method To Avoid Homologous Blood

Woolson and Watt[16] reported that 92 percent of patients who used a combination of predeposit, intraoperative cell salvage, and postoperative salvage did not require homologous transfusion. An average of 408 ml of blood was salvaged and reinfused.[16]

In a study of 233 total hip replacements conducted at HJDOI, we noted that homologous transfusions were required in only 4 percent of patients who predonated 2 units of autologous blood and used the Cell Saver and the postoperative reinfusion device. These results were better than predonation alone or a combination of Cell Saver and postoperative reinfusion devices without predonation.[17]

Blood Loss and Fluid Replacement

An accurate account of the intraoperative blood loss should be performed during the operation, and involves

Weighing of sponges

Determination of blood lost into suction bottles minus irrigation fluids

Measure of blood loss into Cell Saver minus heparinized saline

Estimate of the blood loss onto drapes and the floor

In general, intraoperative hemoglobin and hematocrit values should be obtained to determine the patient's status. If acute blood loss occurs early in the procedure, the autologous blood may have to be given before Cell Saver blood is processed and available. Managing blood and fluid replacement in patients undergoing total joint replacement has become more difficult with the use of the Cell Saver and postoperative reinfusion devices. This occurs because the patient is usually not transfused during the course of the operation but toward the conclusion of the procedure. The patient's Cell Saver blood is administered and then the patient is re-evaluated as to the need for further transfusion. Wound drainage blood will become available for reinfusion as blood is lost into the wound. If the hematocrit level is low and autologous blood is also reinfused, care should be taken that too much volume is not reinfused into the patient too quickly.

Methylmethacrylate Cement

The use of methylmethacrylate cement has been a major advance in orthopedic surgery. However, episodes of vasodilatation, hypotension, hypoxemia, bronchoconstriction, cardiopulmonary reactions, and even cardiac arrest have been reported with its use.[18-25]

Hypoxemia and hypotension are frequent findings.

During the early 1970s, intraoperative deaths were reported during cement insertion in patients with fractured hips.

Kepes et al,[19] who reported two intraoperative deaths in 1972, suggest that air, fat, bone marrow elements, and methylmethacrylate might be responsible.

An autopsy performed on one patient demonstrated "widespread" marrow elements in the pulmonary arteries.

Hypovolemia, trauma, anemia, and underlying medical problems were considered factors that may have contributed to the complications associated with cement application in those early cases, and correction of these has been suggested as a method to decrease the incidence of adverse outcomes.[19]

Systemic complications associated with methylmethacrylate cement insertion have been attributed to

Methylmethacrylate monomer

Bone marrow elements and marrow fat

Thromboplastic elements

Methylmethacrylate Monomer

Methylmethacrylate bone cement results from the mixing of methylmethacrylate liquid monomer with methylmethacrylate powder, which forms into a soft, pliable, dough-like mass.

Mode of Action
This acrylic cement-like substance allows seating and securing of a prosthesis to bone. When the material hardens, it provides for even weight distribution and stresses between the prosthesis and the bone.

As the prosthesis is forced down the cement-filled canal, the bony trabeculae indent the cement and soft cancellous spaces are filled by the cement. No adhesion occurs between the surface of the prosthesis and the cement. The load is transmitted by the cement to the endosteal surface of the femur through the many trabeculae in the form of a honeycomb.

Besides fixing prostheses to bone, the cement is also used for the fixation of pathologic fractures.

It is the forcing and packing of cement into the femoral canal that is thought to be responsible for embolization of cement, fat, and marrow elements to the central circulation.

Warning:

The liquid monomer is highly volatile and flammable. Provide adequate ventilation during mixing.

When the cement is being mixed, it should not be kneaded so long that it is no longer soft and pliable.

Once the cement is placed in the bone and the prosthesis has been inserted, the patient should not be allowed to move until the cement has hardened.

Adverse Reactions

Leakage of the liquid monomer into the circulatory system has been implicated in causing marked hypotension, vasodilatation, hypoxemia, bronchoconstriction, and other cardiopulmonary complications, including cardiac collapse.[18-25] These episodes tend to occur more frequently in patients with elevated blood pressure, hypovolemia, and pre-existing cardiovascular abnormalities. The hypotension may appear within the first 2 to 3 minutes after application of the bone cement.

Episodes of hypotension and hypoxemia appear to occur more frequently when the methylcrylate cement is very liquid and when more monomer is present on the surface of the cement at the time of insertion.

Cement in a more liquid form may be introduced by means of a cement gun into the medullary cavity. This may allow the introduction of more liquid monomer into the circulation, with a greater tendency to hypotension.

It is believed that meticulous cleaning of the medullary cavity before the insertion of the cement may help prevent systemic complications. To decrease the intramedullary pressure generated by packing of the cement into the femoral canal, some surgeons insert a fine catheter into the femoral canal to act as a vent during cement insertion and withdraw it at the time the prosthesis is placed.

Another method to prevent the hypotensive effect from occurring is by avoiding hypovolemia. If persistent hypotension occurs, a vasopressor such as neosynephrine should be administered to counteract the drop in blood pressure.

Bone Marrow Elements

Packing of the femoral canal with cement increases intramedullary pressure and probably results in marrow embolization into the central circulation.

Kallos[23] demonstrated elevated intramedullary pressures and pulmonary embolization of fat and bone marrow emboli when cement was placed in the femoral shaft of dogs. If a hole was drilled in the distal femoral shaft, femoral medullary pressure did not become elevated and embolization was not evident.

In 1974, Herndon et al[22] used ultrasound and femoral vein catheters to document that fat embolism occurs during femoral cementing of total hips or hemi-arthroplasty. The amount of fat emboli was decreased if the femoral canal was vented.

Venting is not very common at present.

Thromboplastic Elements

Modig et al[24] obtained blood samples in the pulmonary artery and found bone marrow elements in mitosis, fat globules, and aggregated platelets and fibrin. By conducting coagulation tests, these authors concluded that it was the thromboplastic elements in the pulmonary circulation that resulted in cardiopulmonary dysfunction and decreases in oxygen saturation.

Decreases in Arterial Oxygenation

Whatever the cause of the cardiopulmonary reactions, there is no question that decreases in arterial oxygenation occur during total joint replacement at the time methylmethacrylate cement is inserted. Measured PaO_2 decreases during femoral cementing, even with increased inspired oxygen concentrations (Fig. 4-1).

A higher arterial oxygenation at the initial time of cementing provides a greater margin of safety should decreases occur. Most important to the anesthesiologist are clinically relevant desaturations that would be evident with pulse oximetry.

Both general and regional anesthesia techniques are associated with desaturations. However, those receiving regional anesthesia tend to start out with a lower PaO_2 because they receive nasal oxygen, which provides a lower F_1O_2 than with general anesthesia, and thus are at an increased risk of suffering a clinically relevant desaturation.[21,26]

Desaturation

At HJDOI, we noticed that patients who had low preoperative oxygen saturations (less than 95 percent) on room air were at higher risk of desaturation while under general anesthesia than patients who entered the operating room

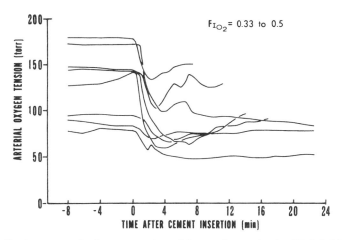

Fig. 4-1. PaO_2 decreases during cementing of femoral prosthesis. High initial PaO_2 values afford some protection against significant desaturations. (From Kallos,[23] with permission.)

with oxygen saturations of 95 percent or higher, even though both groups were placed on FiO_2 of 1.0 during cementing (Fig. 4-2). Desaturations were noted during acetabular cementing, femoral reaming, and femoral cementing.[27]

Although desaturations during cementing had previously been recognized to occur, we also note episodes of desaturation during femoral reaming. These desaturations were clinically relevant and probably result from marrow fat and thromboplastic element embolization. We have also noted desaturations during broaching and reaming of the femoral canal in patients receiving noncemented femoral components.[27]

Recommendations for patients at the time of cementing include

1. Administration of increased inspired oxygen concentrations during acetabular and femoral reaming and femoral cementing. If any desaturation is noted, inspired oxygen should be changed to 100 percent.
2. Observation of oxygen saturation monitors for evidence of desaturation. An arterial blood gas analysis should be obtained if evidence of desaturation occurs.
3. Maintenance of adequate intravascular volume. This can help decrease the side effects of hypotension noted with cementing.

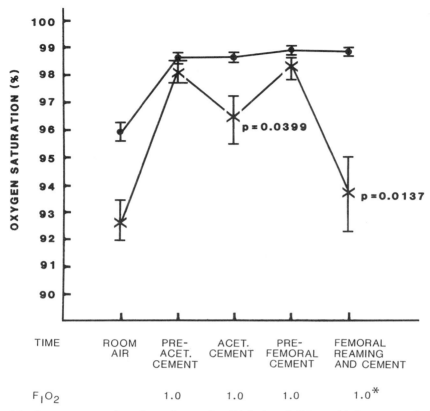

Fig. 4-2. Oxygen saturations in patients who did ($\times$) and did not ($\bullet$) desaturate during cemented hip replacement. P values demonstrate significant decreases in oxygen saturation. *During femoral reaming, F_IO_2 was less than 1.0. (From Rosenberg et al,[27] with permission.)

4. Awareness that hypotension and pulmonary and cardiac dysfunction can occur during the period of cementing.

Injury to the Sciatic Nerve

Congenital Hip Dislocation

The head of the femur rides high on the ilium in congenital hip dislocation, with shortening of the limb and associated soft tissue changes leading to adduction contracture with decrease in the length of nerves and blood vessels. There may not be a proper acetabulum, which may have to be fashioned from the ilium.

The shaft of the femur may be narrow.

Problems

Traction on the femur to gain length during surgery may result in vascular and nerve damage.

Somatosensory evoked potentials (SSEPs) may be used during surgery to determine the status of the sciatic nerve.[28]

Inhalation agents are not used if SSEP monitoring is employed.

Revision Surgery

Besides sciatic nerve injury during repair for congenital hip dislocation, sciatic nerve injury is possible during primary and revision hip surgery.

Case Study

A patient underwent total hip replacement for osteoarthritis secondary to congenital hip dislocation. During surgery, the SSEP monitoring demonstrated prolongation of the latency. A shorter prosthesis was placed, but the motor dysfunction did not resolve during surgery as noted during a wake-up test. Nerve dysfunction was present postoperatively but resolved over a period of time. Sciatic nerve function is frequently tested only after the patient awakens from the anesthesia, and this case demonstrates how intraoperative SSEP monitoring was of value in detection of the problem.

Causes for postoperative foot drop other than trauma to the sciatic nerve must be considered.

Case Study

A 56-year-old man underwent revision of a total hip prosthesis involving a cemented femoral component and noncemented acetabular cup. A normal neurologic examination was noted in the initial postoperative period but deteriorated, and the patient developed signs of peroneal nerve palsy. It was noted that the straps for the abduction pillow that is placed between the legs were too tight around the head of the fibula and resulted in the neurologic dysfunction.

Sudden Hypotension

Sudden hypotension may occur during total hip replacement and is seen at the time of reaming, cementing, or insertion of the prostheses.

Sudden hypotension is caused by

1. Effect of reaming causing embolization of fat, bone marrow, and thromboplastic elements

2. Monomer causing vasodilatation and hypotension
3. Fat emboli reaching the pulmonary vasculature or passing through a patent foramen ovale

Case Study

During cementing of the femoral component of a total hip replacement, sudden marked hypotension and oxygen desaturation were noted. Vasopressors re-established an adequate blood pressure, but maneuvers such as administering 100 percent oxygen and adding positive end-expiratory pressure only increased the PaO_2 into the 80- to 90-mmHg range. The patient remained unstable and was transferred to the intensive care unit. The patient did not awaken after surgery and had massive brain edema postoperatively. The presumptive diagnosis was fat embolism with possible embolization across a probe patent foramen ovale.

4. Venous air emboli with or without paradoxical embolization
   Although not considered an adverse reaction to cement, venous air embolism has been documented during total hip replacement and can occur during reaming and cementing.
   It can result in hemodynamic alterations including hypotension, hypoxemia, and cardiac arrest.
   A case of paradoxical air embolism through a probe patent foramen ovale into a coronary artery, resulting in ST-segment elevation and myocardial infarction, has been reported.[29]
   Open venous sinuses in the femoral shaft have been implicated as the site of air entrainment. Air can enter these sinuses during reaming as a result of cement insertion down the canal or from the lateral decubitus position, which places the operative site above the level of heart.[29]
5. Pulmonary emboli (may come from the pelvic area and reach the lung, leading to hypoxemia and hypotension)
6. Massive occult bleeding (e.g, femoral vessel or pelvic vessel lacerated during surgery)

Treatment

Circulation is supported with vasopressors, and fluid, if needed. One hundred percent oxygen is administered to combat the problems of hypoxemia and hypotension.

BILATERAL TOTAL HIP REPLACEMENTS

Bilateral total hip replacements are usually indicated in patients who can tolerate the procedure and who have contractures of the hips. Replacing one hip and not the other at the same time could lead to a situation in which postoperative physical therapy would be hindered by the contracture on the nonoperated side.

Careful evaluation of the medical status of the patient must be carried out before embarking on bilateral total hip replacements.

Adequate blood must be prepared before these procedures.

Re-evaluation of the patient, including the blood loss from the first side, hemo-dynamic status, hematocrit value, autologous blood used, urine output, and body temperature, must be performed before starting the second side.

REVISION HIP SURGERY

Revision surgery is performed after

1. Failure of internal fixation for hip fractures
2. Previous total hip replacement or joint surgery
3. Surgery for fractured neck of the femur

In some instances after surgery for fractured neck of the femur, blood supply to the femoral head may be inadequate, with osteonecrosis occurring.

Alterations in the status of fixation by the nail and plate may occur, requiring removal and reconstruction with total joint replacement.

If the acetabulum is intact, replacement of the proximal femur may be all that is indicated. If both the femoral and acetabular component are destroyed, total hip replacement may be necessary.

Revision Surgery After Total Joint Replacement

Indications are

1. Loosening of the acetabular component
2. Loosening of the femoral component
3. Loosening of both components
4. Wearing out of the acetabulum
5. Previously placed components in malposition, leading to dislocation
6. Poor placement of femoral component

Revision surgery is more difficult to perform because the prosthesis and cement have to be removed. In some instances, the components come out easily. In other instances, the cement is adherent to the prosthesis but the prosthesis is broken. In revision surgery:

The time for the procedure is lengthened.

Bleeding may be increased.

The chance for neurologic damage may be increased.

The chance for vascular damage may be increased.

In some instances, in which it is suspected that the cement may be impinging on a blood vessel, a preoperative arteriogram should be performed and consultation with a vascular surgeon obtained before the surgical procedure.

Vascular Involvement

Case Study

A 74-year-old man underwent revision of a left total hip replacement. As the acetabulum was removed, it was noted that methylmethacrylate was adherent to a large arterial vessel. A vascular surgeon was contacted, and the methylmethacrylate removed and the artery repaired.

Preparation

Careful evaluation of the patient should be carried out, and the patient should be brought into the best possible condition before surgery because it will be prolonged and blood loss will be increased.

Anesthetic Management

Regional Anesthesia

Spinal Anesthesia

If a simple revision is to take place, spinal anesthesia may be sufficient to provide the necessary time for the surgery.

If the procedure is to be prolonged, epidural anesthesia with a continuous catheter technique may be indicated. If epidural anesthesia is considered, the patient may not be able to tolerate lying on one side for the length of time necessary.

Undue sedation to carry the patient through the procedure should be avoided because hypoxia and hypercarbia may result.

General Anesthesia

General endotracheal anesthesia is usually the anesthesia of choice for revision surgery.

In conjunction with general anesthesia, an epidural catheter may be placed for postoperative pain relief.

Local anesthetics may be added during the procedure to decrease the amount of general anesthesia required.

Position

The patient is placed in the supine or lateral decubitus position, with the side to be operated uppermost.

Monitors

See also Monitoring and Equipment. Total Hip Replacement

ECG

Arterial line for continuous monitoring of the blood pressure and for blood gas determinations

End-tidal carbon dioxide

Pulse oximeter

Body temperature monitoring and method for warming patient

Esophageal stethoscope for heart sounds and breath sounds

Urinary catheter to monitor urinary output

Nerve stimulator

Scale to weigh sponges and volumetric determination of shed blood

Central venous pressure monitor as indicated

Pulmonary artery catheter as indicated

If the Cell Saver is to be used, a method should be instituted to determine the volume of blood loss that has occurred during the procedure because the estimated blood loss may not be readily determined.

PROBLEMS IN THE POSTANESTHESIA CARE UNIT AFTER HIP SURGERY

Special attention should be directed toward fluid, cardiac, pulmonary, and neurologic status. Electrolytes and hemoglobin and hematocrit levels should be obtained.

Care must be taken not to overload the patient with fluid. An accurate assessment of intake and output must be carried out so the patient's fluid status can be ascertained.

Fluids should be reinfused carefully so the patient does not receive too much fluid at one time. Results of the electrolytes and hemoglobin and hematocrit levels are evaluated. The blood products (Cell Saver, postoperative reinfusion, autologous blood, or homologous blood) the patient has received are reviewed. If a transfusion is required, autologous blood must be used if it has been predonated.

After a surgical procedure during which spinal anesthesia was used, patients may develop signs of fluid overload in the PACU.

When the spinal anesthesia level recedes and vasoconstriction occurs in previously vasodilated areas, a relative central hypervolemia occurs, which may result in fluid overload. Avoidance of this is possible by administering vasopressors to counteract hypotension during spinal anesthesia and limiting the volume of fluid administered. In patients with a history of congestive heart failure and a pulmonary artery catheter present, small doses of furosemide may be advantageous if pulmonary artery pressures increase as the spinal anesthetic recedes.

Administration of a diuretic will quickly help to counteract the effects of fluid overload.

Body Temperature

If the patient is hypothermic, warming devices such as the Bair Hugger or heating lamps are used.

Neurologic Problems

The sciatic nerve may be injured during the surgical procedure by traction. Sciatic nerve injury can also occur during acetabular reconstruction. An immediate operation may be necessary to decompress the sciatic nerve.

Before rushing back to the operating room, the straps from the abduction pillow should be checked to be certain they are not compressing the common peroneal nerve at the head of the fibula.

Vascular Problems

Increased bleeding may occur, leading to excessively large amounts of blood in the wound salvage device.

Bleeding may occur into the thigh with massive swelling in the area. The thigh should be checked frequently for this.

Problems associated with massive bleeding include compression of nerves and vessels, leading to a ''compartment syndrome.''

Massive occult bleeding may occur with hypotension and decreased urinary output resulting from hypovolemia, which may not be appreciated unless the wound and thigh are examined.

If hypotension should occur in the immediate postoperative period, the first thought should be excessive hemorrhage into the wound. If this is not the cause of hypotension, other factors must be considered.

Postoperative Pain Control

If a regional anesthetic was administered, epidural or spinal narcotics may provide postoperative pain relief. Alternatively, patient controlled analgesia or intermittent intramuscular injections may be used (see also Ch. 14).

Pulmonary Problems

Some orthopedic surgeons prefer to have their patients in a position with the feet slightly elevated and abducted postoperatively (Charnley position). This may cause respiratory difficulty in the patient with pre-existing pulmonary or cardiac dysfunction.

TOTAL KNEE REPLACEMENT

Indications for Surgery

Total knee replacement is performed in patients in whom significant structural changes in the knee have occurred that result in pain, inability to ambulate, and deformities of the knee joint.

Conditions Leading to Surgery

Rheumatoid arthritis

Osteoarthritis

Varus and valgus deformities with degenerative arthritis

Position

The patient is placed on the operating table in the supine position.

Description of the Operation

A vertical incision is made in the skin over the anterior aspect of the knee joint. The distal end of the femur and the proximal end of the tibia are resected. After preparation and proper alignment, prosthetic devices are placed into the distal end of the femur and the proximal part of the tibia.

Both cemented and noncemented devices are available.

Patella realignment and reconstruction are performed when necessary.

Soft tissue releases are performed as necessary.

Postoperative wound drainage devices are inserted

The subcutaneous tissues and skin are closed.

A bulky dressing is applied with the knee in extension.

Anesthetic Management

Antibiotic Prophylaxis

If intravenous antibiotics are requested by the surgeon, they should be administered at least 5 minutes before tourniquet inflation to achieve an adequate blood level.[30]

Spinal and Epidural Anesthesia

This is an excellent method to provide anesthesia and analgesia for patients undergoing total knee replacement. Patients are in the supine position, can receive adequate sedation, and can be awake and alert shortly after the procedure is finished. If a spinal anesthetic is administered, at least 3 hours of anesthesia will need to be supplied.

The anesthetic level should be to the T8 level to provide adequate pain relief and block tourniquet pain. Narcotics can be administered to help decrease tourniquet pain and provide postoperative pain relief. Intraoperative tourniquet pain can be diminished by small doses of epidural fentanyl (see Ch. 7).

An intrathecal dose of approximately 0.4 or 0.5 mg of morphine is adequate for postoperative pain relief.

Epidural anesthesia enables the anesthetic level to be achieved slowly. Epidural morphine (5 mg) can provide excellent pain relief if an epidural anesthetic is used.

General Anesthesia

General anesthesia is an acceptable technique for patients undergoing total knee replacement. The patient's age and medical condition should be taken into consideration when administering medications.

If general anesthesia is used, postoperative patient controlled analgesia for pain control should be considered.

Use of Tourniquets

Tourniquets may be used during surgery or just applied to the thigh but not inflated (see Ch. 7).

Although tourniquets do provide a dry operative surgical field, some problems might occur during tourniquet inflation.

When the tourniquet is inflated during the procedure, bleeding is not noted but may be profuse after tourniquet release. Be prepared for sudden hypotension.

If little or no bleeding occurs after tourniquet release, it is possible that a major vessel had been injured during the operative procedure while the tourniquet was inflated.

Patients with significant atherosclerotic disease may suffer vascular damage from tourniquet use. This could occur from compression of noncompliant vessels or breaking off of plaques. Preoperative evaluation of pulses should be performed by the surgeon. If significant disease exists, the surgeon should be dissuaded from using a tourniquet. Pulses and temperature must be checked after tourniquet deflation before leaving the operating room.

Control of Hemorrhage After Tourniquet Release

If a tourniquet is used during total knee replacement, the main perioperative blood loss begins at the time of tourniquet deflation and continues through the recovery room stay.

Hemostasis should be obtained by the surgical team.

One can recover blood from the wound and process it in a Cell Saver or use salvage and reinfusion devices.

Blood or fluid is administered as indicated to maintain circulatory stability.

Systemic Effects of Tourniquet Release

Tourniquet release can result in alterations in blood pressure, systemic circulation of metabolic products, and even fat or pulmonary embolism (see Ch. 7).

Intraoperative Management of Major Vascular Injuries

Obtain vascular surgery consultation immediately.

Perform an angiogram in the operating room.

Perform vascular repair immediately to avoid prolonged effects of ischemia.

After vascular repair, continue the orthopedic component of the surgery.

Peroneal Nerve Palsy

Intraoperative factors may predispose patients to postoperative peroneal nerve palsies.[31]

Peroneal palsies should be suspected in patients with

1. Flexion deformities
2. Valgus deformities
3. Nerve stretching during surgery
4. Hematoma formation in the postoperative period

If regional anesthesia is used for total knee replacement, this must be borne in mind if peroneal palsies are noted in the postoperative period.

Postoperative Management

Postoperative management in the PACU should include the following:

Use same considerations as after total hip replacement.

Make certain that the tourniquet and padding have been removed.

Check vascular status.

Check neurologic status.

Observe postoperative wound drainage device for blood loss (300 to 400 ml of blood may be lost in a very short period of time causing hypotension). In contrast to total hip replacements, total knee replacement patients lose a large percentage of their total blood loss in the PACU.

Reinfuse lost blood using a filter.

Bilateral Total Knee Replacement

Bilateral total knee replacement is occasionally performed, especially if adequate postoperative rehabilitation can only be obtained if both knees are corrected at the same time. The operation should be performed on one side and then the other, not simultaneously.

Do not allow the use of bilateral tourniquets simultaneously because serious strain on the heart can occur because of a high afterload.

After the procedure on the first side, wound drainage devices must be observed because large amounts of blood may be lost while the second operation is being carried out. The wound drainage catheter should be hooked up to the Cell Saver suction and the blood processed and reinfused.

Blood being lost into the wound drainage device from the first side is replaced if a sufficient amount is lost while surgery is being performed on the second side. Large amounts of blood can be lost from the wound and from the operative site simultaneously.

When a patient is scheduled for bilateral total knee replacement, there should be a pause to evaluate the status of the patient after completion of the first side. Fitness for tolerating the operation on the second side should be determined at this time.

When patients are scheduled for bilateral total knee replacement, they should be notified that only one side may be performed as determined by their status after surgery on the first side.

TOTAL SHOULDER REPLACEMENT

Total shoulder replacement is performed in patients with degenerative joint disease of the shoulder secondary to

Rheumatoid arthritis

Osteoarthritis

Trauma

Description of the Operation

The operation involves removal of the humeral head and replacement with a prosthetic device inserted into the shaft of the humerus. A prosthetic component is also placed into the repaired glenoid fossa.

Position

The patient is placed in a sitting position toward the edge of the operating table on the side of the surgery.

When the patient is placed in the sitting position, the following should be performed.

1. Maintain the head in the neutral position. The tendency to turn the head away from the operative site may cause traction on the brachial plexus, with neurologic injury.

2. Secure the endotracheal tube carefully.
3. Avoid traction during the surgical manipulations that occur as part of the surgical procedure.
4. Flex the hips and knees to avoid traction on the sciatic nerve in the sitting position.
5. Observe for hypotension because the sitting position also may cause some pelvic pooling with decreased venous return and hypotension.
6. Remember that the blood pressure measured in an arm cuff or in an arterial line transducer placed at the level of the wrist does not register the blood pressure perfusing the cerebral cortex. Place the transducer at the level of the ear to determine the blood pressure perfusing the brain.
7. Remember that venous air embolism may occur because the operative site is above the level of the heart and any incisions into veins may lead to venous air embolism.

Anesthetic Management

Regional Anesthesia

Operations on the shoulder can be performed under interscalene brachial plexus block (see Ch. 6).

General Anesthesia

General endotracheal anesthesia in the sitting position involves problems such as

Hypotension

Air embolism

Dislodgement of the endotracheal tube

Possible hypotension secondary to the use of cement

Postoperative Care

Neurologic status in the extremity is evaluated to ensure that traction or intraoperative injury has not occurred.

REFERENCES

1. Stephen CR: The risk of anesthesia in surgery in the geriatric patient. p. 231. In Krechel SE (ed): Anesthesia in the Geriatric Patient. Grune & Stratton, Orlando, FL, 1984
2. Pettine KA, Aamlid BC, Cabanela ME: Elective total hip arthroplasty in patients older than 80 years of age. Clin Orthop 266:127, 1991

3. Smith TC: Anesthesia and orthopaedic surgery. p. 1215. In Barash PG, Cullen BF, Stoelting RK (eds): Clinical Anesthesia. 2nd Ed. JB Lippincott, Philadelphia, 1992

4. Sculco TP, Ranawat C: The use of spinal anesthesia for total hip replacement arthroplasty. J Bone Joint Surg 57A:173, 1975

5. Goodnough LT, Rudnick S, Price T et al: Increased preoperative collection of autologous blood with recombinant human erythropoietin therapy. N Engl J Med 17:1163, 1989

6. Danersund BG, Hogman C, Milbrink J et al: Physiological response to phlebotomies for autologous transfusion at elective hip-joint surgery. Eur J Haematol 46:136, 1991

7. Toy P, Strauss RG, Stehling LC et al: Predeposited autologous blood for elective surgery. A national multicenter study. N Engl J Med 316:517, 1987

8. McVay PM, Andrews A, Kaplan E et al: Reactions among autologous donors. Transfusion 30:249, 1990

9. Pindyck J, Avorn J, Kuriyan M et al: Blood donation by the elderly: clinical and policy considerations. JAMA 257:1186, 1987

10. Education Program Expert Panel: Special communication. The use of autologous blood—the national blood resource. JAMA 263:414, 1990

11. Toy P: Autologous transfusion. p. 533. In Spiess BD (guest ed): Hemorrhagic Disorders. Vol. 8, No. 3. WB Saunders, Philadelphia, 1990

12. Murray DJ, Gress KG, Weinstein SL: Coagulopathy after reinfusion of autologous scavenged red blood cells. Anesth Analg 75:125, 1992

13. Clements DH, Sculco TP, Burke SW et al: Salvage and reinfusion of postoperative sanguineous wound drainage. J Bone Joint Surg 74(A):646, 1992

14. Bengston JP, Backman L, Stenqvist O et al: Complement activation and reinfusion of wound drainage blood. Anesthesiology 73:376, 1990

15. Woda R, Tetzlaff JE: Upper airway oedema following autologous blood transfusion from a wound drainage system. Can J Anaesth 39:290, 1992

16. Woolson ST, Watt JM: Use of autologous blood in total hip replacement. J Bone Joint Surg 73(A):76, 1991

17. Rosenberg AD, Bernstein D, Ramanathan S: What is the best method to avoid homologous transfusion. Anesthesiology 73:1016, 1990

18. Newens AF, Volz RG: Severe hypotension during prosthetic hip surgery with acrylic bone cement. Anesthesiology 36:298, 1972

19. Kepes ER, Underwood PS, Becsey L: Intraoperative death associated with acrylic bone cement. JAMA 222:576, 1972

20. Pebbles DJ, Ellis RH, Stride SDK et al: Cardiovascular effects of methylmethacrylate cement. Br Med J 1:349, 1972

21. Dhamee MS, Ramic R, Asidao CB: Arterial oxygen tension during application of methylmethacrylate for total hip arthroplasty. Anesth Rev 13:17, 1986

22. Herndon JH, Bechtol CO, Crichenberger DP: Fat embolism during total joint hip replacement. J Bone Joint Surg 56(A):1350, 1974

23. Kallos T: Impaired arterial oxygenation associated with the use of bone cement in the femoral shaft. Anesthesiology 42:210, 1975

24. Modig J, Busch C, Olerud S et al: Arterial hypotension and hypoxemia during total hip replacement: the importance of thromboplastic products, fat embolism and acrylic monomers. Acta Anaesthesiol Scand 19:28, 1975

25. Park WY, Balingit P, Kenmore PI et al: Changes in arterial oxygen tension during total hip replacement. Anesthesiology 39:642, 1973

26. Al-Shaikh B: Effect of inspired oxygen concentration on the incidence of desaturation in patients undergoing total hip replacement. Br J Anaesth 66:580, 1991

27. Rosenberg AD, Bernstein RL, Bernstein DB et al: Oxygen desaturation during cemented hip replacement—who desaturates and when? Anesthesiology 67:551, 1987
28. Black DL, Reckling F, Porter S: Somatosensory-evoked potential monitoring during total hip arthroplasty. Clin Orthop 262:170, 1991
29. Camann WR, Sacks GM, Schools AG et al: Nearly fatal cardiovascular collapse during total hip replacement: probable coronary arterial embolism. Anesth Analg 72:245, 1991
30. Friedman RJ, Friedrich LV, White LR et al: Antibiotic prophylaxis and tourniquet inflation in total knee arthroplasty. Clin Orthop 260:17, 1990
31. Asp JPL, Rand JA: Peroneal nerve palsy after total knee arthroplasty. Clin Orthop 261:233, 1990

Thromboembolism

PREVENTION

Preventing deep vein thrombosis (DVT), pulmonary embolism (PE), and fatal pulmonary embolism (FPE) are major concerns of anesthesiologists and orthopedic surgeons who care for patients undergoing orthopedic surgery.

INCIDENCE

The incidence of DVT after hip surgery has been reported to be as frequent as 68 percent.[1]

DVT is also reported to occur more than 50 percent of the time in other orthopedic procedures performed on the lower extremity.[2]

FPE occurs in up 2 percent of patients undergoing hip joint replacement and in 4 to 7 percent of patients who undergo repair of hip fracture.[3-5]

Because DVT can result in PE and FPE, a major emphasis has been placed on preventing its occurrence. However, studies demonstrate that even in patients receiving prophylaxis, there is still a high incidence of DVT.

HIGH-RISK GROUPS

The following are factors that cause patients to be at high risk for the development of DVT:

Orthopedic surgery on lower limbs

Recent thrombophlebitis

Advanced age

Obesity

Presence of malignancy

Congestive heart failure

Prior DVT or PE

Estrogen use, oral contraceptives, smoking

Trauma

Immobilization

Prolonged bed rest[3,4]

PROPHYLAXIS

Antithromboembolism prophylaxis has helped decrease the incidence of both DVT and FPE.[6-8]

Different methods, both pharmacologic and nonpharmacologic, are available to prevent DVT, PE, and FPE.[9]

Graduated Compression Stockings

Graduated compression stockings provide varying degrees of compression, with the highest at the ankle and a gradual decrease in pressure up the extremity until the midthigh, where the pressure is lowest. These should be avoided in patients with peripheral vascular disease.

Intermittent Pneumatic Compression Boots

Air-filled boots applied to the leg are intermittently compressed by a machine. This compression helps to prevent venous stasis in the legs by applying sequential pressure from the ankle (highest) to the thigh (lowest). This technique increases the blood flow velocity in the legs and also induces the fibrinolytic system.[9] In a randomized trial of patients undergoing total hip replacement, patients receiving intermittent compression had a significantly lower incidence of proximal vein and calf vein thrombosis than controls.[10]

Note: These should be instituted before surgery. Do not institute after surgery when clots may have already developed.[3]

Combined Use

The use of both graduated compression stockings and intermittent pneumatic compression boots together helps to prevent venous stasis as well as to increase the velocity of blood flow in the extremity.[9,11]

Drug Therapy

Low-Dose Heparin

Low-dose heparin (5,000 units subcutaneously) is administered 2 hours before surgery and then every 8 hours.

A reduction in PE has been documented with this technique:

64 percent reduction in FPE

40 percent reduction in nonfatal PE

However, wound hematomas occur, and excessive bleeding is seen.[2,9,12]

Low-Molecular-Weight Heparin

Low-molecular-weight heparin is not available in the United States at this time but is effective when given once daily in preventing DVT in elective hip surgery.[13-15]

Less bleeding occurs with this agent than with regular heparin. There does not appear to be an increased risk of bleeding when used with spinal or epidural anesthesia.[9]

Low-molecular-weight heparin has a longer half-life than standard heparin.[9,16,17]

Case Study

In a prospective study of patients receiving standard heparin three times daily versus patients receiving low-molecular-weight heparin once daily after total hip replacement, those receiving low-molecular-weight heparin had significantly fewer episodes of pulmonary emboli ($P = .016$). Patients in both groups received their first doses preoperatively (the low-molecular-weight heparin group the evening before surgery and the standard heparin group 2 hours before surgery). Although the overall incidence of DVT was not different between the two groups, there was a lower incidence of femoral thrombosis in the low-molecular-weight heparin group ($P = .011$).[15]

Even in this study, in which patients received anticoagulation (standard or low-molecular-weight heparin group), the incidence of PE was still frequent (8 of 65 in the low-molecular-weight heparin group and 19 of 62 in the standard group). Only 3 patients had clinical signs of PE.[15]

Dextran

Dextran is a polysaccharide produced by *Leuconostoc mesenteroides* that is believed to work by decreasing platelet aggregation, diluting clotting factors, and improving rheology.[18] Dextran, which is used by some as a volume expander, increases intravascular volume and may lead to fluid overload in some patients.

Dextran is administered either as dextran 40 (mean molecular weight, 40,000) or dextran 70 (mean molecular weight, 70,000) in a dose of 500 ml (daily or every other day) after surgery until the patient is ambulatory.[18]

However, the drug is given in different dosing regimens by different surgeons because there has not been a real treatment end-point determined. It is not yet known what blood concentration is necessary to provide thromboembolism prophylaxis. The administered volume is usually decreased in patients who cannot tolerate large volume infusions.

The administration of dextran has been associated with dextran-induced anaphylactoid/anaphylactic reactions (DIAR). A study of 1.3 million dextran administrations revealed a 0.013 percent incidence of anaphylactic reactions to dextran 40 and a 0.025 percent incidence of DIAR to dextran 70. Fatal reactions occurred in 0.003 percent of dextran 40 patients and 0.004 percent of dextran 70 patients.[19]

Dextran-reactive antibodies, which are immunoglobulin G, may be present in the body as a result of prior exposure, a different source such as dental plaque, cross-reactivity from bacterial infection, or dextran contaminants in sugar.[19-21]

When a long-chain dextran polymer is administered to a patient, it can react with dextran-reactive antibodies and form an immune complex and possibly result in an anaphylactic-type reaction characterized by the development of urticaria, flushing, wheezing, varying degrees of hypotension, and respiratory or cardiac arrest.[19-21]

This severe reaction can occur after only a few drops of dextran.

Prevention

Administration of Promit, a low-molecular-weight dextran (molecular weight, 1,000) before starting the dextran 40 or dextran 70 appears to diminish the chance of DIAR.

Promit acts as a hapten, binding to the antigenic sites on the dextran-reactive antibodies. As a short-chained molecule, Promit cannot cross-bridge and thus cannot allow immune-complex formation. If adequate Promit is administered and all dextran-reactive binding sites occupied, DIARs should not occur after the large-chain dextran molecule is infused.[18]

Twenty milliliters of Promit should be administered intravenously 5 minutes before a dextran 40 or 70 infusion is begun. When dextran is started, the patient is observed for signs of a dextran reaction. The incidence of reactions has been greatly diminished with the institution of the regimen of Promit before dextran 40 or 70.[18]

We had one case in which an anaphylactic reaction occurred after a few drops of dextran were administered despite prophylactic administration of Promit.[22]

Renal Toxicity

Another side effect of dextran is renal toxicity. Dextran can precipitate in renal tubules and cause renal dysfunction. We avoid its use in patients with significant pre-existing renal disease.

Comparison with Other Drugs

Recently, low-molecular-weight heparin was shown to be more effective than dextran 70 in thromboprophylaxis for patients undergoing elective total hip replacement.[23]

Warfarin

Warfarin can be administered just before surgery in an attempt to decrease the incidence of thromboembolism. Increased bleeding may not be seen intraoperatively because the full warfarin anticoagulation effect has not occurred.

An initial dose administered the evening before surgery or on the morning of surgery will not have taken full effect by the time surgery takes place.

After surgery, the dose can be increased to achieve a prothrombin time 1.5 times the control.[2,24,25]

Bleeding and control of anticoagulation levels so they are neither too elevated or too low are difficulties associated with the use of warfarin.[26]

In patients who are being treated with warfarin for an underlying medical condition or because of a history of DVT, we have used a combination of an initial warfarin dose preoperatively and dextran postoperatively until the warfarin dose is adequate.

Although both warfarin and low-molecular-weight heparin are effective in decreasing DVT, low-molecular-weight heparin has been shown to be more effective than warfarin in decreasing DVT in patients undergoing surgery for fracture of the hip.[3,27]

Anesthetic Technique

It appears that the use of regional anesthesia may decrease the incidence of DVT in patients undergoing lower extremity orthopedic surgery when compared with general anesthesia.[2,28–33]

Reasons for the protective antithrombotic effect of regional anesthesia include vasodilatation of lower extremity veins, improved blood flow, decreased viscosity, alterations in clotting parameters, and a decrease in venous stasis.[2,4]

Hematologic Effect of Local Anesthetics

Some data exist to suggest that regional anesthesia may alter hematologic clotting parameters.[2,28,30] However, alterations in blood viscosity may be secondary to fluid administration during these procedures and not a direct local anesthetic effect.

Increase in Lower Extremity Blood Flow

Regional techniques increase lower extremity blood flow.[32] This effect may only continue as long as the regional anesthesia is in effect. It may continue into the postoperative period if the anesthetic is continued.[32,33]

Anticoagulation

Regional anesthesia should not be administered in an anticoagulated patient receiving a full dose of anticoagulants.

Patients receiving nonsteroidal anti-inflammatory agents or aspirin present a problem. Withholding of these agents for a number of days before surgery may be a good method.[2]

If there is concern, a bleeding time should be obtained.

Consensus

There does not appear to be a uniform consensus among orthopedic surgeons as to the most effective method of providing prophylaxis.

In our institution, different surgeons use aspirin, dextran, warfarin, pneumatic compression boots, or some combination of the above.

It is clear that the best regimen for prophylaxis is not yet finalized.

SIGNS AND SYMPTOMS

Concern exists that patients may arrive in the operating room with a pre-existing DVT or a DVT with subclinical pulmonary emboli already occurring. This is a major consideration in trauma patients and patients who are immobilized, wheelchair bound, or have been at bed rest for a prolonged period of time. If signs and symptoms were not present preoperatively, we are alarmed when we note

A resting tachycardia in a patient without pain that does not decrease with minimal sedation

Hypoxia in room air that does not improve significantly with supplemental oxygen

Dyspnea and increased respiratory rate

Other signs and symptoms include[3,4,34]

Pulmonary
    Shortness of breath
    Tachypnea, dyspnea
    Pleuritic chest pain
    Hypoxemia
    Hypocapnia
    Cyanosis
    Low oxygen saturation on pulse oximeter
    Rales
    Cough, hemoptysis

Cardiac
    Sinus tachycardia
    Nonspecific ST-T wave changes

Neurologic
    Confusion—especially if deterioration from mental status on admission
    Apprehension
    Syncope

Low-grade fever

Additional signs and symptoms
    Phlebitis
    Edema

These signs and symptoms can occur from pulmonary emboli caused by blood or fat. Caution should be exercised before anesthetizing patients with these findings, and consideration should be given to performing a workup for PE, including arterial blood gases, ventilation/perfusion scan, and possibly a pulmonary angiogram, so decisions can be made concerning appropriate anticoagulation should PE be diagnosed.

Note:

It appears that it is very difficult at the present time to propose a unified method of prophylaxis for thromboembolism. Individual orthopedic surgeons have developed their own methods of treating patients.

Anesthesiologists should be aware of the different prophylactic modalities available for preventing DVT and PE, alert for perioperative signs of PE and alert for DVT and PE as possible problems when they visit patients postoperatively.

Below are some cases that have taught us about occult and symptomatic pulmonary emboli and patients at risk.

Case Study

A 24-year-old man who fractured his femur 2 days before surgery arrived in the operating room. Blood pressure was stable, pulse was 110 beats/min, and the patient was complaining of pain in areas of the fracture. The patient was induced into general anesthesia. Procedure continued without problem until acute onset of hypotension, hypoxemia, and cyanosis. The patient had a cardiac arrest and was unable to be resuscitated.

Case Study

A 26-year-old man after repair of anterior portion of spine deformity arrived in the operating room for posterior repair with a pulse of 120 beats/min. The patient was induced into anesthesia and had a cardiac arrest.

Case Study

A 58-year-old man underwent uneventful laminectomy, postoperatively ambulated early, but refused to wear compression stockings. On the day before discharge, the patient complained of shortness of breath and had a respiratory arrest. The patient was unable to be resuscitated.

Case Study

An obese woman underwent arthroscopy of the knee. The patient arrived in the emergency department postoperatively complaining of pain in the chest on inspiration. A ventilation/perfusion scan demonstrated a PE. The patient was admitted to the hospital and received full anticoagulation.

PROPHYLAXIS DURING SPINE SURGERY

Patients undergoing spine surgery are not usually pharmacologically anticoagulated perioperatively for fear of an epidural hematoma and cord compression. Some surgeons use graduated compression stockings or intermittent pneumatic compression boots.

REFERENCES

1. Modig J, Borg T, Karlstrom G et al: Thromboembolism after total hip replacement: role of epidural and general anesthesia. Anesth Analg 62:174, 1983
2. Kaufman BS, Young CC: Deep vein thrombosis in embolism I. p. 823. In Capan L, Miller S (eds): Anesthesiology Clinics of North America Vol. 10, No. 4. WB Saunders, Philadelphia, 1992
3. Hull RD, Raskob GE: Prophylaxis of venous thromboembolic disease following hip and knee surgery. J Bone Joint Surg 68(A):146, 1986
4. Dehring DJ, Arens JF: Pulmonary thromboembolism: disease recognition and patient management. Anesthesiology 73:146, 1990
5. Hull RD, Raskob GE, Hirsh J: Prophylaxis of venous thromboembolism: an overview. Chest 89(suppl):374, 1986
6. Kakkar VV, Corrigan TP, Fossard DP: Prevention of fatal pulmonary embolism by low dose heparin. Lancet 2:45, 1975
7. Bergvist D, Bergentz SE, Fredin H: Thromboembolism in orthopedic surgery. Acta Orthop Scand 55:247, 1984
8. Tryckeri AB: Prophylaxis of postoperative thromboembolism with dextran 70: improvements of efficacy and safety. Orion, Solna, Stockholm, 1983
9. Goldhaber SZ, Morpurgo M: Diagnosis: treatment and prevention of pulmonary embolism. JAMA 268:1727, 1992
10. Hull RD, Raskob GE, Gent M et al: Effectiveness of intermittent pneumatic leg compression for preventing deep vein thrombosis after total hip replacement. JAMA 263:2313 and 264:2072, 1990
11. Scurr JH, Coleridge-Smith PD, Hasty JH: Regimen for improved effectiveness of intermittent pneumatic compression in deep vein thrombosis prophylaxis. Surgery 102:816, 1987
12. Collins R, Scrimgeour A, Yusuf S et al: Reduction in fatal pulmonary embolism and venous thrombosis by perioperative administration of subcutaneous heparin: overview of results of randomized trials in general, orthopedic, and urologic surgery. N Engl J Med 318:1162, 1988
13. Turpie AGG, Levine MN, Hirsh J et al: A randomized controlled trial of low-molecular weight heparin (enoxaparin) to prevent deep vein thrombosis in patients undergoing elective hip surgery. N Engl J Med 315:925, 1986
14. Levine MN, Hirsh J, Gent M et al: Prevention of deep vein thrombosis after elective hip surgery: a randomized trial comparing low molecular weight heparin with standard unfractionated heparin. Ann Intern Med 114:545, 1991
15. Eriksson BI, Lalebo P, Anthmyr B et al: Prevention of deep vein thrombosis and pulmonary embolism after total hip replacement. J Bone Joint Surg 73(A):484, 1991
16. Bara L, Billaud E, Gramond G et al: Comparative pharmacokinetics of a low molecular weight heparin (PK 10 169) and unfractionated heparin after intravenous and subcutaneous administration. Thromb Res 39:631, 1985
17. Braff G, Tornebohm E, Lockner D et al: A human pharmacological study comparing conventional heparin and low molecular weight heparin fragment. Thromb Haemos 53:211, 1985
18. Messmer K, Lungstrom KG, Gruber UF et al: Prevention of dextran-induced anaphylactoid reactions by hapten inhibition. Lancet 1:975, 1980
19. Lungstrom KG, Renck H, Standberg K et al: Adverse recations to dextran in Sweden 1970–1979. Acta Chir Scand 149:256, 1983

20. Richter AW, Hedin HI: Dextran hypersensitivity. Immunol Today 3:132, 1982
21. Hedin H, Richter W: Pathomechanisms of dextran-induced anaphylactoid/anaphylactic reactions in man. Int Arch Allergy Appl Immunol 68:122, 1982
22. Bernstein RL, Rosenberg AD, Pada EY et al: A severe reaction to dextran despite hapten inhibition. Anesthesiology 67:567, 1987
23. The Danish Enoxaparin Study Group: Low-molecular-weight heparin (Enoxaparin) vs dextran 70. Arch Inern Med 151:1621, 1991
24. Francis CW, Marder VJ, Evarts CM et al: Two-step warfarin therapy: prevention of postoperative venous thrombosis without excessive bleeding. JAMA 249:374, 1983
25. Francis CW, Pellegrini VD Jr, Marder VJ et al: Comparison of warfarin and external pneumatic compression in prevention of venous thrombosis after total hip replacement. JAMA 267:2911, 1992
26. Fischer HD: Perioperative medical evaluation and management. p. 575. In Zuckerman JD (ed): Comprehensive Care of Orthopaedic Injuries in the Elderly. Urban & Schwarzenberg, Baltimore, 1990
27. Gerhart TN, Yeff HS, Robertson LK et al: Low molecular-weight heparinoid compound compared with warfarin for prophylaxis of deep-vein thrombosis in patients who are operated on for fracture of the hip. J Bone Joint Surg 73(A):494, 1991
28. Modig J: The role of lumbar epidural anesthesia as antithrombotic prophylaxis in total hip replacement. Acta Chir Scand 151:589, 1985
29. Modig J, Maripuu E, Sahlsteot B: Thromboembolism following total hip replacement: a prospective investigation of 94 patients with emphasis on efficacy of lumbar epidural anaesthesia in prophylaxis. Reg Anaesth 11:72, 1986
30. Modig J, Borg T, Bagge L et al: Role of extradural and of general anaesthesia in fibrinolysis and coagulation after total hip replacement. Br J Anaesth 55:625, 1983
31. Sharrock NE, Haas SB, Hargett MJ et al: Effects of epidural anesthesia on the incidence of deep-vein thrombosis after total knee arthroplasty. J Bone Joint Surg 73(A):502, 1991
32. Modig J, Malmberg P, Karlstrom G: Effect of epidural versus general anaesthesia on calf blood flow. Acta Anaesth Scand 24:305, 1980
33. Lindstrom B, Ahlmar H, Johnson O et al: Influence of anaesthesia on blood flow to the calves during surgery. Acta Anaesth Scand 28:201, 1984
34. Senior RM: Pulmonary embolism. p. 422. In Wyngaarden JB, Smith LH (eds): Cecil Texbook of Medicine. 18th Ed. WB Saunders, Philadelphia, 1988

6

Regional Anesthesia

Some patients do not wish to undergo general anesthesia if surgery is to be performed on an extremity. With the popularity of ambulatory surgery, regional anesthesia is requested by patients who wish to be able to go home as soon as possible. It is therefore important for the anesthesiologist to become expert in regional anesthetic techniques as applied to the practice of orthopedic surgery.

There are certain "rules" that determine whether regional anesthesia will be successful.

Bernstein's Rules of Regional Anesthesia

If the patient wants and requests regional anesthesia, the block will most likely be successful.

If the surgeon agrees that the patient should have regional anesthesia, the block will be successful.

However, if the anesthesiologist is the only one who wants regional anesthesia and finally convinces the surgeon and the patient who grudgingly accept this technique, the possibility that the block will be successful is very slim.

All regional anesthesia should be performed in an unhurried manner, allowing enough time for the block to work. If the block is given at the last minute with the surgeon and assistants standing with the scalpel poised, chances are that the block will not have had time to set, the patient will feel the incision, and the block will have failed.

PREOPERATIVE PATIENT PREPARATION

If the patient is properly prepared during the preoperative visit and accepts the concept of regional anesthesia, there will usually be little problem when the procedure is carried out. It should be explained to the patient what the patient will feel while the block is performed and how the area will feel when it is anesthetized.

Acceptance of regional anesthesia will be enhanced if the patient is informed that sedation will be given during the performance of the block and the surgical procedure.

In this chapter, all nerve blocks are described with the use of a nerve stimulator to locate the nerve. This technique results in a very high success rate.

Because patient responses and cooperation are not required when using the nerve stimulator, sedation is possible during the performance of the procedure. In contradistinction, sedation of the patient who is required to report a paresthesia may obtund the patient enough so that the paresthesia is not reported as soon as it is felt but only after the needle has been withdrawn.

COMPLICATIONS OF REGIONAL ANESTHETIC TECHNIQUES

Nerve Injury Caused by Mechanical Trauma

Nerve injury caused by mechanical trauma by the needle can be avoided by the use of the nerve stimulator if paresthesias are not sought, thus avoiding direct contact of the nerve by the point of the needle. Paresthesias elicited during axillary blocks have been associated with an increased incidence of postblock nerve deficits.[1]

The risk of nerve lesions caused by mechanical trauma is further reduced when a short-beveled needle with a 45-degree angle is used instead of a standard long-beveled 14-degree needle.[2]

Toxic Reactions to Local Anesthetic Agents

Toxic effects of local anesthetics occur if a blood level is achieved that exceeds the threshold that can be tolerated by the patient based on dosage and body weight.

Intravenous and intra-arterial injections are avoided by frequent aspiration. Intra-arterial injections in areas such as the neck, when brachial plexus blocks are performed, may lead to toxicity even with very small amounts of local anesthetic because these may be pushed retrograde into the cerebral circulation.

Signs and Symptoms

The earliest symptoms that are diagnostic of toxicity are

A feeling of light-headedness

Numbness of the tongue and circumoral tissues

Visual disturbances with a sensation that the surroundings are moving

Movement of the eyes back and forth in a manner similar to nystagmus

Tinnitus

Muscular twitching

Unconsciousness, convulsions, and coma

Respiratory arrest and cardiovascular depression[2a]

Even though convulsions occur, the primary effect of the drug on the central nervous system is depression. What is initially noted as stimulation results from depression of higher cortical inhibitory centers. During a toxic reaction, ventilatory assistance should be provided if respiration ceases. Hypoxia must be avoided. If convulsions occur, a short-acting barbiturate should be injected and ventilation supported.

Toxic side effects are usually due to an intravenous injection. If patients complain about numbness of the tongue and circumoral tissues or a funny taste in the mouth, the injection must be stopped immediately. Intravenous injection can occur even though careful aspiration has been carried out because blood may not flow back into the syringe during aspiration.

Local anesthetic toxicity can result by an imbalance between the absorption and disposition of the amount of local anesthetic that has been injected.

Factors Affecting Toxicity

Injection into an area with a rich blood supply enhances rapid absorption.

Toxicity occurs after injection in the following order:

1. Intercostal nerve blocks
2. Epidural injections
3. Peripheral nerve blocks

Rate of absorption also affects toxicity.

1. Accidental intravenous injection leads to onset in 15 to 50 seconds
2. Overdose may not be associated with symptoms until 5 to 20 minutes after injections[2a]

Failed Nerve Block

If a nerve block fails, the block should not be repeated immediately—you should wait at least 1 to 1.5 hours. Because it takes 15 to 20 minutes to assess the success of a block, a repeat block should not be performed while the plasma levels are still rising from the first block. At 45 minutes, you would have the peak effects of the first block plus the absorption from the second block, at which time peak plasma levels may result in toxicity.

Prevention of Toxic Reactions

1. Perform history and physical
    Consider
        Age
        Body weight
        Medical conditions of patient
        Vascularity at site of injection
2. Decrease chance of seizure with premedication—Administer central nervous system depressant such as diazepam or midazolam used in appropriate dosage adjusted for weight and age.[3]
3. Be prepared for adverse reaction
    Secure intravenous access
    Drugs for resuscitation
        Midazolam
        Diazepam
        Thiopental or other ultra-short-acting barbiturate
        Atropine
        Vasopressors
        Muscle relaxants
    Equipment
        Oxygen
        Suction
        Equipment to secure an airway (Table 6-1)
4. Use correct medications
    Check drugs, read labels
    Use only preservative-free solutions for intravenous regional anesthesia
    Do not use epinephrine-containing solutions for intravenous regional anesthesia or distal nerve blocks (fingers, toes, penis)
    Calculate dosages carefully
5. Inject in proper fashion

Table 6-1. Emergency Equipment

Equipment	Medications
Anesthesia machine checked and ready for use	Thiopental
Monitors: ECG, blood pressure, pulse oximeter	Midazolam
Laryngoscopes	Atropine
Endotracheal tubes	Ephedrine
Oral and nasal airways	Epinephrine
Suction	Neosynephrine
	Succinylcholine
	Bretylium

Inject small amount of local anesthetic as a test dose
Aspirate frequently for blood or cerebrospinal fluid
6. Monitor patient
Monitor for changes in heart rate, blood pressure, respiration
Maintain verbal contact with the patient to detect any signs or symptoms of overdose
Observe for clues of toxicity
Make certain patient does not move once needle has been placed in position for block[2a]

Treatment of Acute Toxicity to Local Anesthetics

1. Secure and maintain adequate airway.
2. Apply oxygen by face mask, provide adequate ventilation if patient unable to do so, intubate if necessary.
3. Check blood pressure and administer intravenous fluids or vasoactive medications if necessary.
4. Observe ECG monitor for rhythm.
5. If convulsions occur, use thiopental, midazolam or diazepam until seizures stop. Avoid overdose of central nervous system depressants.
6. Use a muscle relaxant (succinylcholine) to aid in providing ventilation. Muscle relaxants will paralyze patient but will not stop seizure activity when administered alone.
7. Medications
Atropine—0.6 mg IV for bradycardia
Ephedrine—5 to 10 mg-increments IV to restore and maintain blood pressure
Epinephrine—1 mg IV if cardiovascular collapse occurs (repeat depending on status of circulation and initiate advanced cardiac life support if necessary)
For bupivacaine toxicity, bretylium treatment and cardioversion if necessary. (Table 6-2)[2a]

CHOICE OF LOCAL ANESTHETIC

In choosing a local anesthetic agent, the duration of surgery as well as the type of nerve block to be performed should be considered (Table 6-3).

The local anesthetic agent should have a duration of action that will be effective for the length of time needed to prepare, perform the surgical procedure, and place the appropriate dressings. The anesthesiologist must be familiar with the length of time a specific surgeon needs to perform a given procedure.

Table 6-2. Problems Associated with Regional Anesthesia

Signs and Symptoms	Causes	Treatment
Immediate Convulsion	Direct intravascular injection	Oxygenate Stop convulsion Support circulation

Onset 5–15 minutes
  Numbness of tongue
    circumoral tissues
  Visual disturbances
  Tinnitus
  Muscular twitching
  Unconsciousness
  Convulsions
  Coma
	Overdose of local anesthetic
	Rapid systemic absorption
		Oxygenate
		Support circulation
		Stop convulsion

Apprehension
Tachycardia
Hypertension
Headache
	Vasopressor effect	Sedation
		Drugs to decrease heart rate,
		  blood pressure (e.g.,
		  β-blockers)

Bradycardia Hypotension Faintness Pallor	Vasovagal response	Atropine Raise legs

Bradycardia
Hypotension
Hypoventilation
	Inadvertent spinal or epidural
	  block seen in
	    Stellate ganglion block
	    Interscalene block
	    Lumbar sympathetic
	      block
		Oxygenate
		Intubate
		Ventilate
		Support circulation

(Modified from Scott and Cousins,[2a] with permission.)

Table 6-3. Local Anesthetic Agents

Drug	Concentration (%)	Maximum Dose	Onset (min)	Duration (hr)
Chloroprocaine	3	600 mg 650 mg with epinephrine 1:200,000	5–10	1–1.5
Lidocaine	1.5	500 mg with epinephrine 1:200,000	15–20	3–3.5
Mepivacaine	2.0	500 mg with epinephrine 1:200,000	15–20	3–3.5
	1–1.5	500 mg with epinephrine 1:200,000	20	4.5
Etidocaine	0.5–1	400 mg with epinephrine 1:200,000	10–20	6–7
Bupivacaine	0.25–0.5	250 mg with epinephrine 1:200,000	20–25	7–7.5
Ropivicaine	0.5	250 mg with epinephrine 1:200,000	15–30	7–12

(Data from Strichartz and Covino,[3a] Raj,[4] and Winnie.[4a])

For brief procedures such as removal of a pin, carpal tunnel release, or trigger thumb release, a short-acting local anesthetic such as chloroprocaine is sufficient. Chloroprocaine has a rapid onset of action and short duration and is useful for very short procedures where it is desirable for the nerve block to wear off rapidly. A longer-acting local anesthetic such as bupivacaine or etidocaine can be used for more extensive and lengthy procedures.

Bupivacaine and lidocaine can be used for almost all regional blocks. Etidocaine is similar to bupivacaine, but it produces a more profound motor block.

DRUGS ADDED TO LOCAL ANESTHETIC AGENTS

Vasoconstrictors

Vasoconstrictors are added to local anesthetic agents to

Slow absorption

Prolong action

Reduce systemic toxicity

Epinephrine

The epinephrine added to solutions of local anesthetic agents at the time of manufacture is unstable and may lose some of its potency when exposed to light. A stabilizing agent such as sodium metabisulfite is added. This allows epinephrine-containing solutions to be autoclaved one time.[2a]

Epinephrine-containing solutions have a pH of 3 to 4.5 as a result of the added antioxidant as compared with untreated solutions whose pH is 6.5 to 6.8. Local anesthetic solutions with a low pH have a decreased rate of diffusion and an associated decreased rate of onset of block.[2a]

Optimal Dose

The optimal concentration of epinephrine is 1:200,000 (5 μg/ml). Increasing the concentration does not enhance the vasoconstrictor activity appreciably but may lead to toxicity.[2a,5]

Addition of Epinephrine

Epinephrine is added just before use.

A fresh ampule of epinephrine containing 1 mg/ml (1,000 μg/ml) is used. The addition of 0.2 ml (200 μg), measured by a tuberculin syringe, to 40 ml of local anesthetic will provide a solution of 1:200,000 epinephrine with 1 ml of local anesthetic containing 5 μg of epinephrine.

> Take 1 ampule (1 mg/ml) of epinephrine.
>> Withdraw 0.2 ml (200 μg).
>> Add to 40 ml local anesthetic solution.
>> or
>> Withdraw 0.15 ml (150 μg).
>> Add to 30 ml local anesthetic solution.
>
> Concentration becomes 1:200,000.
>
> Dose of epinephrine/ml = 5 μg.

The maximum dose of epinephrine should not exceed 200 to 250 μg.[5,6]

Drugs having intrinsically longer durations of action, such as mepivacaine, etidocaine, and bupivacaine, do not benefit as much from the addition of epinephrine.

Epinephrine usually decreases peak blood levels by decreasing absorption but does not decrease peak blood levels as much when administered with bupivacaine and etidocaine.

Contraindications to Use

In orthopedic patients epinephrine should not be used in the following conditions:

Unstable angina

Serious arrhythmias

Uncontrolled hypertension

Hyperthyroidism

Patients on monoamine oxidase inhibitors and tricyclic antidepressants

For peripheral nerve blocks in areas with poor collateral blood supply—digits, penis, wrist or ankle

Sodium Bicarbonate

Addition of sodium bicarbonate to local anesthetic solutions is said to increase the rate of diffusion and onset of blockade.

The addition of 1 mEq of sodium bicarbonate to each 10 ml of 1.5 percent lidocaine raises the pH to 7.15 and increases onset and spread of sensory blockade.[6a]

The addition of 0.1 ml of 8.4 percent sodium bicarbonate to each 10 ml of 0.5 percent bupivacaine with epinephrine 1:200,000 reduced the latency of sciatic nerve block from 25 to 12.5 minutes and prolonged the duration of analgesia from 14.1 to 18.3 hours.[7]

In our opinion, freshly prepared epinephrine-containing solutions (pH 6.5 to 6.8) do not require the addition of sodium bicarbonate.

PATIENT PREPARATION

Check equipment and supplies.

Apply blood pressure cuff, electrocardiogram (ECG) electrodes, and pulse oximeter.

Obtain intravenous access.

Inject midazolam intravenously in 0.5 mg increments slowly to achieve adequate sedation.

Place nasal oxygen cannula at 4 L/min flow.

Monitor ventilation and observe pulse oximeter while nerve block is being performed.

SEDATION

Titrate narcotics, benzodiazepines, propofol, or barbiturates are used to provide *adequate* sedation. Very large amounts of barbiturates, narcotics, and sedatives to make the patient accept the block are avoided because hypoventilation, hypoxia, and hypercarbia can result in serious consequences.

TECHNIQUES FOR SUCCESSFUL NERVE BLOCKS

It is imperative that the anatomy, landmarks, and nerve distribution of the areas to be blocked are well known.

Placement of local anesthetic solution in the area of the nerve or nerves to be blocked requires that the needle be in as close proximity to the nerve as possible.

Methods used to place the needle near the nerve are either by obtaining a paresthesia, which necessitates the needle actually coming into contact with the nerve, or locating the nerve by means of a nerve stimulator. We recommend the use of a nerve stimulator.

NERVE STIMULATOR

Advantages

1. Cooperation of the patient is not necessary as it is when trying to elicit a paresthesia.
2. Patients can be sedated while undergoing a nerve block.
3. Nerve block can be performed under general anesthesia, if necessary, for postoperative pain relief.
4. Nerve injury by needle while seeking a paresthesia is avoided.

Characteristics

The nerve stimulator should

1. Be small, battery-operated, and easily mounted
2. Have an accurate dial for current adjustment
3. Have a digital read-out
4. Have a range from 0.1 to 10 mA
5. Provide impulses at one per second[7a,8]

Use

The peripheral nerve stimulator can be used to locate any nerve that has a motor component.[8]

The nerve stimulator works by producing a current to stimulate the nerve through a needle placed in close proximity to that nerve.

Stimulation leads to motor activity (twitches) of muscles innervated by that nerve. Motor fibers are stimulated at a lower milliamperage than pain fibers, allowing a twitch response without pain.[8]

The stimulator should provide a low-frequency, pulse-generated current that can be incrementally adjusted during the procedure.

The greatest motor activity at the lowest current (0.1 to 0.3 mA) indicates that the needle is in as close proximity to the nerve as possible. Frequently, muscle twitches can be obtained even when the needle is outside the fascial sheath that envelops the nerve. Only by being at low milliamperage levels can one assume they are as close to the nerve as possible. Attention to this will help improve the success rate.

The nerve stimulator used at our institution is one that can be used to monitor neuromuscular blockade when used with high output and for nerve stimulation

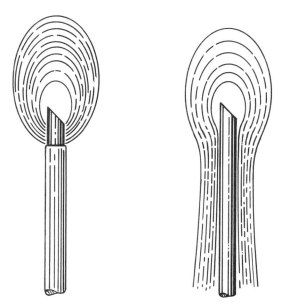

Fig. 6-1. Electric current is concentrated at tip of insulated needle but is diffuse in uninsulated needle.

for regional anesthesia with low output. This is accomplished by inserting the output jack into the low output terminal. The black (−) lead is connected to the needle; the red (+) lead is connected to the ground (ECG pad).

Insulated Needle

Special insulated needles should be available in 1.5, 3.5, and 5-in. sizes. These needles are insulated from a few millimeters proximal to the tip along the entire shaft to the hub. The current passes from the stimulating electrode to the tip of the needle without any current coming from the shaft. With the current concentrated at the tip of the needle, precise localization of the nerve is achieved (Fig. 6-1).[8]

Equipment

Nerve stimulator

ECG pads

Insulated needles—1.5, 3.5, and 5 in.

Antiseptic solution

Gauze sponges

Drapes

Extension tubing

2 20-ml syringes

1 3-ml syringe

1 tuberculin syringe

1 needle (18 × 2.5 cm) (1 in.)

1 needle (25 × 1.25 cm) (0.5 in.)

1 three-way stopcock

Resuscitation equipment (Table 6-1)

Standard Technique

Perform block in a quiet area, and avoid noise from instrument set-up.

Have assistance available.

Explain block to patient.

Provide adequate sedation but do not overdose.

Monitor adequacy of ventilation.

The nerve stimulator set-up is shown in Figure 6-2. The standard technique for use of a nerve stimulator is as follows:

Attach the positive lead to a ground electrode (ECG pad) on the patient opposite the area where the block is to be performed.

Determine the proper landmark—use marking pen.

Prepare and drape the skin.

Raise a skin wheal in the area through which needle is to be passed.

Enlarge opening through skin wheal with 18-gauge needle.

Pass insulated needle through skin wheal.

Attach negative electrode to connector or metal hub of insulated needle.

Connect tubing to hub of needle from syringe with local anesthetic.

Direct needle toward nerve.

Turn stimulator to 1.5 to 2 mA. Use lower current for upper extremity blocks and higher current for sciatic blocks.

Observe muscles supplied by nerve for twitches.

Advance needle in small steps toward nerve until maximum twitch is achieved.

Decrease current so that maximum twitch is achieved with lowest amperage.

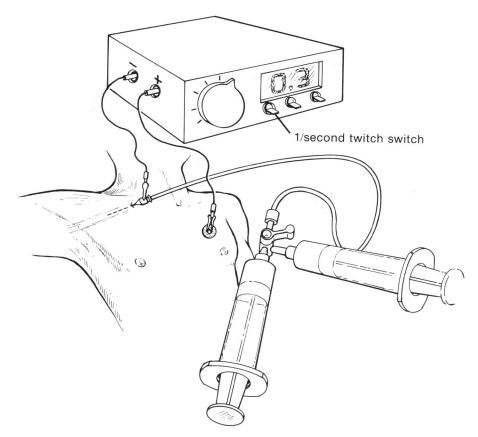

Fig. 6-2. Nerve stimulator set-up. Block needle is attached to negative electrode of nerve stimulator; ground to positive terminal. Injection is performed where maximal twitches are obtained at lowest amperage.

Remember that the point of the needle is closest to the nerve when maximum twitch is achieved with the lowest current.

Remember that greatest success is achieved when 0.1 to 0.2 mA elicits maximum twitches of the muscles (Table 6-4).

Do not move needle and change current at the same time because it will be impossible to determine where the needle is at any point.

When maximum twitch obtained, stabilize needle, aspirate, and inject 2 ml of local anesthetic.

Stimulation at the same mA should not produce twitches after injection of 2 ml of local anesthetic.

Inject remainder of local anesthetic with aspiration every few milliliters, while keeping needle stable.

Table 6-4. Rate of Successful Block as a Function of Decreasing Stimulating Current

Block	Milliamps	No. Successful Blocks (%)
Interscalene	0.6–1.0	4/11 (36)
	0.5	39/47 (82)
	0.4	16/19 (84)
	≤0.3	53/57 (93)
Axillary	0.6–1.0	1/4 (25)
	0.5	24/30 (80)
	0.3–0.4	12/21 (81)
	≤0.2	34/37 (92)

(Data from Albert DB, personal communication.)

THE BLOCK IS GIVEN—WHAT NEXT?

After administering the local anesthetic agent, allow some time for the block to "take" before starting to check for its adequacy.

Assure the patient that adequate anesthesia will be present for the surgical procedure.

Keep the surgeon away from the patient.
> The surgeon should refrain from constantly "checking" the block before incision.

Assess the block.
> For brachial plexus blocks, check
>> The median nerve in the palm proximal to the index finger
>> The ulnar nerve near the fifth finger
>> Extension of elbow for radial nerve
>> Flexion of elbow for musculocutaneous nerve

Sedate the patient.
> The patient can be given more sedation, if needed, while the skin preparation and draping are being performed. Before the incision, propofol or thiopental can be injected intravenously to provide sedation. The patient usually becomes drowsy and awakens to ask when the operation is going to begin, at which time the surgeon is deeply involved in the procedure.

UPPER EXTREMITY NERVE BLOCKS

Brachial Plexus Anatomy

1. The brachial plexus is formed from the anterior primary rami of the fifth, sixth, seventh, and eighth cervical and first thoracic nerves, with contributions from the fourth cervical and second thoracic nerves.[4,4a,5,10a]

The brachial plexus supplies all the motor and almost all the sensory functions of the upper extremity.

The skin over the shoulder is supplied by the branches of the cervical plexus.

The posterior medial aspect of the arm is supplied by the intercostobrachial branch of the second intercostal nerve.

2. The nerve roots forming the brachial plexus emerge between the anterior and middle scalene muscles, where they form three trunks. They lie superior and posterior to the second and third parts of the subclavian artery.

3. These trunks pass from the interscalene space and go over the upper surface of the first rib. The trunks are arranged in a vertical manner in a configuration, where they are seen as superior, middle, and inferior. These trunks pass together with the subclavian artery through the scalene fascia, forming a subclavian perivascular sheath.

4. Each trunk divides into an anterior and posterior division at the edge of the rib. These divisions pass inferior to the midportion of the clavicle to enter the axilla.

5. In the axilla, the lateral, medial, and posterior cords are formed and oc-

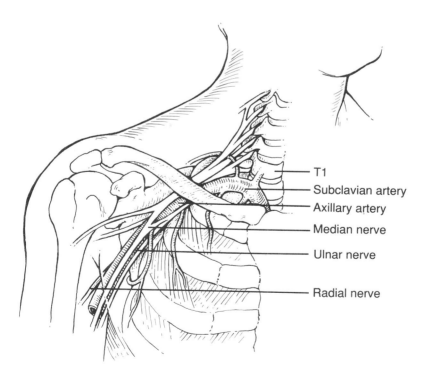

Fig. 6-3. Diagram showing the anatomic relationship of the brachial plexus.

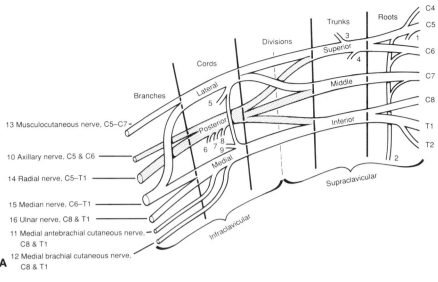

13 Musculocutaneous nerve, C5–C7

10 Axillary nerve, C5 & C6

14 Radial nerve, C5–T1

15 Median nerve, C6–T1
16 Ulnar nerve, C8 & T1
11 Medial antebrachial cutaneous nerve, C8 & T1
12 Medial brachial cutaneous nerve, C8 & T1

A

Branches
Cords
Lateral
5
Posterior
6 7 8 9
Medial
Infraclavicular

Divisions
Superior
3
4
Middle
Inferior
Supraclavicular

Trunks
Roots
C4
C5
1
C6
C7
C8
T1
T2
2

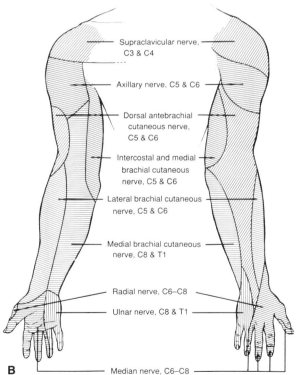

Supraclavicular nerve, C3 & C4

Axillary nerve, C5 & C6

Dorsal antebrachial cutaneous nerve, C5 & C6

Intercostal and medial brachial cutaneous nerve, C5 & C6

Lateral brachial cutaneous nerve, C5 & C6

Medial brachial cutaneous nerve, C8 & T1

Radial nerve, C6–C8

Ulnar nerve, C8 & T1

B

Median nerve, C6–C8

Fig. 6-4. **(A)** Diagram showing brachial plexus nerves. Brachial plexus is blocked above clavicle with interscalene or perivascular subclavian approaches and below clavicle with infraclavicular and axillary approaches. Branches from roots: 1, dorsal scapular; 2, long

Table 6-5. Choice of Blocks for Upper Extremity Surgical Procedures[a]

	Interscalene	Perivascular Subclavian	Infraclavicular	Axillary
Arthroscopy of shoulder	✓			
Closed reduction dislocation of shoulder	✓			
Total shoulder replacement	✓			
Resection distal end clavicle	✓			
Arthroplasty of shoulder for chronic dislocation	✓			
Elbow surgery		✓	✓	✓
Ulnar nerve transposition		✓	✓	✓
Open reduction internal fixation olecranon		✓	✓	✓
Procedure on 4th and 5th digits		✓	✓	✓
Excision distal end of ulna		✓	✓	✓
Carpal tunnel release	✓	✓	✓	✓
deQuervain's release	✓	✓	✓	
Volar ganglion resection	✓	✓	✓	
Dupuytren's contracture				✓
Excision ganglion dorsum wrist		✓	✓	
Radial collateral ligament repair	✓	✓	✓	
Arthroplasty of thumb	✓	✓	✓	
Open reduction internal fixation fracture radius	✓	✓	✓	
Excision distal radius	✓	✓	✓	
Procedures on digits			✓	

[a] Ask the surgeon where the incision is going to be.

cupy these positions around the second part of the axillary artery in the fascia, which is the axillary sheath.

6. At the lateral border of the pectoralis minor, the three cords give rise to the peripheral nerves of the upper extremity (Figs. 6-3 and 6-4).

General Considerations

The choice of block depends on the site of surgery (Tables 6-5 and 6-6).

Interscalene Block

Good for shoulder surgery

Poor for surgery on medial aspect of arm and forearm because the inferior cord, which is the origin of the ulnar nerve, may not be blocked

←

thoracic; branches from trunks: 3, nerve to subclavian; 4, supraclavicular; branches from cords: 5, lateral pectoral; 6, upper scapular; 7, thoracodorsal; 8, lower scapular; 9, medial pectoral; 10, axillary; 11, medial antebrachial cutaneous; 12, medial brachial cutaneous; terminal nerves: 13, musculocutaneous nerve; 14, radial nerve; 15, median nerve; 16, ulnar nerve. **(B)** Diagram showing dermatomal distribution of nerves of arm and shoulder to help guide in choosing correct block for procedure.

Table 6-6. Choice of Anesthesia for the Purist

Shoulder	Interscalene
C3–C6	
Elbow	Infraclavicular
C5–C8 T1 and T2	Subclavian perivascular
Medial aspect	
C8–T2	
Lateral aspect	
Posterolateral aspect	
C5–8	
Forearm	
C5–C7	Infraclavicular
Musculocutaneous nerve	Subclavian pedrivascular
C6–T1	
Median nerve	
C8 and T1	
Ulnar nerve	
C5–C8	
Posterior cutaneous nerve	
C8 and T1	
Medial cutaneous nerve (radial nerve)	
and median nerve	
Wrist and hand	
Wrist snuff box	Subclavian perivascular
Median nerve	Interscalene
Radial nerve	
Musculocutaneous nerve	
Hand and digits	Axillary
Ulnar and digits	
Median nerve decompression	

Frequent phrenic nerve blockade

Epidural, intrathecal, and vertebral artery injections avoided by careful aspiration

Axillary Block

Must have ability to abduct arm to 90 degrees

Good for surgery on hand and wrist, especially in ulnar nerve distribution

May not provide good anesthesia in distribution in area supplied by radial nerve in lateral aspect of hand and forearm

May not block musculocutaneous nerve—to snuff box

Not good for much above elbow, but may work at elbow

Brachial plexus block by the axillary technique associated with greater sensory block and poorer motor block

Infraclavicular Block

With the infraclavicular block, anesthesia can usually be provided for all procedures on the upper extremity below the shoulder.

Note: Brachial plexus block by the interscalene, supraclavicular, or infraclavicular technique leads to a motor block earlier than the sensory block.

Supraclavicular Block

The classical supraclavicular approach is not emphasized here because of the possibility of developing a pneumothorax. Success with this block requires extensive experience and practice.

Anesthetic Agents

Dosage

In general, the dose of anesthetic required for a good surgical block of the brachial plexus is 10 ml/nerve. Because there are four nerves, a total of 40 ml is used.[4]

Choice

For sensory and motor block of the brachial plexus, recommended agents include

0.5 percent bupivacaine

1 percent etidocaine

1.5 percent lidocaine

1.5 percent mepivacaine

3.0 percent chloroprocaine

Sensory Block Only

Sensory block alone may be required if a surgeon wishes to have the patient move the extremity during the surgery. For sensory block alone, lesser concentrations of local anesthetic should be used, such as 1 percent lidocaine.

Factors Influencing Brachial Plexus Anesthesia

Effect of Exercise and Pain

The effect of pain and muscular exercise on the efficacy of brachial plexus blockade has been studied. Patients who sustained acute trauma of the upper limb and underwent brachial plexus blockade showed a significantly decreased latency for both onset of analgesia and partial or complete motor paralysis as compared with a control group. Another group of patients who were free of pain but were asked to do muscular exercise for 5 minutes after injection of local anesthetic was found to have onset of analgesia and partial and complete muscle paralysis significantly sooner than in the control and pain groups. Changes in the duration of the block were not significant. It was concluded that pain and muscular exercise enhanced the onset of brachial plexus block. It is believed that the rapid onset of analgesia in the pain and exercise groups can be explained by the high stimulation frequencies that open the sodium channels, allowing the local anesthetic to reach the receptors rapidly. Therefore, a more rapid onset can be achieved if the patient is asked to exercise the arm after the block.[8a]

Effects of Warming Local Anesthetic Solution

The effect on onset time of warming local anesthetic solutions was investigated. It was found that the latency of onset of subclavian perivascular brachial plexus blocks was significantly more rapid in patients in whom the local anesthetic was warmed to 37°C than those in whom the local anesthetic was at room temperature. The local anesthetic agents used were 0.5 ml/kg of solution prepared by mixing equal volumes of 0.5 percent bupivacaine with epinephrine 1:200,000 and 1 percent prilocaine. The time until an adequate sensory block could be confidently predicted was reduced almost 50 percent by using prewarmed local anesthetic solutions.[9]

Shoulder Surgery

Innervation is as follows:

C3–C6

C3 and C4 cervical plexus—skin on top of the shoulder

C5 and C6 brachial plexus—skin and deeper tissues

C5 and C6—axillary nerve

C5—deep scapular nerve

C5 and C6—suprascapular nerve

Interscalene Brachial Plexus Block

Nerves from the cervical plexus, C3 and C4, and the brachial plexus, C5 and C6, exit between the anterior and medial interscalene muscles and can be blocked in the interscalene groove. In this block, the volume of solution injected spreads above and below the injection site to block both the cervical plexus as well as the brachial plexus.[4a,10]

In some instances, a block of T1 and T2 may be necessary for complete shoulder anesthesia. The T1 and T2 nerves are blocked at the posterior axillary line.

Equipment

Peripheral nerve stimulator

ECG pad for ground electrode

22-gauge 3.5-in. insulated needle

2 20-ml syringes

Extension set

Three-way stopcock

1 2-ml syringe

1 25-gauge needle

Drugs

1. Lidocaine 1.5 percent, 40 ml with epinephrine 1:200,000
2. Bupivacaine 0.5 percent, 40 ml
3. Etidocaine 1.0 percent, 40 ml
4. Lidocaine 2.0 percent, 20 ml with epinephrine 1:200,000
   Bupivacaine 0.5 percent, 20 ml
5. Chloroprocaine 3.0 percent, 40 ml

Position

The patient lies in the supine position with the head turned in the opposite direction. The arm lies against the side of the patient.

Landmarks

1. Cricoid cartilage
2. Posterior border of the sternocleidomastoid muscle
3. Anterior and middle scalene muscles

The posterior border of the sternocleidomastoid muscle is palpated. It can be accentuated by asking the patient to raise the head.[4,4a,10a]

The index and middle fingers are then rolled over the posterior border to the anterior scalene muscle.

The fingers are then moved laterally to the groove between the anterior and middle scalene muscle.

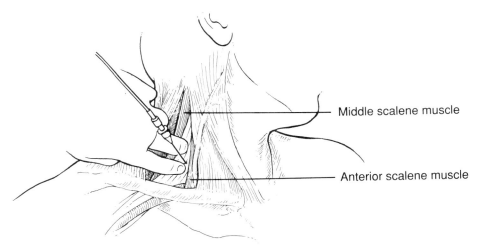

Fig. 6-5. Interscalene brachial plexus block. Needle is inserted between anterior and middle scalene muscles. Needle is directed caudad, mesiad, and posterior.

The interscalene groove can be accentuated by raising the patient's head against resistance.

The needle is inserted between the anterior and middle scalene muscles at the point where the external jugular vein crosses.[4] The external jugular vein can be accentuated by having the patient perform the Valsalva maneuver (Fig. 6-5).

Procedure

Prepare and drape the neck in the usual manner.

Identify the interscalene groove.

Place two fingers at the level of the cricoid cartilage in the interscalene groove.

Spread the fingers apart. Raise a skin wheal between the two fingers.

Pierce the skin wheal with an 18-gauge needle to create an opening in the skin through which the 3.5-in. insulated needle is passed.

Attach the alligator clip from the negative pole of the nerve stimulator to the needle.

Attach the positive alligator clip to the ECG electrode pad.

As the needle is passed into the interscalene groove, set the nerve stimulator at 1.5 mA. Pulses of 1/sec are generated. Twitches are sought in the muscles innervated by the brachial plexus in the upper aspect of the arm and shoulder.

Note whether contractions of the entire upper portion of the body are occurring, which indicates that the diaphragm is probably being stimulated. This means that the needle is on the anterior scalene muscle and is stimulating the phrenic nerve; move it more lateral.

When appropriate muscular twitches are noted, reduce the stimulating current without moving the needle to determine the greatest twitch at the lowest current.

Acceptable twitches before injection should be at 0.2 to 0.3 mA. When this is achieved, inject 2 ml of local anesthetic after aspiration. This should stop the twitches.

Then inject the remainder of the 38 ml of local anesthetic while exerting pressure on the lower border of the interscalene groove to force the volume of solution to the upper portion of the interscalene groove.[4]

Aspirate intermittently.

Anesthesia of the skin of the neck, upper arm, and shoulder is obtained with adequate anesthesia for shoulder surgery.

Note: A high incidence of hemidiaphragmatic paralysis has been noted in patients after interscalene brachial plexus blocks.[11]

Surgery of the Elbow Region

Operations at the region of the elbow include ulnar nerve transposition, reduction of fractures, arthroscopy of the elbow, and excision of radial head.

Innervation is as follows:

C5–C8

T1 and T2

Block of C5–C8 is needed for lateral or posterolateral aspect of the elbow. Block of C8 and T1 and T2 is important for operations on the medial aspect of the elbow.

If tourniquet use is anticipated the superficial branches of C5–C8 and T1 and T2 must be blocked. The infiltration should be subcutaneously across the inner aspect of the arm in axilla for T1 and T2.

Note:

The interscalene block may not consistently block C8 and T1 nerve roots.

The axillary block may miss the musculocutaneous nerve and muscular branches to the upper arm.

Block of Choice

The block of choice is the infraclavicular block or subclavian perivascular block.

Infraclavicular Brachial Plexus Block

The infraclavicular brachial plexus block provides anesthesia from the hand to the shoulder. The cords and branches of the brachial plexus are blocked, providing anesthesia of the musculocutaneous and axillary nerves. The ulnar segment of the medial cord is blocked, as well as the intercostobrachial nerve, which is involved in tourniquet pain.[4,12]

Anatomy

In the axilla, the lateral, medial, and posterior cords are formed. The three cords give rise to the peripheral nerves at the lateral border of the pectoralis minor muscle.

Equipment

Peripheral nerve stimulator
ECG pad for ground electrode
22-gauge 3.5-in. insulated needle
2 20-ml syringes
Extension set
Three-way stopcock
1 2-ml syringe
1 25-gauge needle
1 18-gauge needle

Drug

A dose of 40 ml of 1.5 percent lidocaine with epinephrine 1:200,000 is used.

Use alternative medications based on duration of procedure (Table 6-3).

Position

The patient lies on the operating table in a supine position.

The anesthesiologist stands on the side opposite the one to be blocked.

Landmarks

1. Midpoint of the clavicle
2. Axillary artery

The midpoint of the clavicle is located midway between the prominence of the top of the shoulder and the sternal end of the clavicle. The midpoint of the clavicle is also identified by feeling for the pulsations of the subclavian artery

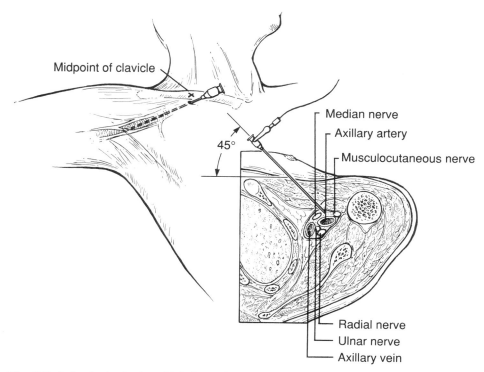

Midpoint of clavicle

45°

Median nerve

Axillary artery

Musculocutaneous nerve

Radial nerve

Ulnar nerve

Axillary vein

Fig. 6-6. Infraclavicular brachial plexus block. Operator stands on side opposite one to be blocked. Needle is inserted 1 in. below midpoint of the clavicle at a 45-degree angle and directed toward pulsations of axillary artery.

where it goes below the clavicle. If this is not possible, the midpoint of the clavicle can be identified by palpation midway between the tip of the shoulder and the insertion of the sternocleidomastoid muscle.

The axillary artery is located by palpation in the axilla. The needle is directed from the midpoint of the clavicle toward the axillary artery (Fig. 6-6).

Procedure

Place a mark on the skin 1 in. below the midpoint of the clavicle.

Prepare and drape the area in the usual manner.

Raise a skin wheal at the mark.

Insert an 18-gauge needle through the wheal.

Through this wheal, pass the 3.5-in. insulated needle. (Use longer needle in muscular individuals.)

Attach the stimulating electrode (negative lead) to the needle, and attach the indifferent electrode to the ECG ground pad.

Identify the axillary artery in the axilla.

Direct the needle at a 45-degree angle with the skin toward the axillary artery.

Turn on the nerve stimulator to 1.5 to 2.0 mA.

Then advance the needle at the 45-degree angle through the skin toward the axillary artery in the axilla while keeping a finger on the artery.

As the needle passes through the pectoralis muscles, contraction of these muscles will occur.

Note that the contractions of the pectoralis muscles cease as you advance the needle.

As the needle is advanced toward the brachial plexus, observe for movement of the muscles of the forearm and hand with flexion or extension of the elbow, wrist, or digits.

At this point, decrease the current; obtain the maximal contraction of the muscles with the current at 0.2 to 0.3 mA. This is evidence that the needle tip is close to the brachial plexus.

To be certain that the needle is in the sheath when maximal twitches are obtained with the lowest current, pass the needle beyond this area, and the twitches should be abolished.

Withdraw the needle back and obtain maximal twitches again at the lowest current. The needle is in the axillary sheath at this time.

Occasionally, while advancing the needle, external rotation of the upper extremity may position the brachial plexus in the axilla so that twitches are more easily obtained. Medially directed pressure on the contents of the axilla can help bring the brachial plexus closer to the advancing needle. Maintain medial pressure during injection in order to prevent the brachial plexus from moving away from the needle.

If muscle movement corresponding to just the musculocutaneous nerve is noted, you may be too superficial (Fig 6-6).

Inject 2 ml of solution after aspiration to abolish the twitches.

Inject the remainder of the local anesthetic solution after careful aspiration.[4]

Subclavian Perivascular Brachial Plexus Block

Anatomy

The trunks of the brachial plexus pass from the interscalene space and are arranged in a superior, middle, and inferior position. These trunks pass with the subclavian artery through the scalene fascia, which forms a subclavian perivascular sheath.[4,4a,13]

Equipment
Peripheral nerve stimulator

ECG pad for ground electrode

22-gauge 1.5-in. insulated needle

2 20-ml syringes

Extension set

Three-way stopcock

1 2-ml syringe

1 25-gauge needle

1 18-gauge needle

Drug
A dose of 40 ml of 1.5 percent lidocaine with epinephrine 1:200,000 is commonly used.

Choose medication based on length of procedure (Table 6-3).

Position
The patient is positioned supine, with head turned to the side opposite the one to be blocked.

Landmarks
1. Midpoint of clavicle at level of C7
2. Pulsation of subclavian artery and interscalene groove

The midpoint of the clavicle is located between the prominence at the top of the shoulder and the sternal end of the clavicle.

The pulsations of the subclavian artery in the interscalene groove above the midpoint of the clavicle are palpated (Fig. 6-7).

Procedure
Raise a skin wheal above the clavicle at the level of C7 in the interscalene groove, where the pulsations of the subclavian artery are felt.

Pass an 18-gauge needle through the skin wheal.

Through this wheal, pass a 1.5-in. insulated needle directly caudad with the needle lying on the skin on a line from the tip of the ear to the midpoint of the clavicle.[4,4a]

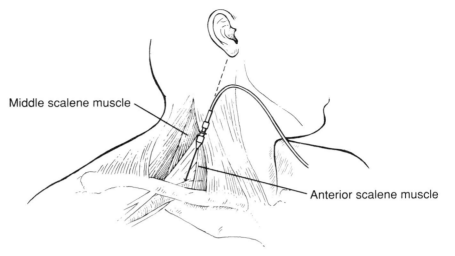

Middle scalene muscle

Anterior scalene muscle

Fig. 6-7. Subclavian perivascular brachial plexus block. Needle is inserted on a line between mastoid process and midpoint of clavicle. Needle should be parallel to skin of neck.

Attach the negative lead from nerve stimulator to the needle, and the positive lead to the ground.

Turn on the nerve stimulator to 2 mA.

Direct the needle caudad until twitches in the muscles of the upper extremity are noted.

Seek the maximum twitch at the lowest current, 0.2 mA.

Inject 2 ml of local anesthetic after aspiration. The twitches should be abolished.

Inject the remainder of the local anesthetic while aspirating to make certain that an intravascular injection is not occurring.

Problems

Puncture of the subclavian artery

Puncture of the lung with pneumothorax

Block of the stellate ganglion

Block of the phrenic nerve

Hematoma[4]

These problems can be avoided by

Using a short 1.5-in. needle

Passing the needle along the border of the middle scalene muscle, which inserts on the first rib making contact with the plexus before the needle reaches the rib

Surgery of the Forearm Region

Surgery of the forearm region requires blocking of all the branches of the brachial plexus formed by C5–T1 nerve roots.

Lateral aspect
    Musculocutaneous nerve—C5–C7

Anteromedial aspect
    Median nerve—C6–T1
    Ulnar nerve—C8 and T1

Posterior cutaneous nerve of forearm—C5–C8

Medial cutaneous nerve of forearm—C8 and T1

Block of Choice

The infraclavicular approach to the brachial plexus will provide anesthesia for surgery of the forearm region because all the nerves involved in this area can be blocked (see p. 184).

Wrist and Hand Surgery

Surgery of the wrist and hand is performed for

Median nerve decompression

Excision of ganglia of the hand

Tendon and nerve repair

Fractures

Surgery at the base of the thumb requires anesthesia of the median nerve, the radial nerve, and the musculocutaneous nerve. (These nerves may be missed and not blocked when using the axillary approach.)

The infraclavicular approach, the interscalene approach, and the subclavian perivascular approach are good techniques for surgery at the base of the thumb.

Axillary Brachial Plexus Block

The axillary brachial plexus block is used for

Surgery on ulnar aspect of wrist

Median nerve decompression—carpal tunnel release

Surgery on digits

Surgery on hand

A fascial sheath surrounds the axillary artery and nerves of the brachial plexus in the axilla.

Anatomic cross-section (Fig. 6-8) demonstrates the position of the nerves in the axilla, with the ulnar nerve medial, the median nerve anterior, and the radial nerve posterior. Note that at this level the musculocutaneous nerve, which is anterior to the axillary artery, as is the median nerve, has already branched off the brachial plexus, exited from the sheath, and runs within the coracobrachialis muscle.[4,4a,10a]

Single or Multiple Injections
Questions have arisen whether multiple injections are necessary to secure anesthesia when doing an axillary block because of the possibility of septa separating the different nerves.

One study carried out on cadavers noted that there are septa. However, these septa are incomplete, and injection of dye into one area spreads throughout other areas.

In the study, a "pop" was not obtained when the sheath was entered but when the needle went through fat. Merely obtaining a pop is not adequate evidence of being within the sheath. We believe that multiple injections should not be performed because one may impale a nerve if multiple attempts are made after the local anesthetic has been given. Nerve damage may result from these multiple attempts in anesthetized nerves. The study also pointed out that because many different techniques are advocated, one is not markedly better than the other.

Because there are connections within the sheath, Partridge et al[14] do not support the need for multiple injections when performing axillary blocks.

Equipment
Peripheral nerve stimulator

ECG pad for ground electrode

22-gauge 3.5-in. insulated needle

2 20-ml syringes

Extension set

Three-way stopcock

1 2-ml syringe

1 25-gauge needle

1 18-gauge needle

Drug

A dose of 40 ml of 1.5 percent lidocaine with epinephrine 1:200,000 is used.

Choose medication based on length of procedure (Table 6-3).

Position

The patient is placed in the supine position with the arm abducted to 90 degrees, the elbow flexed, the forearm externally rotated, and the dorsum of the hand on the table next to the patient's head in the saluting position.[4,4a,10a] Patients with rheumatoid arthritis with shoulder involvement and other patients who cannot abduct to 90 degrees are not candidates for an axillary nerve block.

Landmarks

The landmark is the axillary artery at the highest point in the axilla, just below the coracobrachialis muscle and just lateral to the pectoralis major muscle (Fig. 6-8).

Procedure

Palpate the axillary artery just below the coracobrachialis muscle and lateral to the pectoralis major muscle with the index and middle fingers.

Separate the fingers and raise a skin wheal between them just above the axillary artery.

Through this wheal, use an 18-gauge needle to create a hole for passage of the sheathed stimulating needle.

Insert the stimulating needle through the skin at an angle of 10 to 20 degrees with the artery directed toward the axilla.

Attach the negative electrode to the needle and the positive electrode to the ECG pad placed on the opposite shoulder.

Set the stimulating current at 1.5 mA. Apply digital pressure on the axillary artery distal to the site of needle insertion. This will help prevent distal spread of local anesthetic and may facilitate enough proximal spread to block the musculocutaneous nerve. If the pressure is applied prior to injection of any local anesthetic, then anatomic relationships will not be altered once the maximal twitch response is obtained.

Advance the needle toward the artery, and observe for twitches in the elbow, wrist, or digits of the hand.

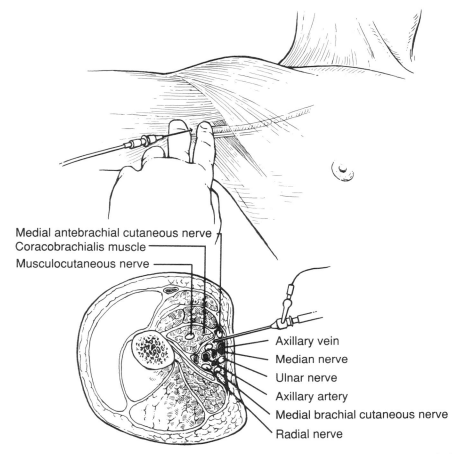

Fig. 6-8. Axillary brachial plexus block. Arm is abducted to 90 degrees. Needle is inserted between two fingers at pulsation of axillary artery as high in axilla as possible and directed medially. Insert shows cross-section view of path of needle.

At the point where the twitch is highest at the lowest level of stimulation (at 0.1 to 0.2 mA) inject 2 ml of local anesthetic after aspiration, and the twitches should be abolished. If twitches are obtained above 0.2 mA you may still be outside the sheath.

Once the twitch is abolished after careful aspiration, inject the remainder of the anesthetic.

On withdrawal of the needle, inject a few milliliters of local anesthetic into the coracobrachialis muscle to block the musculocutaneous nerve.

Bring the arm down to the side to prevent the downward spread of the local anesthetic while compressing the axilla with the fingers of the hand.

Block the intercostobrachial nerve when a tourniquet is used. This is accomplished by infiltrating a band of anesthesia across the medial aspect of the upper arm.[4,4a]

Continuous Brachial Plexus Block

Continuous brachial plexus block is useful in procedures such as reimplantation of digits and other operations that may require prolonged surgery and anesthesia.[13a,14a,15,15a]

Continuous block is also useful in the postoperative period to provide pain relief and to help maintain improved blood supply to reimplanted digits.[14a,15a,16]

Continuous brachial plexus anesthesia kits are available. These contain a needle introducer with a catheter that can be slipped off the needle once the needle has been placed into the axillary sheath.

Equipment
Burron continuous brachial plexus anesthesia kit

Local anesthetic agents

Procedure
Place the patient on the operating room table in the supine position, with the shoulder abducted and the arm flexed, with the hand near the head of the patient.

Prepare and drape the axilla in the usual manner.

Raise a skin wheal four fingers below the axilla in the groove below the coracobrachialis muscle.

By rolling the fingers in this area, you can actually feel the axillary sheath, and in some instances, the pressure of the fingers can elicit mild paresthesias.

Through this skin wheal, use an 18-gauge needle to make a hole.

Pass the blunt needle-catheter introducer through the hole in the skin wheal.

Advance the needle toward the neurovascular bundle at an angle of about 10 to 20 degrees.

When the axillary sheath is reached, an increase in the tissue resistance will be felt.

Advance the needle until the sheath is punctured. Aspirate for possible intravascular placement.

Advance the Teflon cannula, which should now be in the axillary perivascular space over the introducer needle, until its hub has reached the skin. Remove the introducer needle. Insert the catheter to the desired depth. Hold the catheter in place and remove the cannula.

After setting up the connectors, aspirate and introduce local anesthetic agent.

Tape or suture catheter into place securely.

Use of Continuous Brachial Plexus Kit with Nerve Stimulator

Kits are available to perform continuous brachial plexus blocks and other blocks with the use of the nerve stimulator. A metal needle within the plastic cannula aids in locating the nerve with the use of a nerve stimulator as above. When the nerve is located, the cannula is slid off the needle and sutured securely in place. Additional local anesthetic can be added as needed.

Nerves Blocks at the Elbow

Blocks can be performed at the elbow to obtain anesthesia for surgical procedures on the hand as well as for supplementing a brachial plexus block.[4]

Anatomy
Median nerve
> Medial to biceps tendon and brachial artery (Fig. 6-9)

Radial nerve
> Lateral to biceps tendon
> Between brachialis and brachioradialis muscles
> Anterior to lateral condyle of humerus (Fig. 6-9)

Musculocutaneous nerve
> Located on lateral aspect of elbow (Fig. 6-9)
> Superficial to biceps tendon

Ulnar nerve
> Passes in the cubital tunnel between the medial epicondyle and the olecranon process posterior to the medial condyle[16a,17]

Drug
A dose of 5 ml of 1.5 percent lidocaine with epinephrine 1:200,000 is used.

Landmarks
The elbow is flexed 90 degrees to define the elbow crease and to aid in identification of the biceps tendon and brachioradialis muscle.

A perpendicular line is dropped along the volar aspect of the forearm to a point

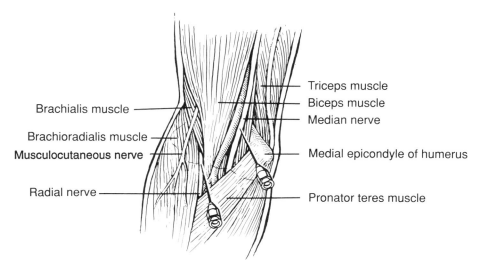

Triceps muscle
Biceps muscle
Median nerve

Brachialis muscle

Brachioradialis muscle
Musculocutaneous nerve

Medial epicondyle of humerus

Radial nerve

Pronator teres muscle

Fig. 6-9. Nerve blocks at the elbow. Median, radial, and musculocutaneous nerves are blocked 2 in. above elbow.

on the volar surface of the arm. This is about four fingers above the elbow and is the level at which the blocks are performed.

Procedure

Perform median, radial, and musculocutaneous nerve blocks (Fig. 6-9).[4]

Prepare the skin of the elbow area in the usual manner.

Median Nerve

Palpate the brachial artery medial to insertion of the biceps tendon.

Insert the needle medial to the brachial artery.

Turn on the nerve stimulator and obtain twitches of muscles in the area supplied by median nerve in hand.

Inject 5 ml of 1.5 percent lidocaine with epinephrine 1:200,000.

Radial Nerve

Palpate the biceps tendon on the lateral aspect of the elbow medial to the brachioradialis muscles.

Insert needle, inject 5 ml of 1.5 percent lidocaine with epinephrine 1:200,000.

Alternate method

Identify the lateral condyle of the humerus.

Mark a point four fingerbreadths proximal to this along the humerus[5].

Insert an insulated needle, turn on the nerve stimulator and advance toward the humerus.

Maximal twitches may be best obtained if the needle is moved anteriorly along the lateral humerus.

At maximal twitch response, after aspiration, administer 5 ml 1.5 percent lidocaine with epinephrine 1:200,000.

Musculocutaneous Nerve

Palpate the biceps tendon.

Insert the needle 1 cm lateral to the biceps tendon in the subcutaneous area.

Inject 5 ml of 1.5 percent lidocaine with epinephrine 1:200,000.

Ulnar Nerve

With the elbow slightly flexed and the arm across the chest, the ulnar nerve is palpated within the groove between the medial epicondyle and the olecranon process (Fig. 6-10).[4,10a]

Raise a skin wheal 3 cm above the level of the condyle. Through this wheal, pass an insulated needle.

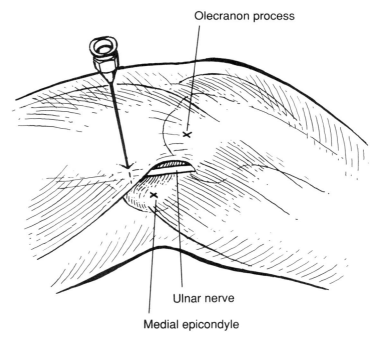

Olecranon process

Ulnar nerve

Medial epicondyle

Fig. 6-10. Ulnar nerve block at elbow proximal to the medial epicondyle.

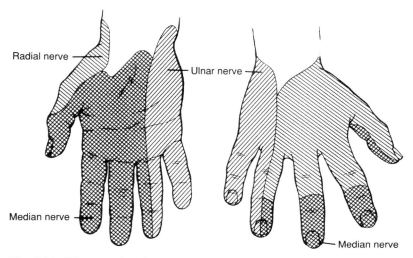

Radial nerve

Ulnar nerve

Median nerve

Median nerve

Fig. 6-11. Diagram showing anatomic distribution of nerves at the wrist.

Attach the nerve stimulator to the needle.

Observe for twitches in muscles supplied by the ulnar nerve.

Obtain maximum twitches at 0.1 to 0.2 mA.

Perform injection.

Do not inject directly into the area of the epicondyle because it may cause damage to the nerve.

Nerve Blocks at the Wrist

Nerve blocks at the wrist are useful for surgical procedure on the distal hand and digits or to reinforce a more proximal block (Fig. 6-11).

Epinephrine should not be used.

Landmarks

The landmark for nerve blocks at the wrist is the ulna styloid and the palmar crease.

Median Nerve Block

Anatomy

The median nerve is medial to the flexor carpi radialis tendon and just lateral and deep to the palmaris longus tendon.

The palmaris longus tendon can be identified by asking the patient to oppose

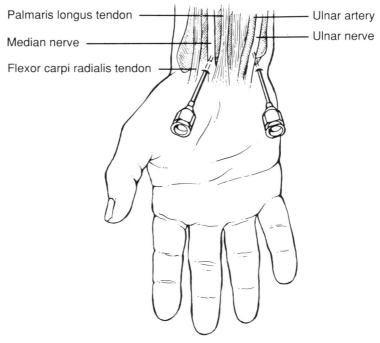

Palmaris longus tendon ——

Median nerve ——

Flexor carpi radialis tendon ——

—— Ulnar artery

—— Ulnar nerve

Fig. 6-12. Median and ulnar nerve blocks at wrist. Median nerve is lateral to palmaris longus tendon; ulnar nerve is adjacent to ulnar artery. Blocks are performed at level of ulna styloid.

the thumb and small finger or by making a fist and slightly flexing the wrist. In some patients, the palmaris longus tendon is absent, and an alternate method of finding the nerve is to inject medial to the flexor carpi radialis at the level of the ulna styloid (Fig. 6-12).

Procedure

Identify the palmaris longus tendon at the wrist.

Raise a skin wheal lateral to the palmaris longus tendon.

Inject 3 ml of local anesthetic through wheal at a depth of 0.5 cm.

Ulnar Nerve Block

Anatomy

The ulnar nerve lies under the flexor carpi ulnaris tendon on the medial side of the ulnar artery and deep to it (Fig. 6-12).

Procedure

Raise a skin wheal on the volar surface of the wrist on the lateral side of the flexor carpi ulnaris tendon.

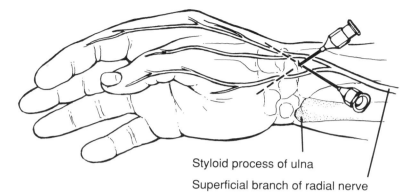

Styloid process of ulna

Superficial branch of radial nerve

Fig. 6-13. Radial nerve block at wrist. Skin on dorsal and volar surface is infiltrated to block superficial branches of radial nerves.

Through this wheal, pass a needle under the tendon to inject 3 to 5 ml of local anesthetic.

Alternate Technique

Make a wheal on the medial side of the flexor carpi ulnaris.

Through this wheal, direct a needle laterally to pass under the tendon to inject 3 to 5 ml of local anesthetic.

Block the superficial branches of the cutaneous portion of the nerve by infiltrating local anesthetic on the dorsal and volar surface of the wrist at the level of the lateral skin wheal.

Radial Nerve Block

The radial nerve at the wrist consists of superficial branches and is blocked by an infiltration technique on the lateral aspect of the wrist at the level of the ulna styloid. Both dorsal and volar infiltration of the skin will block this nerve (Fig. 6-13).

Digital Nerve Block

Digital nerve block is used for procedures on the finger. It can also be used if the finger lacks anesthesia after a more proximal block has been performed.

Anatomy

The nerve supply to the fingers on the palmar aspect of the hand arises from the median and ulnar nerves. Usually the median nerve innervates the lateral three and one-half fingers and ulnar nerve the little finger and medial aspect of the ring finger. The sensory innervation supplying the dorsum of the hand is somewhat variable, but in general the ulnar nerve supplies the medial one and one-half fingers and the radial nerve supplies the remainder with variable innervation to the tips of the fingers, which may be supplied by the median nerve (Fig. 6-11). Nerves to individual digits are derived from common digital nerves which divide at the level of the metacarpal heads. After dividing between two fingers, the digital nerve supplies the lateral aspect of the more medial digit and the medial aspect of the more lateral digit.

Equipment

1 23-gauge, 1.5-in needle.

1 3-ml syringe

Drug

A dose of 1 to 2 ml of local anesthetic is used. Use of more than 1 or 2 ml is contraindicated since the injection is occurring in a closed space and too high of a volume can interfere with blood supply to the fingers.[4]

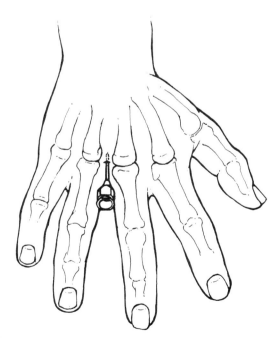

Fig. 6-14. Digital nerve block. Needle is inserted in space between fingers directly between metacarpal heads. A dose of 1 to 2 ml local anesthetic is used. Epinephrine is not used.

Landmarks

Heads of the metacarpal bones

Procedure

Raise a skin wheal on the dorsal surface of the hand between the metacarpals at the level of the head of the metacarpal (Fig. 6-14).

Introduce a 23-gauge 1.5-in needle into the web space to the level of the heads of the metacarpals.

Warning:

Do not use epinephrine.

Do not inject the local anesthetic if pain is felt with the injection.

LOWER EXTREMITY NERVE BLOCKS

Hip Surgery

The two main operations in this area are hip arthroplasty and operations for fracture of the neck of the femur. Spinal and epidural anesthesia are the regional anesthetic techniques of choice for these operations. Lumbar plexus blocks may be useful for surgery for fractures of the femoral neck (See p. 215). Femoral nerve and lateral femoral cutaneous nerve blocks have been used on occasion for repair of fractures of the head of the femur.

To produce anesthesia of the hip, the T10–S2 nerve roots or their peripheral branches proximal to the hip have to be blocked.

Knee Surgery

Arthroscopy, menisectomy, ligament repair, patella surgery, and total knee replacement are the surgical procedures in this area.

The innervation is from L2–S2 (Fig. 6-15).

If tourniquets are used, the L1 nerve root must be blocked as well. Besides spinal and epidural anesthesia for knee surgery, lower extremity peripheral nerve blocks can be performed.

When peripheral nerve blocks are used, the sciatic, femoral, obturator, and lateral femoral cutaneous nerves need to be blocked.

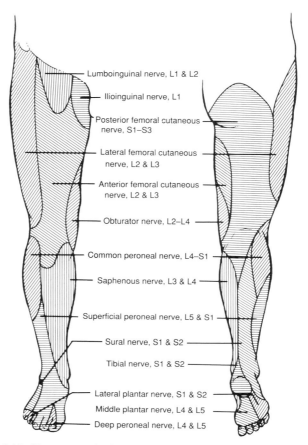

Fig. 6-15. Dermatomal distribution of nerves of lower extremity.

The femoral nerve (L2–L4) supplies the skin over the anterior surface of the thigh. It supplies motor innervation to the quadriceps group and the knee joint. The saphenous nerve supplies the medial part of the calf down to the medial malleolus. The femoral nerve can be blocked in patients with a fracture of the shaft of the femur who are in severe pain and are awaiting transfer to the operating table.

The lateral femoral cutaneous nerve of the thigh (L2 and L3) supplies the antero-lateral and lateral aspect up to the middle of the thigh. It also provides a branch to the patella. The lateral femoral cutaneous nerve of the thigh can be blocked in patients with fracture of the hip to reduce the pain before moving.

The obturator nerve (L2–L4) innervates the adductor muscles and the skin over the medial aspect of the thigh. It sends a branch to the knee joint. Obturator nerve block can be performed for diagnosis and evaluation in patients in whom a obturator neurectomy is contemplated for adductor spasm secondary to neuromuscular disorders.

The sciatic nerve (L4 and L5, S1–S3) innervates the posterior part of the thigh and all areas below the knee joint except the medial aspect up to the medial malleolus, which is supplied by the saphenous nerve. Block of the sciatic nerve is usually performed in combination with other nerve blocks of the lower extremity.

Leg Surgery

For surgical procedures in the leg, spinal or epidural anesthesia is satisfactory.

A combined sciatic and femoral block can be used for anesthesia in the leg.

Block of nerves around the knee such as saphenous, tibial, and common peroneal nerves, can be performed. However, complications, such as neuropathies, as well as intravascular injections are higher at this level.

If a tourniquet is to be used, L1–L4 nerves need to be blocked as well.

Femoral Nerve Block

Equipment

Peripheral nerve stimulator

ECG pad for ground electrode

22-gauge 1.5-in. insulated needle

1 10-ml syringe

Extension set

1 2-ml syringe

1 25-gauge needle

1 18-gauge needle

Drug

A dose of 10 ml of 1.5 percent lidocaine with 1:200,000 epinephrine is used.

Choose medication based on duration of procedure (Table 6-3).

Landmarks

Inguinal ligament (Poupart's ligament)—extends from the anterior superior illiac spine to the pubic tubercle

Femoral artery

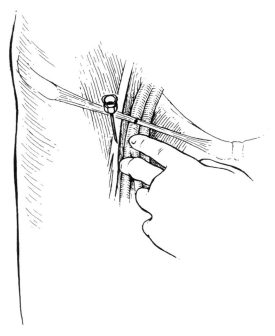

Fig. 6-16. Femoral nerve block. Femoral artery is palpated below inguinal ligament. Needle is inserted perpendicular to skin lateral to femoral artery.

Procedure

Place the patient on the operating table in the supine position (Fig. 6-16).

Palpate the inguinal ligament.

At the midpoint of the inguinal ligament, palpate the femoral artery.

With the fingers on the femoral artery, raise a skin wheal just lateral to the pulsations, approximately 2 cm below the inguinal ligament.

Through this wheal, pass an 18-gauge needle.

Insert the sheathed needle through this wheal.

Make the connections to the nerve stimulator and to the ground electrode.

Pass the needle perpendicular to the skin.

Set the nerve stimulator at 1.5 mA.

Remember that this nerve lies about 1 cm below the skin and is encountered almost immediately.

When you note twitches of the muscles of the thigh, decrease the stimulating current until maximum twitches are obtained at 0.2 to 0.3 mA.

Inject 2 ml of local anesthesia after aspiration.

If the twitch disappears, inject the remainder of the drug after aspiration.

When this block is used to provide pain relief for patients with fracture of the femur, start with a very low current because violent contractions of the muscles using a high current can lead to severe pain.

Lateral Femoral Cutaneous Nerve Block

Indications

1. Surgical anesthesia of the lateral aspect of the thigh—useful for anesthesia of skin for repair of fracture of the hip
2. Treatment of meralgia paresthetica
3. Surgery on or above the area of knee in conjunction with femoral and sciatic nerve blocks
4. Anesthesia for muscle biopsy

Anatomy

This nerve arises from the lumbar plexus, courses medial to the anterior superior iliac spine, and passes through the fascia lata 3 to 4 cm below the inguinal ligament to supply cutaneous innervation to the lateral aspect of the thigh.

Equipment

1 25-gauge needle for skin wheal

1 22-gauge 3-in. needle

Drug

A dose of 7 ml of 1.5 percent lidocaine with epinephrine 1:200,000 is used.

Position

The patient is placed in the supine position.

Procedure

Raise a skin wheal 2.5 cm medial and 2.5 cm inferior to the anterior superior iliac spine (Fig. 6-17).

Introduce a 22-gauge 3-in needle superiorly and laterally through the skin wheal and toward the iliac crest until the needle approaches the inner side of the iliac crest.

Perform a fanwise injection of 5 to 7 ml of local anesthesia in this area.

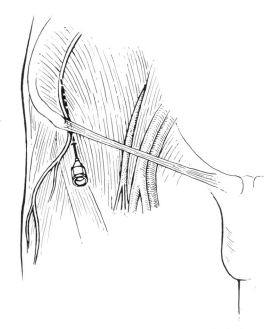

Fig. 6-17. Lateral femoral cutaneous nerve block. Needle is inserted 1 in. medial and 1 in. inferior to anterior superior iliac spine. Anesthetic solution is infiltrated in a fanwise direction.

Anesthesia of the lateral aspect of the thigh down to the knee area results from this block.

Obturator Nerve Block

Indications

1. Diagnosis of painful conditions of the hip
2. Relief of adductor spasm of the hip
3. Supplement to sciatic-femoral and lateral femoral cutaneous nerve blocks for surgery on or above the knee

Anatomy

The obturator nerve (L2–L4) passes through the obturator foramen along the obturator groove with the obturator vessels. The obturator nerve supplies the hip and knee joints, the adductor muscles, and cutaneous branches to the lower inner thigh. Its innervation to the knee joint may be significant in patients undergoing knee surgery.[4,10a]

Equipment

Peripheral nerve stimulator

ECG pad for ground electrode

22-gauge 3.5-in. insulated needle

1 10-ml syringe

Extension set

1 2-ml syringe

1 25-gauge needle

1 18-gauge needle

Drug

A dose of 7 ml of 1.5 percent lidocaine with epinephrine 1:200,000 is used.

Position

The patient is placed on the operating room table in the supine position with the leg to be blocked in slight abduction.

Landmarks

The pubic tubercle is the landmark for an obturator nerve block.

Procedure

Prepare and drape area in the usual manner and isolate the genitalia so they do not come in contact with antiseptic solution (Fig. 6-18).

Palpate the pubic tubercle.

Raise a skin wheal 1 to 2 cm below and 1 to 2 cm lateral to the pubic tubercle.

Introduce a 3.5-in. insulated needle through the skin wheal.

Attach the negative electrode to the needle and the positive electrode to the ground pad.

Direct the needle in a medial direction to strike the ramus of the pubis.

Withdraw and redirect the needle at a 45-degree angle in the cephalad direction to define the superior portion of the obturator canal.

Then withdraw and direct the needle laterally and inferiorly to pass into the obturator canal.

With the nerve stimulator set at 2 mA observe for muscular movement on the medial aspect of the thigh.

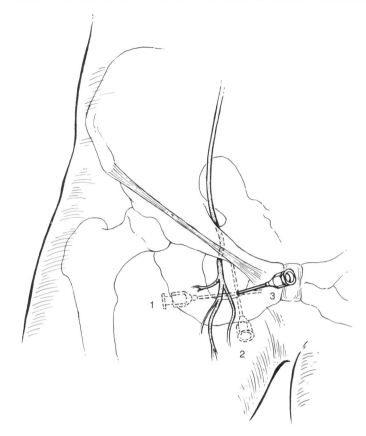

Fig. 6-18. Obturator nerve block. Needle is inserted 1 to 2 cm below and 1 to 2 cm lateral to the pubic tubercle. 1, medial direction—identity ramus of pubis; 2, 45 degrees cephalad—superior portion of canal; 3, lateral and inferior—into canal.

When the muscular movement is greatest at a stimulating current of 0.1 to 0.2 mA, inject the local anesthetic after aspiration.[4,10a]

Caution: Aspirate carefully before injection to be certain that the obturator vessels have not been entered.

Inguinal Paravascular Block

This involves an approach to the psoas compartment to block the three nerves of the lumbar plexus, the femoral nerve, the lateral femoral cutaneous nerve, and the obturator nerve.[17a]

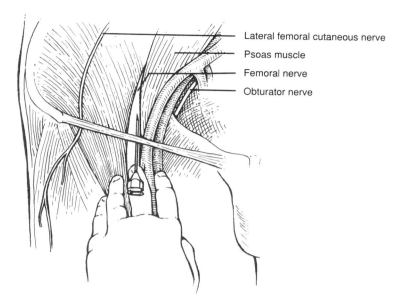

Fig. 6-19. Inguinal paravascular block. Needle is inserted as in femoral nerve block. Digital pressure is applied distal to needle insertion while performing injection.

Landmarks

Anterior superior iliac spine, pubic tubercle

Femoral artery

Procedure

Place the patient in the supine position (Fig. 6-19).

Prepare and drape the inguinal area in the usual manner.

Apply a ground pad.

Raise a skin wheal medial to the femoral artery 1 in. inferior to the inguinal ligament.

Through this wheal, insert an 18-gauge needle.

Then pass an insulated needle through the wheal.

Attach the stimulating electrode negative lead to the needle and the ground electrode to the ECG pad.

Turn the nerve stimulator to 2 mA.

Apply pressure to the femoral sheath below the level of the site of needle insertion to help force the local anesthetic agent cephalad to the lumbar plexus. It is important to apply pressure before the maximal twitch is obtained in order not to alter position of the needle.

Insert the needle perpendicular to the skin and observe for twitches in the muscles supplied by the femoral nerve.

When the maximum twitches are achieved at 0.2 mA, direct the needle cephalad. Assure that maximal twitches persist.

Inject 2 ml of local anesthetic to abolish the twitches.

After aspiration, inject 35 to 40 ml of local anesthetic solution while maintaining pressure below the site of injection. This should anesthetize the three nerves.

Note: If the obturator and lateral femoral cutaneous nerves are not blocked a separate block of these nerves may be necessary.

Sciatic Nerve Block

Anatomy

The sciatic nerve (L4 and L5, S1–S3) exits into the thigh between the greater trochanter and the ischial tuberosity. It supplies motor innervation to the hamstring muscles and all muscles below the knee.

The sciatic nerve supplies sensory innervation to the posterior thigh and entire leg and foot from just below the knee, except for medial aspect, which is supplied by saphenous nerve.

Equipment

Peripheral nerve stimulator

ECG pad for ground electrode

22-gauge 3.5-in. insulated needle

1 20-ml syringe

Extension set

Three-way stopcock

1 2-ml syringe

1 25-gauge needle

1 18-gauge needle

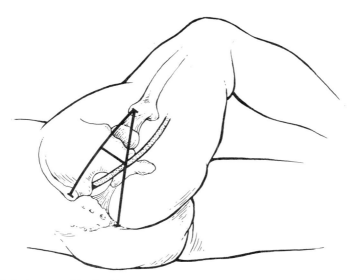

Fig. 6-20. Sciatic nerve block (Sims position). Lines are drawn between posterior superior iliac spine and tip of coccyx to greater trochanter. Perpendicular line connecting midpoint of first line overlies sciatic nerve at intersection of second line.

Posterior Approach of Labat

Drug

A dose of 20 ml of 1.5 percent lidocaine with epinephrine 1:200,000 is used.

Position

The patient is placed on the operating table in the Sims position (Fig. 6-20) on the side opposite the one to be blocked. the hip and knee are flexed with the knee on the side to be blocked touching the operating table.[18]

Landmarks

The posterior superior iliac spine, the greater trochanter and the tip of the coccyx are the landmarks.

Procedure

Prepare and drape the area in the usual manner.

Apply the ground pad.

Identify the posterior superior iliac spine and the greater trochanter.

Draw a line between these two structures.

Draw another line between the tip of the coccyx and the greater trochanter.

Draw a perpendicular line from the line between the posterior superior iliac spine and greater trochanter and project it onto the line between the greater trochanter and the tip of the coccyx.

At this point, raise a skin wheal.

Make a hole in the wheal with an 18-gauge needle.

Through this wheal pass a 3.5-in. insulated needle through the skin.

Turn the nerve stimulator to 3 mA and advance the needle. As the needle passes through the gluteal muscles, there will be direct muscle stimulation. Continue to advance the needle since this is not stimulation of the sciatic nerve.

Look for twitches in the area of muscles supplied by the sciatic nerve (muscles of knee, calf, or ankle).

When you have achieved the maximum twitch at the lowest current (0.2–0.4 mA) inject 2 ml of local anesthetic after aspiration, which should abolish the twitches.

Inject the remainder of the anesthetic after aspiration.

Supine Approach of Raj

Position

The patient is placed on the operating table in the supine position (Fig. 6-21), the hip is flexed to 90 degrees, and the knee is flexed to 90 degrees. The leg can be placed on a padded stand to maintain this position.[18a]

Procedure

Prepare and drape the area between the greater trochanter and ischial tuberosity.

Apply the ground pad.

Raise a skin wheal on a line between these two landmarks somewhat closer to the ischial tuberosity then midway between the two landmarks.

Make a hole in the wheal with an 18-gauge needle.

Pass the sheathed needle through this wheal and direct the needle perpendicular to the skin.

Turn the twitch monitor to 3 mA. Superficial muscular twitches may be noted at first, but these are to be disregarded.

Then pass the needle farther toward the sciatic nerve, observing for twitching in the muscles of the knee, calf, or ankle.

Note dorsal and plantar flexion or eversion and inversion of the ankle.

When you have obtained the lowest current for the maximal twitch, inject 2

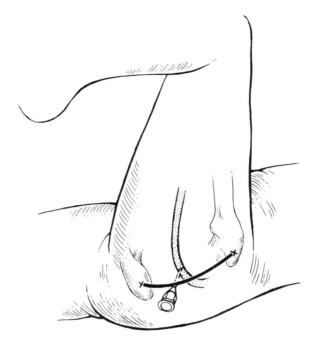

Fig. 6-21. Supine approach sciatic nerve block. Needle is inserted between ischial tuberosity and greater trochanter and advanced. Needle is kept parallel to table.

ml of local anesthetic solution after careful aspiration. This should abolish the twitches.

Inject the remainder of the local anesthetic after aspiration.

Anterior Approach of Beck

This block is used when

The lower extremity cannot be moved

The patient has a cast or cannot be turned

Position
The patient is placed on the operating table in a supine position.[19]

Landmarks
The landmark is the inguinal ligament from the anterior superior iliac spine to the pubic tubercle. A parallel line to this line is drawn at the level of the greater trochanter.

Procedure

Prepare and drape the area in the usual manner.

Place a ground pad.

Draw a line from the medial one-third of the line that represents the inguinal ligament perpendicular to the line drawn at the level of the greater trochanter (Fig. 6-22).

At the point where these two lines intersect, raise a skin wheal.

Make a hole in the skin wheal with an 18-gauge needle.

Through this wheal, pass a 5-in. sheathed needle until it contacts the femur at the level of the lesser trochanter.

Then redirect the needle off the femur in a more medial direction.

Attach the nerve stimulator to the sheathed needle.

Turn current to 2 to 3 mA.

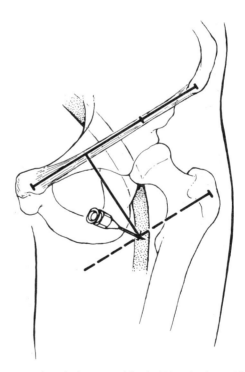

Fig. 6-22. Anterior approach sciatic nerve block. Line is drawn from anterior superior iliac spine to pubic tubercle. Second line is drawn parallel to this line from greater trochanter. A perpendicular line is dropped from inner one-third of first line to second line. At the point of intersection, needle is inserted in a perpendicular fashion.

Advance the needle while stimulating until the maximal twitch response is obtained at the lowest current.

When you obtain the maximum twitches at the lowest current (0.2 to 0.4 mA), inject 2 ml of local anesthetic after aspiration, and the twitches should disappear.

Inject the remaining 18 ml of local anesthetic solution after aspiration.

Lateral Approach of Ichiyanagi

Position

The patient is placed on the operating table in the supine position.[19a]

Place a small pillow behind the knees.

Landmark

The posterior border of the greater trochanter is the landmark.

Procedure

Raise a skin wheal 1 in. posterior to the greater trochanter (Fig. 6-23).

Through this wheal, insert an 18-gauge needle to enlarge the hole.

Through this hole, pass the sheathed 5-in. stimulating needle perpendicular to the skin and attach it to a nerve stimulator.

Turn the current to 2 to 3 mA.

Direct the needle medially and slightly anteriorly.

Seek maximal twitches at 0.2 mA.

Inject 2 ml of local anesthetic after careful aspiration, the twitches should be abolished.

After careful aspiration, inject 18 ml of local anesthetic.

Lumbar Plexus Block

Anatomy

The lumbar plexus is formed from the roots of L2–L4. These roots form the lateral femoral cutaneous nerve, the femoral nerve, and the obturator nerve (Fig. 6-24).

The roots of the lumbar plexus lie between the psoas and the quadratus lumborum muscles. This block can be performed at the level of the roots.

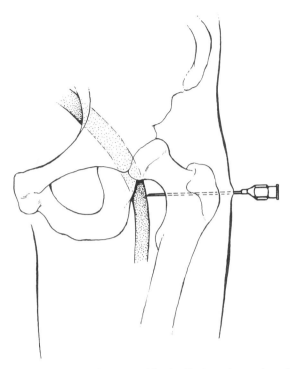

Fig. 6-23. Lateral approach sciatic nerve block. Patient is supine. Needle is passed medially from a point 1 in. posterior to greater trochanter.

Equipment

Peripheral nerve stimulator
ECG pad for ground electrode
1 22-gauge 5-in. insulated needle
2 20-ml syringes
Extension set
Three-way stopcock
1 2-ml syringe
1 25-gauge needle
1 18-gauge needle

Drug

A dose of 40 ml of 1.5 percent lidocaine with epinephrine 1:200,000 is used.

Position

The patient is placed in the lateral position with a folded sheet under the ribs to straighten out the vertebral column.

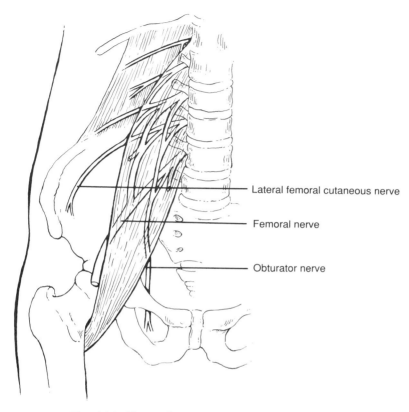

Lateral femoral cutaneous nerve

Femoral nerve

Obturator nerve

Fig. 6-24. Illustration showing anatomy of lumbar plexus.

Landmarks

Marks are placed on the spinous processes of the lumbar vertebra. The spinous process of each lumbar vertebra coincides with the level of the transverse process of that vertebra.

Procedure

Place a mark 5 cm lateral to the spinous process of the third lumbar vertebra (Fig. 6-25).

Place a ground pad.

Prepare and drape the area.

Raise a skin wheal at the site of the marker.

Insert an 18-gauge needle through the skin wheal.

Through this wheal, advance a 5-in. insulated needle perpendicular to the skin until the transverse process is encountered.

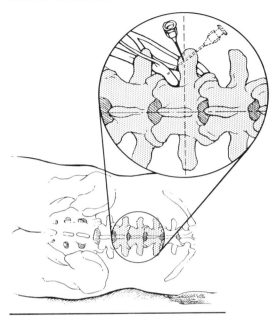

Fig. 6-25. Lumbar plexus block. Patient is placed in lateral position. Needle is inserted until transverse process is encountered and redirected deeper while observing for twitches.

Then slide the needle inferiorly off the transverse process and direct it deeper.

Attach a nerve stimulator to the hub of the needle.

Set the stimulator at 2 mA.

Advance the needle while stimulating.

Remember that when twitches on the anterior aspect of the thigh are noted, the needle is in the correct plane.

Note that the nerve roots should lie at a depth between 7 and 10 cm.

Inject 2 ml of local anesthetic after aspiration. The twitches should cease.

After aspiration, inject the remainder of the local anesthetic.

Psoas Compartment Block of Chayen

In the psoas compartment block of Chayen,[20] the patient is placed on the side with the operative limb uppermost and the thighs flexed on the trunk. The fourth lumbar spine is identified by a line passing through the iliac crest. A point 3 cm caudad and 5 cm laterally is marked. A wheal is raised on the skin in this area. A 15-cm 20-gauge needle is inserted through the wheal perpendicular to the skin until it encounters the fifth lumbar transverse process. The course of the needle is then changed to a slightly cephalad direction until it glides above the transverse process. A 20-ml syringe containing air is attached to the needle, which is advanced 1 to 2 cm to enter the quadratus lumborum muscle. The needle is advanced 1 cm at a time while light tapping on the plunger of a syringe attached to the needle is carried out until loss of resistance is obtained. Chayen noted this to be at a depth of about 12 cm. If the needle is further advanced, it enters the psoas muscle, and resistance is once again felt on tapping the plunger. Air is injected to expand the compartment, and 30 ml of the anesthetic solution is added.

A nerve stimulator can be used for this approach.

Lumbar Plexus Block of Winnie Using Nerve Stimulator

In the lumbar plexus block of Winnie, the site of puncture is marked at the intersection of the intercristal line (the line between the iliac crests) and a perpendicular line dropped from the posterior superior iliac spine. The needle is passed through the skin, and the nerve stimulator is attached until twitches are noted. If the iliac bone or the vertebral body of the fifth lumbar vertebra is contacted a few millimeters beyond the skin, the needle is withdrawn and reinserted either more medially or laterally.[20a]

Tibial Nerve Block at the Knee

Anatomy

The tibial nerve passes vertically through the middle of the popliteal fossa which is formed by the semi-membranosus muscle medially, the biceps femoris muscle laterally, and the two heads of the gastrocnemius muscle inferiorly. The popliteal artery is medial to the nerve in the popliteal fossa.[4]

Equipment

Peripheral nerve stimulator

ECG pad for ground electrode

22-gauge 3.5-in. insulated needle

1 10-ml syringe

Extension set

1 2-ml syringe

1 25-gauge needle

1 18-gauge needle

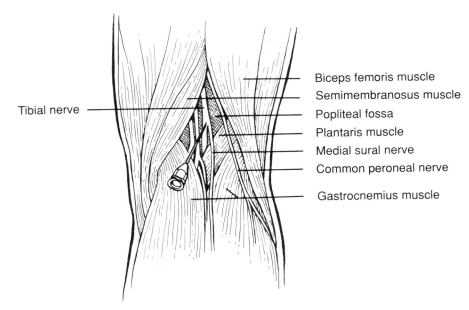

Tibial nerve

Biceps femoris muscle
Semimembranosus muscle
Popliteal fossa
Plantaris muscle
Medial sural nerve
Common peroneal nerve

Gastrocnemius muscle

Fig. 6-26. Tibial nerve block at knee. Needle is placed between semimembranosus and biceps femoris muscle and gastrocnemius muscle.

Position

The patient is placed in the prone position with the knee extended. The pulsations of the popliteal artery are felt at the bend of the knee.

Procedure

Identify the crease of the knee (Fig. 6-26).

Raise a skin wheal in the midpoint of the fossa at the crease lateral to the pulsations of the popliteal artery.

Make a hole in the wheal with an 18-gauge needle.

Through this wheal, pass the needle.

Attach the nerve stimulator.

Direct the needle perpendicular to the skin until motor twitches are seen in the ankle or calf.

Inject 5 to 8 ml of local anesthetic.

Common Peroneal Nerve Block at the Knee

Anatomy

The common peroneal nerve is a branch of the sciatic nerve. It divides into the superficial and deep peroneal nerves. The superficial peroneal nerve crosses the neck of the fibula.

Equipment

Peripheral nerve stimulator

ECG pad for ground electrode

22-gauge 1.5-in. insulated needle

1 10-ml syringe

Extension set

1 2-ml syringe

1 25-gauge needle

1 18-gauge needle

Drug

A dose of 6 ml of 1.5 percent lidocaine with epinephrine 1:200,000 is used.

Position

The patient is placed in the supine position.

Procedure

Raise a skin wheal at the neck of the fibula (Fig. 6-27).

Make a hole through this wheal with an 18-gauge needle.

Through this wheal, pass the nerve stimulating needle.

Remember that twitching of the leg muscles causes movement of the ankle.

When the maximal twitch is attained at the lowest current, (0.1 to 0.2 mA), inject 5 to 6 ml of local anesthetic.

For this block, avoid a side-port needle because the nerve is so superficial that the needle tip may be stimulating the nerve when the side port is just subcutaneous.

Saphenous Nerve Block at the Knee

Anatomy

The saphenous nerve is a continuation of the femoral nerve. It lies between the tendons of the sartorius muscle and the gracilis muscle along the medial femoral condyle.[4]

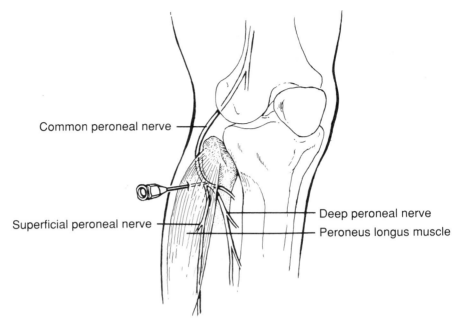

Fig. 6-27. Common peroneal nerve block at knee. A skin wheal is raised at neck of fibula. Needle is passed while observing for twitches.

Equipment

Equipment is one 5-ml syringe and one 27 gauge 1.5-in. needle.

Drug

A dose of 5 ml of 1.5 percent lidocaine with epinephrine 1:200,000 is used.

Procedure

Place a needle on the medial condyle of the femur between the tendons of the sartorius muscle and the gracilis muscle. Local infiltration in this area will block the saphenous nerve (Fig. 6-28).

Ankle Block

Indications for ankle block include

Bunionectomies

Forefoot reconstruction

Hammertoe correction

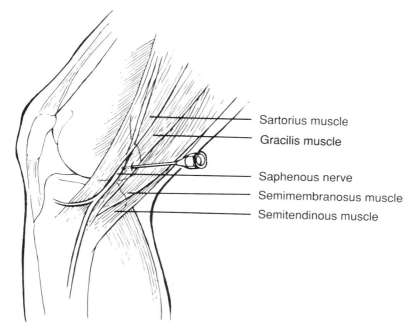

Fig. 6-28. Saphenous nerve block at knee. Needle is inserted on medial condyle between tendons of the sartorius and gracilis muscles. This is a sensory nerve only.

Fractures of the metatarsals

Surgery on the sole of the foot

If a tourniquet is needed for short procedures, an Esmarch's bandage can be tightly placed above the level of the malleoli.

A ringblock of anesthesia can be placed by infiltrating the skin in the area of the tourniquet before its application.

Anatomy

Five nerves innervate the foot below the ankle (Fig. 6-29).[4,21] Also see Figure 6-15 for cutaneous innervation.

Deep Peroneal Nerve

The deep peroneal nerve lies adjacent to the anterior tibial artery on the anterior surface of the distal tibia at the level of the malleoli. It is located lateral to the tendon of the extensor hallucis longus. Its cutaneous innervation is to the web

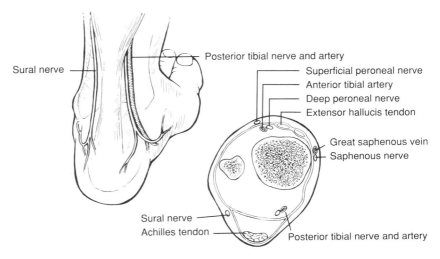

Fig. 6-29. Ankle block anatomy. Posterior tibial nerve is blocked between medial malleolus and Achilles tendon. Sural nerve is blocked lateral to Achilles tendon.

space between the great and second toe. The other four nerves course in the superficial fascia of the foot.

Sural Nerve

The sural nerve passes behind the lateral malleolus between the Achilles tendon and the lateral malleous to innervate the lateral side of the foot.

Saphenous Nerve

The saphenous nerve is a distal sensory branch of the femoral nerve. It supplies the medial aspect of the dorsum of the ankle and some of the medial aspect of the foot. It is adjacent to the saphenous vein.

Superficial Peroneal Nerve

The superficial peroneal nerve supplies innervation to the dorsum of the foot between the areas supplied by the sural nerve and deep peroneal nerve.

Posterior Tibial Nerve

The posterior tibial nerve is situated between the medial malleolus and the Achilles tendon. It is adjacent and posterior to the posterior tibial artery and descends into the foot to innervate muscles and skin on the sole of the foot.

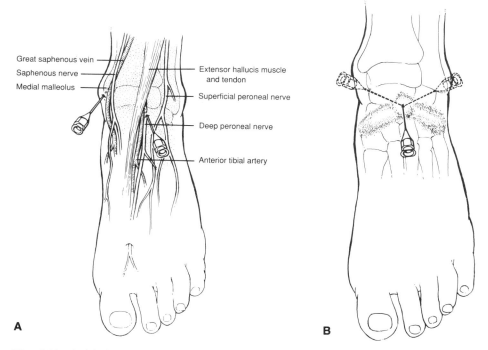

Great saphenous vein
Saphenous nerve
Medial malleolus

Extensor hallucis muscle
and tendon
Superficial peroneal nerve

Deep peroneal nerve

Anterior tibial artery

A   B

Fig. 6-30. Ankle block. **(A)** Block of deep peroneal and saphenous nerves. **(B)** Block of superficial nerves. These nerves are very superficial and are blocked by infiltrating skin.

Landmarks

The major landmarks for the ankle block are the medial and lateral malleoli (Figs. 6-30 and 6-31).

Procedure

Do not use epinephrine in any of the blocks.

Raise a skin wheal at the level of the malleoli on the anterior aspect of the ankle lateral to the tendon of the extensor hallicus longus and the pulsations of the anterior tibial artery.

Identify the extensor hallicus longus by having the patient dorsiflex the great toe.

Deep Peroneal Nerve Block

Insert a 27-gauge needle through this wheal and direct it in a perpendicular fashion until it hits the bone.

Inject 5 ml of local anesthetic after aspiration (Fig. 6-30).

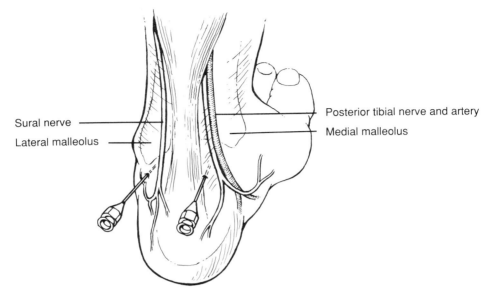

Sural nerve

Lateral malleolus

Posterior tibial nerve and artery

Medial malleolus

Fig. 6-31. Sural nerve and posterior tibial nerve block.

Sural Nerve Block

Raise a skin wheal between the lateral malleolus and the Achilles tendon.

Through this wheal, pass a needle and inject 5 ml of local anesthetic solution (Fig. 6-31).

Saphenous Nerve Block

Raise a skin wheal anterior to the medial malleolus in the area of the saphenous vein.

Through this wheal, pass a needle subcutaneously and inject 5 ml of local anesthetic solution (Fig. 6-30)[4,21].

Superficial Peroneal Nerve Block

Lay a wall of anesthesia in the subcutaneous tissue in a medial and lateral direction from the site of the injection of the deep peroneal nerve.

Note: All the superficial nerves can be blocked by extending the anesthesia from the area of the deep peroneal nerve by placing a wall of anesthesia in a medial and lateral direction (see Fig. 6-30B).

Posterior Tibial Nerve Block

Raise a skin wheal midway between the medial malleolus and the Achilles tendon (Fig. 6-31).

Through this wheal, pass a needle toward the pulsations of the posterior tibial artery.

Detect twitching of the sole of the foot when a nerve stimulator is used. Do not use a side-port stimulating needle because the nerve is very superficial. Inject 5 to 6 ml of local anesthetic solution after careful aspiration.

INTRAVENOUS REGIONAL ANESTHESIA

Intravenous regional anesthesia is a technique in which an intravenous injection of local anesthetic is administered into an extremity that has been exsanguinated and has had the arterial blood supply occluded by a tourniquet.

This technique is easy to perform and provides a rapid onset of analgesia and muscular relaxation.

The duration of anesthesia depends on the length of time that the tourniquet is inflated.

After the tourniquet is released, normal sensation and motor power return rapidly.

Contraindications

Contraindications to intravenous regional anesthesia include

Infection

Allergy to local anesthetic

Conditions precluding use of tourniquet
    Scleroderma
    Sickle cell disease (possible)
    Raynaud's disease
    Malignancy
    Increased intracranial pressure
    Thrombophlebitis or deep vein thrombosis
    Vascular insufficiency

Equipment

Pneumatic tourniquet control apparatus (calibrated against a standard before each use).

Double pneumatic tourniquet (tourniquet with a proximal and distal chamber that can be inflated separately)

Esmarch's bandage

1 50-ml syringe

1 20-gauge cannula with an appropriately sized stylet

Local anesthetic solution (lidocaine—3 mg/kg of 0.5 percent solution [up to 40 ml])

> Use 0.5 percent lidocaine from a factory-sealed fresh bottle to avoid the necessity for dilution of other concentrations to 0.5 percent
>
> **Note:** Check carefully. *The local anesthetic solution should not contain vasoconstrictors such as epinephrine or preservatives.*

Solution Temperature

The effects of injected solution temperature on intravenous regional anesthesia were studied. Injections of 40 ml of 0.5 percent prilocaine were performed at a solution temperature of 0°C, 22°C, or 37°C. There were no differences between the three different methods in the rate of development or in the quality of the block. There was a significant difference in the comfort of injection. Cold solutions caused more discomfort than warm solutions.[21a]

Alkalinization of Solutions

The role of alkalinization was studied to determine whether there was any difference in the blocks. It was found that the group that received the alkalinized solution had significantly less pain on injection, during surgery, and 5 minutes after the tourniquet was deflated than the other group. There was no difference in the time between injection and commencement of surgery in either group.[22]

Comment:

We do not notice any pain on injection when non-alkalinized solutions are used.

Exsanguination Technique

The effect of the technique of exsanguination of the arm for intravenous regional anesthesia was evaluated in two groups of patients; one group had the arm exsanguinated using an Esmarch's bandage as compared with the other group who had the arm exsanguinated using elevation of the arm for 2 minutes plus arterial occlusion by compression of the brachial artery. It was found that the injection pressure was significantly higher in the elevation group than in the exsanguinated group. The quality of anesthesia did not differ in the two groups. There was a higher cubital vein pressure when elevation plus compression was used for exsanguination as compared with the exsanguination by means of an Esmarch's bandage. However, the individual peak pressure (98 mmHg) was below the tourniquet occlusion pressure of 300 mmHg. The main difference between the two techniques is the excess of blood that remains in the arm when elevation is used.[22a]

Comment:

We exsanguinate by use of Esmarch's bandage after elevation of the extremity.

Upper Extremity

Drug

Lidocaine (3 mg/kg of 0.5 percent solution) is used.

Procedure

Check the tourniquet and tourniquet control box, the switch, and all connections to determine that they are secure and will not pop off when the tourniquet is inflated (Fig. 6-32).

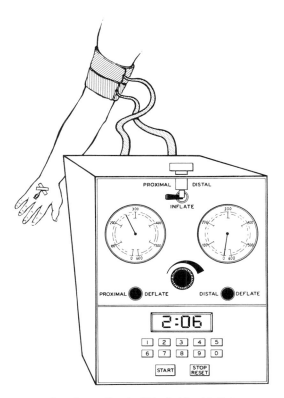

Fig. 6-32. Intravenous regional anesthesia (Bier's block). Intravenous cannula is placed on dorsum of hand. Extremity is exsanguinated; proximal tourniquet is inflated. Anesthetic agent is injected *slowly*. Cannula is removed. Twenty minutes later, distal tourniquet is inflated, and then proximal one is deflated.

Place the patient on the operating table.

Start an intravenous line in the hand opposite the hand to be blocked.

Apply a blood pressure cuff.

Determine the systolic blood pressure.

Apply ECG electrodes and pulse oximeter.

Wrap Webril padding around the arm to be blocked, as high in the axilla as possible. Avoid any creases.

Check both compartments of the double tourniquet before application to see that they inflate properly and maintain the pressure without leaks.

Apply the double tourniquet as snugly as possible with the tubing from the tourniquet positioned so that it does not end up in the axilla of the patient.

Select a suitable vein on the dorsum of the hand. The closer to the hand the better the analgesia for hand surgery.

Insert a 20-gauge cannula into the vein.

Insert a 20-gauge stylet into the cannula.

Tape cannula securely.

Elevate the extremity as high as possible to promote gravity drainage.

Exsanguinate the blood from the arm using an Esmarch's bandage. Start the bandaging at the tips of the fingers. Take care not to dislodge the cannula. Wrap the bandage as tightly as possible, overlapping the previous turn. Apply the wrapping until the distal end of the tourniquet is covered.

Inflate the proximal tourniquet. Palpate to make sure that the pressure in the tourniquet holds.

Set the pressure to 50 mmHg above the patient's systolic blood pressure. Some clinicians set the pressure slightly higher.

Remove the Esmarch's bandage.

Palpate for a radial pulse, which should no longer be present.

Grasp the hub of the needle with the thumb and forefinger of the left hand.

Remove the stylet from the cannula. Do not dislodge the cannula.

Attach the 50-ml syringe to the cannula. Use extension tubing.

Apply a rubber tourniquet around the forearm. This tourniquet ensures that the local anesthetic is concentrated in the area of the hand where the surgery is to be performed.

Inject the local anesthetic over a period of 3 minutes. *Rapid injection can lead to pressures high enough to cause passage of drug under the tourniquet into the general circulation.*

After the injection of a portion of the drug, release the tourniquet around the forearm. While the local anesthetic is being injected, feel the proximally inflated tourniquet to make certain that it does not suddenly deflate.

Remove the needle from the dorsum of the hand at the completion of the injection.

Place a gauze sponge over the needle puncture site and elevate the arm to prevent leakage of fluid from the injection site while the anesthesia is developing.

Start an elapsed time clock. Do not deflate tourniquet until 20 minutes have elapsed.

After a period of 2 to 3 minutes, place the arm on the operating table.

Then allow the preparing and draping of the extremity to progress. By the time the preparing and draping is completed, surgical anesthesia and muscle relaxation of the arm is present.

Remember that the reason for the double tourniquet is to allow local anesthetic to enter the arm underneath the uninflated distal tourniquet. After 20 minutes—no more, no less—inflate the distal tourniquet and palpate to ensure inflation and deflate the proximal tourniquet in that order. This will provide an area of anesthesia under the tourniquet to prevent tourniquet pain.

Keep the tourniquet inflated for at least 20 minutes, although the operation may have ended sooner. This is to avoid the release of local anesthetic into the circulation.

Remember that deflation should occur by a series of deflations and inflations. The deflation should last 30 seconds. Then reinflate the tourniquet, keep it reinflated for 30 seconds, and repeat the cycle several times so the local anesthetic can be washed into the circulation slowly.

Note that after tourniquet release, sensory and motor function should return very rapidly.

Intravenous Regional Anesthesia in Patients with Large Arms

One may encounter difficulty performing successful intravenous regional techniques on obese patients or patients with large arms. We have found in these patients that the combined tourniquet does not perform well because it does not properly wrap around the arm or occlude the arterial supply when inflated. Use of two individual tourniquets has been more successful.

Forearm Tourniquets

Intravenous regional anesthesia with a tourniquet placed on the forearm has been recommended for surgery of the hand, wrist, and distal forearm. The use of the tourniquet on the forearm rather than on the arm was investigated to determine whether it would be possible to decrease the volume of local anesthetic used and possibly decrease the toxicity of this technique.

A double tourniquet was placed on the forearm a few centimeters below the elbow. Exsanguination was performed by means of an Esmarch's bandage after a suitable vein was cannulated on the dorsum of the wrist. The dose of 0.5 percent lidocaine was 2 mg/kg. The total amount was 25 ml (125 mg) in one group.[23,24]

In the study by Chan, despite slow intravenous injection of the lidocaine over 2 minutes in an attempt to minimize abrupt elevation of the venous pressure, leakage past a properly functioning tourniquet still occurred in 6 of the 11 patients. This was stated to be similar to the leakage rate of 67.5 percent reported by Kalso et al.[25]

In seven hypertensive patients, in the study by Chan, with blood pressures greater than 190/100 mmHg, three showed venous congestion of the forearm below the tourniquet.

Advice: Do not use forearm tourniquets. Proper occlusion cannot be achieved because blood vessels run on the interosseous membrane between the radius and ulna.

Continuous Intravenous Regional Anesthesia

Procedure

Insert a catheter in the proximal forearm for administration of the drug.

During the operation, let down the tourniquet and allow the blood supply to the extremity to be re-established.

After this, an Esmarch's bandage is applied by the surgeon.

Reinflate the tourniquet.

Administer one-half of the previous dose of drug through the cannula. The operation then proceeds until it is time for the tourniquet to be released again.[26]

Lower Extremity

Equipment

A pneumatic tourniquet control apparatus (calibrated against a standard before each use)

Double tourniquet large enough for the lower extremity (tourniquet with one proximal and one distal chamber that can be inflated separately)

Esmarch's bandage

2 50-ml syringes

1 20-gauge cannula with an appropriately sized stylet

Local anesthetic solution (lidocaine—0.375 percent solution [up to 100 ml]—25 ml saline without preservative added to 75 ml 0.5 percent solution of lidocaine)

Note: Check carefully. *The local anesthetic agent should not contain vaso-constrictors such as epinephrine or preservatives.*

Double tourniquets for the lower extremity are available. Two separate thigh tourniquets can be used as well.

Drug

A dose of 100 ml of 0.375 percent lidocaine is used.

Do not use epinephrine or preservatives.

Procedure

Apply the tourniquets to the thigh as high as possible after placing adequate Webril padding and making certain that the padding does not have creases.

Find a suitable vein in the dorsum of the foot (this may be the most difficult part of the anesthesia). Nitroglycerin ointment may be helpful to dilate the veins.

Insert a 20-gauge cannula into the vein and place a 20-gauge stylet.

Elevate the limb.

Exsanguinate the limb by wrapping an Esmarch's bandage in a tight fashion, starting from the toes up to the distal end of the tourniquet.

Inflate the proximal tourniquet to at least 50 mmHg above the patient's systolic pressure. Some clinicians use slightly higher pressures. The pulse should be absent in the foot.

Remove the Esmarch's bandage. Do not dislodge the cannula. Remove the stylet from the cannula.

Use an extension tube, three-way stopcock, double syringe technique in order to not dislodge the cannula in the vein by frequent syringe changes.

Inject the anesthetic slowly to avoid passage of local anesthesia under the tourniquet.

Check the pressure in the proximal tourniquet during the injection. Stop the injection if the tourniquet deflates.

After completing the injection, remove the cannula.

Place a sterile gauze pad over the site of the injection and raise the extremity for 3 minutes to avoid any leakage of fluid from the cannula site.

The operation can proceed as soon as preparing and draping have occurred; adequate anesthesia and relaxation will be present at this time.

After 20 minutes, inflate the distal tourniquet and deflate the proximal tourniquet in that order to avoid tourniquet pain.

Note: Do not deflate tourniquet until 20 minutes have elapsed.

At the conclusion of surgery, release and then reinflate the tourniquet. The deflation should last approximately 30 seconds; then reinflate the tourniquet and keep it inflated for approximately 30 seconds. Repeat the cycle several times so that the local anesthetic can be washed into the circulation slowly.

Complications

The most common complication is a toxic reaction to the local anesthetic. This can result from accidental loss of tourniquet pressure before the anesthetic has had time to fix to the tissues. Therefore, the tourniquet should be checked for leaks before application and all connections should be secure.

It is necessary to keep the tourniquet inflated for at least 20 minutes after the injection.

Toxic reactions can occur when the tourniquet is deflated at the end of the procedure. To minimize chances of this occuring the tourniquet should be deflated, reinflated, deflated, and reinflated to allow the drug to enter the circulation slowly.

See chapter 7 for complications associated with the use of a tourniquet.

PEDIATRIC ORTHOPEDIC SURGERY

Peripheral nerve blocks of the extremities as well as spinal and caudal techniques can provide both anesthesia for surgical procedures and postoperative pain relief.

All blocks should be performed with resuscitation equipment and medications available.

An intravenous line should be started before any procedure is performed.

Monitors used include

ECG
Blood pressure
Pulse oximeter
Method to monitor temperature

Nerve Blocks Under General Anesthesia

Many procedures are performed with the aid of "light" general anesthesia in order to decrease the anesthetic requirements for the procedure as well as to provide postoperative analgesia. This is especially important in patients in whom squirming or moving about because of pain in the postoperative period may disrupt skin grafts or tendon repairs.

Nerve Blocks With Sedation

Operations under nerve blocks with sedation may be necessary in situations such as a supracondylar fracture of the forearm with a compromise of the vascular supply, in a patient with a full stomach, in children with severely compromised respiratory function, or in severe cardiovascular disease.

Extremity Blocks

Children are less likely to cooperate while their block is being performed while they are awake than are adults. Children may not be able to report the presence of a paresthesia; therefore the use of a nerve stimulator is essential in pediatric extremity blocks (see p. 172).

Upper Extremity Blocks

Upper extremity blocks can be used for reduction of fractures and anesthesia for repair of lacerations and débridement of open wounds. The anesthetic agents used by Broadman are a combination of

Lidocaine 0.5 percent
Tetracaine 0.12 to 0.2 percent
Epinephrine 1:200,000

These will provide anesthesia and analgesia for 6 to 8 hours.[27]

Brachial Plexus Block

Brachial plexus blocks are performed with the use of a nerve stimulator to locate the nerves (see pp. 172, 180, and 189). A dose of 0.33 ml/kg of local anesthetic solution is used for axillary blocks and 0.25 ml/kg for interscalene blocks.[27]

Lower Extremity Blocks

Sciatic Nerve Block

The sciatic nerve is blocked by having the patient placed in the lateral or Sims position. The greater trochanter and the ischial tuberosity are located by palpation. The sciatic nerve lies midway between these two points.[27]

A 22-gauge 3.5-in. insulated needle connected to a nerve stimulator is inserted midway between these landmarks and advanced until dorsiflexion and plantar flexion of the foot is noticed. Direct gluteal muscle stimulation may occur during insertion of the needle. If nerve stimulation corresponding to the distribution of the sciatic nerve is not noted, the needle should be advanced further. A dose of 1 ml of local anesthetic solution is injected once appropriate twitches are noted. If the twitch is abolished, the needle tip is in the correct position. The remainder of the anesthetic can then be injected with intermittent aspiration for blood. A dose of 0.15–0.2 ml/kg is used.[27]

Sciatic Nerve Block—Anterior Approach

McNicol utilized sciatic nerve block by the anterior approach to provide postoperative pain relief in children undergoing orthopedic procedures on the lower limb in the area innervated by the sciatic nerve. After induction of general anesthesia, the block was performed. (For technique see p. 213.) A dose of 1 mg/kg of 0.5 percent bupivacaine with epinephrine 1:200,000 was used. A nerve stimulator can be used for this approach.[28–33]

Femoral Nerve Block

The femoral nerve lies lateral to the femoral artery. A skin wheal is raised at this point 1–in. below the inguinal ligament, and the needle is passed through this skin wheal, the nerve stimulator is turned on, and twitches of the quadriceps muscle reveal that the needle is in close proximity to the femoral nerve. After aspirating and injecting 1 or 2 ml of local anesthetic, the twitches should be abolished. If this occurs, the remainder of the solution is injected. A dose of 0.5 ml/kg of the "Broadman" local anesthetic solutions is used.[27]

McNicol[28] utilized femoral and lateral femoral cutaneous nerve blocks in 50 patients with a 96 percent success rate for postoperative pain relief. 0.5 percent bupivacaine (0.05–1.0 mg/kg for each block) was utilized with epinephrine 1:200,000 to speed onset of analgesia.

Oral pain medications were instituted early to avoid postoperative pain after the block subsided.

Spinal Anesthesia in Infants

Preparation

While no sedation is used in infants less than 52 weeks' conceptual age, Broadman[27] recommends ketamine (1 to 2 mg/kg IM) and atropine (0.015 to 0.02 mg/kg) in infants older than 52 weeks' conceptual age.

Equipment

A 22-gauge or 25 gauge 1.5-in. disposable spinal needle is used.

Drugs and Dosages

In children weighing less than 10 kg, Yaster[34] uses 1.5–2.0 mg of hyperbaric tetracaine (1 ml of 1 percent tetracaine in 1 ml 10 percent dextrose) and he administers 0.3–0.4 ml in children less than 10 kg and 0.2–0.3 mg/kg in children weighing more than 10 kg.

Cook recommends 0.4 mg/kg of tetracaine or 1 mg per year of age with a minimal dose of 1.5–2.0 mg.[39]

Ecoffey describes the use of 0.5 percent tetracaine with 5 percent dextrose (0.13 ml/kg in infants less than 4 kg and 0.7 ml/kg in infants greater than 4 kg) but utilizes 0.5 percent isobaric bupivacaine (0.75 ml for infants weighing between 2 and 5 kg and 1 ml for infants weighing more than 5 kg).[35,36]

Position

The child is turned into the lateral position, and the neck is extended. Flexion of neck can lead to airway compromise. Broadman[37] prefers to perform the spinal in the sitting position in infants less than 52 weeks' conceptual age to decrease the incidence of a dry tap.

Landmarks

The site of injection is either L4–L5 or L5–S1 to minimize the risk of spinal cord injury. Remember that the spinal cord extends lower in neonates and infants than in adults.

Procedure

Prepare and drape the back in the usual manner.

Pass the needle through the L4–L5 or L5–S1 interspace in the midline. A ''pop'' may be felt with dural puncture but this is not always a constant finding.

Advance the needle slowly and remove the stylet often to observe for cerebrospinal fluid. Cerebrospinal fluid is usually obtained at about a depth of 1 cm.[27,34]

Caudal Anesthesia

Caudal anesthesia is performed with the patient under general anesthesia.[39a]

Drugs

Broadman et al[38] performed more than 1,150 consecutive caudals using bupivacaine and did not detect any toxic side effects with doses of 0.056 ml/kg/spinal segment up to 3 mg/kg.[39]

Yaster[34] uses 1 ml/kg (maximum of dose 30 ml) 0.25 percent bupivacaine with epinephrine 1:200,000 prior to surgery and 1 ml/kg 0.125 percent bupivacaine at the conclusion of surgery for pain relief.

Cook[39] recommends 0.25 percent bupivacaine 1 ml/kg with epinephrine 1:200,000 with a maximum dose of 3 mg/kg.

Ecoffey[35] uses 0.25 percent bupivacaine 0.5 ml/kg for lumbosacral procedures and 1 ml/kg for thoracolumbar procedures. Postoperative pain relief is prolonged with epinephrine 1:200,000.

Position

The child is turned into the lateral position.

Landmarks

The sacral hiatus is palpated. The upper margin of the sacral hiatus is bounded by the sacral cornua.

Procedure

Prepare and drape the skin in the usual manner.

Insert a 23-gauge hypodermic needle at an angle of 60 degrees through the sacrococcygeal membrane. Note a distinct ''pop'' as the needle enters the sacral canal.

Then advance the needle an additional 2.0 mm into the sacral canal. Aspirate before injecting the local anesthetic agent.[27]

INTRAVENOUS REGIONAL ANESTHESIA IN CHILDREN

Intravenous regional anesthesia can be used in children. Equipment must be checked carefully (see pp. 227–234; see ch. 7). Be prepared to treat the toxic side effects associated with an inadvertent premature tourniquet release.

Olney et al[40] performed intravenous regional anesthesia on 400 extremities in 3-16-year-old children who had sustained fractures and dislocations. Utilizing 3 mg/kg lidocaine, they reported a successful reduction rate of 97 percent and adequate analgesia in 90 percent. Determination of serum lidocaine levels after tourniquet deflation revealed variable release into the circulation with peak lidocaine levels in some children occurring after 15 minutes.

In another series Farrell et al[41] successfully used a "mini-dose" Bier block of 0.5 percent lidocaine 1–1.5 mg/kg in 29 children 2-13-years old. If adequate anesthesia was not obtained as determined by gentle manipulation after 15 minutes, then an additional 0.5 mg/kg was injected into an intravenous catheter that was kept in the injured extremity. Farrell et al[41] believe that the mini-dose Bier block technique decreases the chance of toxic side effects that may be seen with a 3 mg/kg dose.

REFERENCES

1. Selander D, Edshage S, Wolff T: Paresthesia or no paresthesia? Nerve lesions after axillary blocks. Acta Anaesthesiol Scand 23:27, 1979
2. Selander D, Dhuner KG, Lundborg G: Peripheral nerve injury due to injection needles used for regional anaesthesia. Acta Anaesthesiol Scand 21:182, 1977
2a. Scott DB, Cousins MJ: Clinical pharmacology of local anesthetic agents. p. 86. In Cousins MJ, Bridenbaugh PO (eds): Neural Blockade in Clinical Anesthesia and Management of Pain. JB Lippincott, Philadelphia, 1980
3. de Jong RH, Heavner JE: Diazepam prevents local anesthetic seizures. Anesthesiology 34:523, 1971
3a. Strichartz GR, Covino BG: Local anesthetics. p. 437. In Miller RD (ed): Anesthesia. 3rd Ed. Churchill Livingstone, New York, 1990
4. Raj, PP, Rai U, Rawal N: Technique of Regional Anesthesia in Adults. In Raj PP (ed): Clinical Practice of Regional Anesthesia. Churchill Livingstone, New York, 1991
4a. Winnie AP: Plexus Anesthesia: Perivascular Techniques of Brachial Plexus Block. Vol 1. WB Saunders, Philadelphia, 1983
5. Moore DC: Regional Block: A Handbook for Use in Clinical Practice of Medicine and Surgery. 4th Ed. CC Thomas, Springfield, 1979

6. Katz RL, Epstein RA: The interaction of anesthetic agents and adrenergic drugs to produce cardiac arrhythmias. Anesthesiology 29:763, 1968

6a. DiFazio CA, Carron HO, Grosslight KR et al: Comparison of pH adjusted lidocaine solutions for epidural anesthesia. Anesth Analg 65:760, 1986

7. Coventry DM, Todd JG: Alkalinisation of bupivacaine for sciatic nerve blockade. Anaesthesia 44:467, 1989

7a. Raj PP, Rosenblatt R, Montgomery SJ: Use of the nerve stimulator for peripheral blocks. Reg Anaesth 5:19, 1980

8. Pither C: Nerve Stimulation. p. 161. In Raj PP (ed): Clinical Practice of Regional Anesthesia. Churchill Livingstone, New York, 1991

8a. Okasha AS, El-Attar AM: Enhanced brachial plexus blockade. Effect of pain and muscular exercises on the efficiency of brachial plexus blockade. Anaesthesia 43: 427, 1988

9. Heath PJ, Brownlie GS, Herrick MJ: Latency of brachial plexus block. The effect on onset time of warming local anesthetic solutions. Anaesthesia 45:297, 1990

10. Winnie AP: Interscalene brachial plexus block. Anesth Analg 49:455, 1970

10a. Berry FR, Bridenbaugh LD: The upper extremity: somatic blockade. p. 297. In Cousins MJ, Bridenbaugh PO (eds): Neural Blockade in Clinical Anesthesia and Management of Pain. JB Lippincott, Philadelphia, 1980

11. Urmey WF, Talts KH, Sharrock NE: One hundred percent incidence of hemidiaphragmatic paresis associated with interscalene brachial plexus anesthesia or diagnosed by ultrasonograph. Anesth Analg 72:498, 1991

12. Raj PP, Montgomery SJ, Nettles D et al: Infraclavicular brachial plexus block. A new approach. Anesth Analg 52:897, 1973

13. Winnie AP, Collins VJ: The subclavian perivascular technique of brachial plexus anesthesia. Anesthesiology 25:353, 1964

13a. Ang ET, Lassale B, Goldfarb G: Continuous axillary brachial plexus block—A clinical and anatomic study. Anesth Analg 63:680, 1984

14. Partridge BL, Katz J, Benirschke K: Functional anatomy of the brachial plexus sheath. Implications for anesthesia. Anesthesiology 66:743, 1987

14a. Berger A, Tizian C, Zenz M: Continuous plexus blockade for improved circulation in microvasculasr surgery. Ann Plast Surg 14:16, 1985

15. Selander D: Catheter technique in axillary plexus block: presentation of a new method. Acta Anaesth Scand 21:324, 1977

15a. Matsuda M, Kato N, Aosoi M: Continuous brachial plexus block for reimplantation in the upper extremity. The Hand 14:129, 1982

16. Rosenblatt R, Rockwell FP, McKillop MJ: Continuous axillary analgesia for traumatic hand injury. Anesthesiology 51:565, 1979

16a. Wadsworth TG, Williams JR: Cubital tunnel external compression syndrome. Br Med J 1:662, 1973

17. Stoelting RK: Postoperative Ulnar Nerve Palsy—Is it a preventable complication? Anesth Analg 76:7, 1993

17a. Winnie AP, Ramamurthy S, Durrani Z: The inguinal paravascular technique of lumbar plexus anesthesia: the "3-in-1 block." Anesth Analg 52:989, 1973

18. Labat G: Regional Anesthesia. Its Technique and Clinical Applications. WB Saunders, Philadelphia, 1928

18a. Raj PP, Parks RI, Watson TD et al: New single position supine approach to sciatic-femoral nerve block. Anesth Analg 54:489, 1975

19. Beck GP: Anterior approach to sciatic nerve block. Anesthesiology 24:222, 1963

19a. Ichiyanagi K: Sciatic nerve block: lateral approach with patient supine. Anesthesiology 20:601, 1959

20. Chayen B, Nathan H, Chayan M: The psoas compartment block. Anesthesiology 45:95, 1976

20a. Winnie AP, Ramamurthy S, Durani Z et al: Plexus blocks for lower extremity surgery. Anesthesiol Rev 1:11, 1974

21. Bridenbaugh PO: The lower extremity: somatic blockade. p. 321. In Cousins MJ, Bridenbaugh PO (eds): Neural Blockade in Clinical Anesthesia and Management of Pain. JB Lippincott, Philadelphia, 1980

21a. Paul DL, Logan MR, Wildsmith JAW: The effects of injected solution temperature on intravenous regional anaesthesia. Anaesthesia 43:362, 1988

22. Armstrong P, Watters J, Whitfield A: Alkalinisation of prilocaine for intravenous regional anaesthesia. Suitability for clinical use. Anaesthesia 45:935, 1990

22a. Haasio J, Hippala S, Rosenberg PH: Intravenous regional anaesthesia of the arm. Effect of the technique of exsanguination on the quality of anaesthesia and prilocaine plasma concentration. Anaesthesia 44:19, 1989

23. Chan CS, Pun WK, Chan YM et al: Intravenous regional analgesia with a forearm tourniquet. Can J Anaesth 34:121, 1987

24. Plourde G, Barry PP, Tardis L et al: Decreasing the toxic potential of intravenous regional anaesthesia. Can J Anaesth 36:498, 1989

25. Kalso E, Tuominen M, Rosenberg PH et al: Bupivacaine blood levels after eight intravenous regional anaesthesia of the arm. Reg Anaesth 5:81, 1982

26. Brown EM, Weissman F: A case report: prolonged intravenous regional anesthesia. Anesth Analg 45:319, 1966

27. Broadman LM: Pediatric regional anesthesia and postoperative analgesia. p. 43. In Barash PG (ed): American Society of Anesthesiologists Refresher Courses in Anesthesiology. Vol. 14. JB Lippincott, Philadelphia, 1986

28. McNicol LR: Lower limb blocks in children. Anaesthesia 41:27, 1986

29. McNicol LR: Sciatic nerve block for children. Anaesthesia 40:410, 1985

30. McNicol LR: Anterior approach to sciatic nerve block in children: loss of resistance or nerve stimulator for identifying the neurovascular compartment. Anesth Analg 66:11, 1987

31. Magora F, Pessachovitch B, Shoham I: Sciatic nerve block by the anterior approach for operations on the lower extremity. Br J Anaesth 46:121, 1974

32. Bashein G, Haschke RH, Ready LB: Electrical nerve location: numerical and electrophoretic comparison of insulated and uninsulated needles. Anesth Analg 63:919, 1984

33. Ford DJ, Pither C, Raj PP: Comparison of insulated and uninsulated needles for locating peripheral nerves with a peripheral nerve stimulator. Anesth Analg 63:925, 1984

34. Yaster M: Pediatric regional anesthesia. p. 235. In Barash PG (ed). ASA Refresher Course. The American Society of Anesthesiologists, Park Ridge, IL, 1992

35. Ecoffey C, McIlvaine WB: Techniques of regional anesthesia in children. Ch. '3. In Raj PP (ed): Clinical Practice of Regional Anesthesia. Churchill Livingstone. New York, 1991

36. Mahe V, Ecoffey C: Spinal anesthesia with isobaric bupivacaine in infants. Anesthesiology 68:601, 1988

37. Broadman L: Regional analgesia in children in 1992. p. 68. International Anesthesia Research Society (ed): Review Course Lectures. IARS. Cleveland, OH, 1992

38. Broadman LM, Hannallah RS, Norden JM et al: "Kiddie caudals" experience with 1154 consecutive cases without complications. Anesth Analg 66:S18, 1987

39. Cook DR: Pediatric anesthesia. Ch. 48. In Barash PG, Cullen BF, Stoelting RK (eds): Clinical Anesthesia. 2nd Ed. JB Lippincott, Philadelphia, 1992

39a. Takasaki M, Dohi S, Kawabata Y et al: Dosage of lidocaine for caudal anesthesia in infants and children. Anesthesiology 47:527, 1977

40. Olney BW, Lugg PC, Turner PL et al: Outpatient treatment of upper extremity injuries in childhood using intravenous regional anesthesia. J Ped Orthop 8:576, 1988

41. Farrell RG, Swanson SL, Walter JR: Safe and effective IV regional anesthesia for use in the emergency department. Ann Emer Med 14:239, 1985

7

Tourniquets

A tourniquet is used to temporarily arrest the circulation to an extremity to provide a bloodless field for proper operating conditions.

EQUIPMENT

1. Pneumatic cuff
2. Method of inflating the cuff
3. Gauge to determine the pressure
4. Padding, which is placed on the extremity underneath the pneumatic portion of the tourniquet
5. Tourniquet pressure test device

Warning:

All connections should be secure. Avoid connections that depend on the bare end of the rubber tubing connecting with a nipple. They slip off and lead to problems.

PROCEDURE

1. Check the accuracy of the pressure gauge by comparing it with a test manometer or a mercury blood pressure manometer.
2. Assemble the tourniquet and pressure source and inflate the tourniquet before applying it to the patient to test all connections for leaks.
3. Make certain all connections are securely joined to each other and that there are no cracks in the rubber tubing that may leak.
4. Wrap several layers of padding around the extremity as high as possible. Avoid any creases, folds, or ridges because they may cause pressure on the skin.
5. Apply the cuff as snugly as possible over the previously applied padding as high in the extremity as possible.
6. Connect the tubing from the cuff to the tourniquet device. Make certain that the connection between the tubing and the cuff is secure.
7. Check all connections of the system to make certain that they are tight and that the rubber is not rotted.
8. If any questions exists, obtain a different tourniquet apparatus.

SIZE

It is suggested that the width of the cuff should be approximately the diameter of the area to which it is applied.

INFLATION PRESSURE AND DURATION OF INFLATION

Damage to the involved extremity can occur because of elevations of inflation pressure or duration of inflation.[1]

Setting Inflation Pressure

Inflation pressure should be set at 50 mmHg above the patient's systolic blood pressure for the arms and 100 mmHg for the thigh.[1] However, slightly higher inflation pressures are often used without deleterious effects.

If major changes occur in the blood pressure during surgery, adjustments should be made in the setting of the tourniquet pressure gauge.

Settings that are too high may cause undue pressure, resulting in ischemia and possible paralysis.

Settings that are too low may lead to venous but not arterial occlusion with arterial blood flow into the extremity without venous drainage. This results in major swelling and obliteration of the surgical site by blood.

Creeping Deflation

A small continuous tourniquet leak may allow for arterial inflow into the limb while obstructing venous outflow. This may result in the development of a postoperative compartment syndrome.[2]

If signs of bleeding occur, the tourniquet should be released and the equipment checked and changed if necessary. A new tourniquet should be applied, and exsanguination and inflation of the pneumatic cuff performed. Pressures are then checked.

Tourniquet Time

Absolute limits of tourniquet ischemia are not firmly established. Safe limits of tourniquet inflation range from 45 minutes to 4 hours.[3,4]

Two-Hour Limit

Based on data concerning pathologic ischemic changes and metabolic acidosis that occurs with tourniquet use, up to 2 hours is considered a safe period for tourniquet inflation.[5] Flatt[6] documented only two complications in 1,500 patients undergoing hand surgery who had ischemia time limited to 2 hours, and those resulted from elevated tourniquet pressure.

At the end of the first hour, we inform the surgeon of the tourniquet time. We then inform them at 1.5 hours of tourniquet time and a few times as the 2-hour point approaches. After 2 hours, we discuss whether the tourniquet is needed any longer, and if so, we deflate it for at least 15 minutes before reinflating.

Wilgis[7] showed that an increase in acidosis occurred in venous blood distal to the tourniquet directly related to the duration of tourniquet occlusion. At 120 minutes of inflation, the pH in the venous blood distal to the tourniquet was 6.90.[7]

The recovery time needed for the pH to be readjusted toward normal between successful deflations and inflations of the tourniquet increases with time. After 30 minutes, it takes 3 to 5 minutes and after 120 minutes, it takes 15 to 20 minutes.

Tissue Damage

1. Nerve—more susceptible to mechanical pressure
2. Muscle—more vulnerable to ischemia

Postoperative Edema

There may be an increase in postoperative edema after hand operations in which the tourniquet is used. This has also been noted after tourniquet use for plating of tibial plateau fractures. The possible etiologies for postoperative edema are reactive hyperemia, postoperative hematoma, or postanoxic edema.[8]

Post-Tourniquet Paralysis

Paralysis after tourniquet use is related to the pressure beneath the tourniquet, which interferes with the blood supply to the nerve beneath the cuff.

Patients with Atherosclerotic Disease

Caution should be employed if a tourniquet is used in the presence of atherosclerotic disease. Reports of damage to vessel walls and ischemic limbs have been noted after tourniquet release.

All patients who have a tourniquet used intraoperatively should have their pulses checked after tourniquet deflation and before leaving the operating room.

If a patient with severe atherosclerotic disease does have a tourniquet used, pulses should be documented preoperatively.

Skin Damage from Preparation Solutions

The accumulation of preparation solution beneath the tourniquet should be avoided. This solution may remain under the tourniquet and cause skin damage, blisters, and burns. A towel should be placed around the tourniquet to make certain that no solution leaks beneath the tourniquet during the preparation.

Tourniquet Puncture

During the draping procedure, puncturing the pneumatic cuff or tubing with towel clips should be avoided.

Pulmonary Embolism

Immobilized patients who present for surgery may have developed deep vein thrombosis. Limb exsanguination and tourniquet inflation may result in pulmonary embolism in these patients.[9-11]

Maximizing Tourniquet Time

As soon as the tourniquet is inflated, surgery should begin. All discussions and conferences about the operation as well as skin markings should be carried out before tourniquet inflation.

As soon as tourniquet inflation occurs, a time clock should be started. The time of inflation is noted on the anesthesia record. Many surgeons wish to be informed of tourniquet time every 30 minutes. The anesthesiologist should comply. We ask the surgeon to compress the tourniquet right after inflation, which will be reflected in the pressure readings as a slight "bounce" of the reading with each compression. This informs the operating team that the connection between the tourniquet and the pressure gauge is complete and that no kinks are present preventing the desired inflation pressure from having its affect on the limb.

After the completion of the procedure the tourniquet should be released, and if everything is satisfactory, it should be removed with the underlying padding. The underlying padding can actually act as a tourniquet itself and cause venous distention and lead to edema. No circumferential items should be around the limb at the end of the procedure except the dressings applied by the surgeon.

TOURNIQUET PAIN

Anesthetic records of patients who have undergone surgery with a tourniquet inflated demonstrate an increase in blood pressure and heart rate after the tourniquet has been inflated for about 1 hour or sometimes sooner.[1]

These hemodynamic changes are frequently noted during orthopedic surgery and are considered a "tourniquet effect" attributed to pain from ischemia or activation of pain fibers from the presence of an inflated tourniquet. Deflation of the tourniquet is followed by resolution of the hemodynamic alterations.[12]

The phenomenon of tourniquet pain was studied on volunteers. The pattern of tourniquet pain was followed by a visual analog scale (VAS) score and blood pressure changes. As time progressed, the VAS score increased, with its highest point just before tourniquet deflation (Fig. 7-1).

Increases in blood pressure were noted just after inflation (5.0 mmHg increase) and before deflation (9.5 mmHg above baseline levels)[13].

Chasing the blood pressure and heart rate in patients receiving general anesthesia with high-dose, long-acting narcotics may not be successful.[1,14] Short-acting intravenous agents or inhalation agents that can be decreased just before tourniquet deflation are better than medications that will have a persistent systemic effect after tourniquet pain is gone.

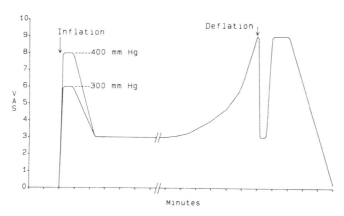

Fig. 7-1. Typical VAS curve. Note difference in VAS scores with inflation to 300 and to 400 mmHg. After a variable time, pain again increases up to moment of deflation. Deflation provides only temporary relief, after which the pain, although different in nature, usually peaks at about the predeflation VAS value. It then recedes within minutes to about zero. (From Hagenouw et al,[13] with permission.)

If the blood pressure rise is of such magnitude that it is believed that the hemodynamic status of the patient may be compromised because of increased afterload, administration of a vasodilator to control the high blood pressure should be considered.

Tourniquet pain in the patient receiving regional anesthesia manifests itself as

1. A direct complaint that the tourniquet hurts
2. Patient acting fidgety and restless
3. Nonspecific complaints of pain in the area of the tourniquet

This is also very difficult to treat and may require intravenous sedation. To help alleviate this pain, we occasionally administer 25 to 50 μg of fentanyl epidurally, with good results during lower extremity surgery.

Others have found 100 μg of epidural fentanyl to be effective for tourniquet pain during orthopedic surgery.[15]

Tuominen et al[16] were able to provide significant tourniquet pain relief by administering 0.3 mg of morphine intrathecally with hyperbaric bupivacaine to patients undergoing lower extremity orthopedic surgery.

Propofol by infusion or low-dose bolus and alfentanil in 250-μg doses also helps alleviate discomfort. The "very" awake complaining patient requiring significant sedation may become very somnolent and even require respiratory assistance after the tourniquet is released and discomfort is relieved.[1]

Etiology of Tourniquet Pain

Chabel et al[17] were concerned about the etiology of severe tourniquet pain despite what appeared to be adequate anesthesia.

Several possible etiologies for pain exists including activity from small-diameter pain fibers (A-δ or C fibers) or pain pathways involving large myelinated fibers.[1,17,18]

A rat model for tourniquet-induced ischemia demonstrated that shortly after tourniquet inflation, firing of fibers in the C-fiber range occurs.

These fibers are not active before tourniquet inflation and are not affected by movement, anesthesia, or cold block distal to the tourniquet. However, if nerve block was performed just proximal to the tourniquet or deflation of the tourniquet was performed, the fiber firing was abolished. Elevations in blood pressure were noted with tourniquet inflation even if surgery was not performed.[17]

The work of Chabel and others[17] lends a physiologic basis for tourniquet pain and why just increasing the depth of anesthesia may not be adequate treatment.

EFFECTS ON PATIENTS WITH INCREASED INTRACRANIAL PRESSURE

Elevation in blood pressure after tourniquet inflation may be detrimental to patients with head injury because increases in intracranial pressure have been noted at this time.

Another detrimental side effect of tourniquet use in head-injured patients is elevations in $PaCO_2$, $PETCO_2$, and intracranial pressure that occur with tourniquet release[19] (Fig. 7-2).

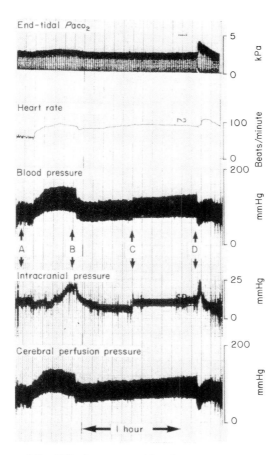

Fig. 7-2. Recordings of $PETCO_2$, heart rate, blood pressure, intracranial pressure, and cerebral perfusion pressure. Event A, application of tourniquet: B, administration of thiopentone 250 mg; C, change in height of operating table; D, tourniquet release. (From Eldridge and Williams,[19] with permission.)

TOURNIQUET EFFECTS ON BODY TEMPERATURE

Elevated Body Temperature In Pediatric Patients During Tourniquet Inflation

Temperature elevation has been noted in pediatric patients during tourniquet inflation. Also, pediatric patients with bilateral tourniquets had significantly greater increases in temperature than those patients undergoing surgery with one tourniquet. A decrease in distal skin surface area available for heat loss, and maintenance of heat in the central compartment are explanations for the temperature elevation. It is suggested that pediatric patients requiring tourniquets for surgery not receive "aggressive" warming because their temperature will rise as a result of the tourniquet[20] (Fig. 7-3).

Temperature Decrease after Tourniquet Release

Temperature release allows for recirculation of blood into a cold extremity. This mixing results in a lowering of core temperature. In 20 patients undergoing knee surgery, tourniquet release was associated with a 0.78°C (mean) temperature decrease. Reis[21] suggests possible causes of decreasing temperature as

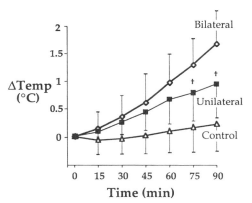

Fig. 7-3. Change in nasopharyngeal temperature in patients given unilateral leg tourniquets, bilateral leg tourniquets, or no tourniquets (control) during 90 elapsed minutes. Time zero was the time as soon after induction of anesthesia as possible at which the first central temperature was recorded. Initial temperatures after induction of anesthesia (elapsed time zero) were 36.6 ± 0.4°C in unilateral tourniquet group, 36.4 ± 0.4°C in bilateral group, and 36.5 ± 0.6°C in control group. Patients in control group remained nearly normothermic. By contrast, central temperatures increased 1.0 ± 0.6°C in 90 minutes in patients with unilateral tourniquets and 1.7 ± 0.6°C in those with bilateral tourniquets. Central temperatures in each treatment group were significantly greater than values at time zero after 15 elapsed minutes. Central temperature increases in both tourniquet groups significantly exceeded values in control patients at all times after each 15 minute interval. Increases in bilateral tourniquet group were significantly greater than those in unilateral group at 75 and 90 elapsed minutes (†). (From Bloch et al,[20] with permission.)

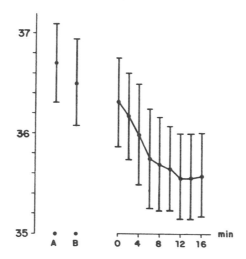

Fig. 7-4. Esophageal temperature (mean ± SD) during general anesthesia for knee surgery in 20 patients. *A*, immediately after induction; *B*, tourniquet inflated; *0*, tourniquet deflated. (From dos Reis Junior,[21] with permission.)

1. Cooling effect of blood from ischemic extremity flowing centrally
2. Cooling of systemic blood flowing through ischemic extremity
3. Reactive hyperemia after tourniquet deflation with increased heat loss from extremity (Fig. 7-4)

SYSTEMIC EFFECTS OF TOURNIQUET RELEASE

Metabolic Changes

After the release of a tourniquet, especially in the lower extremity, there is a rise in acid metabolites that enter the circulation. Plasma bicarbonate buffers the acid metabolites, and this results in an elevation of $PaCO_2$. This can be noted as elevations in $PETCO_2$. As the elevated $PaCO_2$ circulates centrally, it stimulates the respiratory center and may result in increases in respiratory rate or depth. We have noted a sudden deep breath after release of the tourniquet. Dickson et al[22] demonstrated significant increases in $PETCO_2$ after tourniquet release from both upper and lower extremities with increases in lower extremity $PETCO_2$, demonstrating the most significant change (Table 7-1).

Concern exists that release of metabolic products might cause an undesirable systemic reaction. Studies appear to have allayed such fears in healthy patients.[1]

Table 7-1. $P_{ET}CO_2$ Values Immediately before Tourniquet Release and 1 to 5 Minutes after Tourniquet Release in Patients Undergoing Upper and Lower Extremity Surgery

Time	$P_{ET}CO_2$ (mmHg [mean ± SEM)]	
	Upper Extremity[a]	Lower Extremity[a]
BTR	29.7 ± 1.3	31.7 ± 1.1
1 min ATR[b]	31.6 ± 1.5	37.8 ± 0.9
2 min ATR[b]	32.5 ± 1.6	40.1 ± 1.0
3 min ATR[b]	32.2 ± 1.7	40.5 ± 1.1
4 min ATR[b]	31.8 ± 1.6	39.6 ± 1.0
5 min ATR[b]	32.1 ± 1.6	38.3 ± 1.0

ATR, after tourniquet release; BTR, immediately before tourniquet release; $P_{ET}CO_2$, end-tidal partial pressure of carbon dioxide.

[a] ATR increases in PCO_2 in lower extremity group are significantly greater than increases in upper extremity group ($P < .05$, multifactor analysis of variance).

[b] Significantly different when compared with BTR ($P < .05$, multifactor analysis of variance).

(From Dickson et al,[22] with permision.)

Klenerman et al[23] sampled blood from the right atrium and found it to be buffered so that no significant rise in metabolic products was noted with the samples obtained.

Pulmonary Embolism

Although tourniquet use is generally considered safe, there are times when significant systemic alterations occur after tourniquet release. Pulmonary embolism with marked hemodynamic alterations and even cardiac arrest have been noted after tourniquet release from the lower extremity. The source of the pulmonary embolism may be deep vein thrombosis or fat and marrow elements that have accumulated in the veins distal to the tourniquet. After tourniquet deflation, these elements travel to the central circulation and cause systemic reactions. McGrath et al[11] described two cases of massive pulmonary embolism approximately 5 to 6 minutes after tourniquet deflation. In one case, the pulmonary embolism was noted by transesophageal echocardiography. Chest compressions, cardioversion, and high-dose vasoconstrictors and inotropes were used to obtain an adequate blood pressure.[11]

Besides pulmonary embolism, elevations in right-sided heart pressures may result in opening a patent foramen ovale and paradoxical embolism.[24]

Case Study

A 60-year-old woman with rheumatoid arthritis and a history of tuberculosis presented for right total knee replacement. The patient underwent uneventful induction of general anesthesia with fentanyl, vecuronium, and propofol. Vital signs were stable except that the blood pressure increased from its baseline of 100/60 mmHg to 150/90 mmHg after 1 hour of tourniquet inflation.

Approximately 10 minutes after tourniquet deflation, the blood pressure suddenly decreased to 50/30 mmHg. Ephedrine and neosynephrine were administered without result. High-dose infusions of neosynephrine, epinephrine, and dopamine were started. An arterial blood gas analysis on an FIO_2 of 1.0 revealed pH, 7.36; PCO_2, 43 mmHg; PO_2, 130 mmHg. After 15 minutes of the infusion of the vasopressors, the blood pressure slowly rose to 110/70 mmHg. Arterial blood gases revealed pH, 7.36; PCO_2, 40 mmHg; PO_2, 380 mmHg. The vasoactive drips were discontinued, the pressure remained stable, and the patient awoke without sequelae. The ventilation/perfusion scan was read as low to intermediate probability.

Comment

This case appears to be a classic example of pulmonary embolism after tourniquet deflation. Fortunately, the low blood pressure and relative hypoxemia resolved after about 15 minutes.

Effect on Asthmatics

Be alert during tourniquet release in patients who are prone to asthmatic attacks. We have noted an asthmatic attack developing in a known asthmatic patient on the release of a tourniquet. This attack was probably brought on by the increase in acid metabolites in the circulation.

USE OF TOURNIQUETS ON BOTH EXTREMITIES SIMULTANEOUSLY

Inflation of tourniquets simultaneously on both lower extremities is a dangerous procedure and should never be carried out. This maneuver leads to a very high afterload, which may be dangerous to the cardiovascular system, especially in those patients in whom there is some cardiovascular compromise and who cannot tolerate sudden increased afterload.

Case Study

It was reported to us that at another hospital, a 67-year-old woman who was a known hypertensive and suffered from arteriosclerotic heart disease was scheduled to undergo bilateral simultaneous bunionectomies under tourniquet control. When the tourniquets were inflated, the patient developed acute pulmonary edema and an acute myocardial infarction. The patient died on the operating table.

COMPLICATIONS OF TOURNIQUETS ON THE FOREARM OR CALF

In the forearm or calf, the vessels are located on the interosseus membranes and are not able to be compressed as in the thigh or arm. Use of tourniquets in these areas may not adequately occlude the blood supply and may lead to leakage into the wound with poor visualization and inability to perform the surgical procedure in a completely bloodless field. There may also be postoperative edema as a result of the inflow of arterial blood with venous occlusion.

Tourniquet application on the calf may cause pressure on the common peroneal nerve near the head of the fibula.

CONTRAINDICATIONS

Infection

Tourniquets should not be used in patients in whom there is infection in the extremity. Case reports of acute pulmonary edema and cardiac arrest have been reported after tourniquet release in septic patients.[25,26]

Tumors

Exsanguination and tourniquet inflation in an extremity with a tumor is not recommended because tumor cells may be squeezed into the circulation.

Sickle Cell Disease

Sickling may occur in a limb that has been occluded by a tourniquet for a period of time as a result of the accumulation of acidotic products as well as the associated anoxia. Although we do not use nor recommend tourniquets in patients with sickle cell disease, Stein and Urbaniak[27] believed that sickle cell disease was not a contraindication to the use of a tourniquet.

Sickle Cell Trait

Use of a tourniquet is not contraindicated in patients with sickle cell trait.[28] Care must be exercised in this patient population.

REFERENCES

1. Smith TC: Anesthesia and orthopaedic surgery. p. 1215. In Barash PG, Cullen BF, Stoelting RK (eds): Clinical Anesthesia. 2nd Ed. JB Lippincott, Philadelphia, 1992
2. O'Neil D, Sheppard JE: Transient compartment syndrome of the forearm resulting from venous congestion from a tourniquet. J Hand Surg 14A:894, 1989
3. Eckhoff NL: Tourniquet paralysis. Lancet 2:343, 1931
4. Wolff LH, Adkins TF: Tourniquet problems in war injuries. Bull US Army Med Dept 87:77, 1945
5. Green DP (ed): Operative Hand Surgery. 3rd Ed. Churchill Livingstone, New York, 1993

6. Flatt A: Tourniquet time in hand surgery. Arch Surg 104:190, 1972
7. Wilgis EFS: Observations on the effects of tourniquet ischemia. J Bone Joint Surg 53(A):1343, 1971
8. Salam AA, Eyres KS, Cleary J et al: The use of tourniquet when plating tibial plateau fractures. J Bone Joint Surg 73(B):86, 1991
9. Hofmann AA, Wyatt RW: Fatal pulmonary embolism following tourniquet inflation. J Bone Joint Surg 67(A):633, 1985
10. San Juan AC, Stanley TH: Pulmonary embolism after tourniquet inflation. Anesth Analg 63:371, 1984
11. McGrath BJ, Hsia J, Epstein B: Massive pulmonary embolism following tourniquet deflation. Anesthesiology 74:618, 1991
12. Tartiere J, Berthelin C, Jehan C et al: Hemodynamic changes during total knee replacement surgery with total condylar prosthesis. Anesthesiology 67:838, 1987
13. Hagenouw RPRM, Bridenbaugh PO, van Egmond J et al: Tourniquet pain: a volunteer study. Anesth Analg 65:1175, 1986
14. Kaufman RD, Walts LF: Tourniquet induced hypertension. Br J Anaesth 54:333, 1982
15. Solanki DR: Epidural fentanyl for relief of lower extremity tourniquet. Anesth Analg 66:S161, 1987
16. Tuominen M, Valli H, Kalso E et al: Efficacy of 0.3 mg morphine intrathecally in preventing tourniquet pain during spinal anaesthesia with hyperbaric bupivacaine. Acta Anaesthesiol Scand 32:113, 1988
17. Chabel C, Russell LC, Lee R: Tourniquet-induced limb ischemia: a neurophysiologic animal model. Anesthesiology 72:1038, 1990
18. Iggo A: Pain receptors. p. 3. In Bonica JJ, Procaccip P, Pagni CA (eds): Recent Advances in Pain: Pathophysiology and Clinical Aspects. Charles C Thomas, Springfield, IL, 1974
19. Eldridge PR, Williams SS: Effect of limb tourniquet on cerebral perfusion pressure in a head injured patient. Anaesthesia 44:973, 1989
20. Bloch EC, Ginsberg B, Binner RA et al: Limb tourniquets and central temperature in anesthetized children. Anesth Analg 74:486, 1992
21. dos Reis Junior A: Tourniquet use and intraoperative hypothermia. Anesth Analg 69:548, 1989
22. Dickson M, White H, Kinney W et al: Extremity tourniquet deflation increases end tidal PCO_2. Anesth Analg 70:457, 1990
23. Klenerman L, Meenakshi B, Hulands GH et al: Systemic and local effects of the application of a tourniquet. J Bone Joint Surg 62(B):385, 1980
24. Coleman SA, Wilson-MacDonald J: Fatal paradoxical pulmonary embolism during anaesthesia. Anaesthesia 43:213, 1988
25. O'Leary AM, Veall G, Butler P et al: Acute pulmonary edema after tourniquet release. Can J Anaesth 37:826, 1990
26. Gielen M: Cardiac arrest after tourniquet release. Can J Anaesth 38:541, 1991
27. Stein RE, Urbaniak J: Use of tourniquet during surgery in patients with sickle cell hemoglobinopathies. Clin Orthop 151:231, 1980
28. Searle JF: Anaesthesia in sickle cell states: a review. Anaesthesia 2848, 1973

8

Special Considerations in Surgery of the Extremities

HAND SURGERY

The general categories of conditions addressed in hand surgery are listed below.

Traumatic
    Crush injuries with bone, muscle, skin, nerve, and vascular involvement
    Amputations of parts of digits, digits, or loss of entire hand
    Fractures—open or closed
    Lacerations of skin
    Nerve injuries

Neoplastic
    Tumors of bone
    Tumors of connective tissue
    Tumors of blood vessels
    Tumors of nerves

Reconstructive
    Congenital—syndactyly as well as other anomalous conditions
    Arthritis—reconstruction for rheumatoid arthritis, including capsulotomies, synovectomy, tendon releases, and joint reconstruction
    Tendon transfers
    Abnormalities of skin and underlying connective tissue such as Dupuytren's contracture
    Nerve entrapment syndrome such as carpal tunnel syndrome, decompression of ulnar nerve at wrist in canal of Guyon

Infection
    Incision and drainage of infections

Hand surgery can easily be performed under general or regional anesthesia. It appears natural that regional anesthesia is an effective method (see Ch. 6).

Special Considerations in Choosing Regional Anesthesia

Infection

If infection is present, axillary brachial plexus block should be avoided. Interscalene block, subclavian perivascular block, and infraclavicular block may be used.

257

Tumor

If tumor is present, axillary block should be avoided.

Position

The patient is placed on the operating table in the supine position.

A special hand table is placed adjacent to the operating table and may be hooked to the side rails of the operating table or placed under the mattress of the operating table.

The padding on the hand table should be equal in height to that of the operating table. Otherwise, if the arm is placed on the hand table, traction would be exerted on the brachial plexus because of the difference in height between the operating table and the hand table.

The padding should be soft to avoid pressure on the patient's arm.

Once the patient's arm is on the hand table, the height of the hand table should be adjusted when the height of the operating table is changed. This is especially important if the hand table is equipped with its own legs and does not move when the regular operating table moves.

Postoperative Ulnar Nerve Neuropathy

Ulnar nerve injury can occur from pressure in the area of the elbow during hand surgery. This can occur on the operative and nonoperative side.

Case Study

After a surgical procedure on the hand not involving nerves, the patient complained of numbness in the distribution of the ulnar nerve. Examination revealed ulnar nerve injury at the elbow. It was believed that ulnar nerve compression had occurred during the surgical procedure because of the position of the arm on an inadequately padded hand table.

Besides padding, proper positioning of both the surgical and nonoperative arm and hand is important to help decrease the incidence of postoperative ulnar nerve palsy. Pronation of the hand exposes the ulnar nerve at the elbow to possible injury from compression, whereas supination of the hand protects the nerve from direct compression injury.[1-3]

In a recent review, Stoelting[1] points out that all postoperative ulnar nerve neuropathy is not preventable and can occur without apparent etiology. A pre-existing subclinical neuropathy caused by diabetes, vitamin deficiency, cancer, alcoholism, degenerative arthritis, trauma, occupational use, or other etiologies may become evident during the postoperative period. This may occur for unknown reasons or because additional factors such as positioning, use of a blood pressure cuff, and alterations in blood flow to the ulnar nerve may occur.[1]

Tourniquet Use

Most hand surgery is performed under tourniquet control to provide a bloodless field for the procedure (see Ch. 7).

If a tourniquet is used, even for a short procedure, the most stoic of patients may require some sedation to tolerate the tourniquet pain. Adequate sedation in the operating room for tourniquet pain may result in oversedation once the tourniquet is deflated and the source of pain is no longer present.[4]

Quick Cases

"I won't be too long, just give him a whiff" is a statement that might be heard in some cases, such as trigger finger releases and release of stenosing tenosynovitis (DeQuervain's), that appear to lend themselves to anesthesia by mask.

The anesthesiologist should not be lulled into a false sense of security and perform all those cases with a mask. All precautions should have been taken to avoid aspiration. A mask should not be used for these short cases in any situation in which aspiration may occur.

If aspiration is a major concern in a minor peripheral surgical procedure, the use of local anesthesia should be considered. Minimum, if any, sedation is provided.

For minor cases in which local anesthesia is administered and the patient is not at risk of aspiration, sedation with alfentanil and propofol is a very successful and satisfying technique.

Bilateral Simultaneous Procedures—The Two-Team Approach

Place an intravenous line in the lower extremity.

Place a blood pressure cuff on the thigh.

Place a pulse oximeter on the toe.

Set up all lines so there is access to them at the head of the table.

Avoid bilateral simultaneous regional anesthesia. The dosages necessary may exceed the toxic level and should not be used.

Bone Grafts

Some surgical procedures require a bone graft, which may be obtained from local areas such as the radius or from the iliac crest. The surgeon should always be consulted before administering regional anesthesia as to whether a bone graft from the iliac crest may be necessary. In this instance, the contralateral iliac crest is used for the graft. The patient is positioned with that side slightly elevated to provide access to the iliac crest.

General anesthesia is usually administered when iliac bone grafts are to be taken.

REIMPLANTATION

Reimplantation of single digits, multiple digits, forearms, or arms have been performed.

Digits

Implantation of a digit involves suturing a number of arteries and veins using a microscope. This is a long and tedious procedure.

Anesthetic Technique

General anesthesia can be used, but it should be remembered that the patient probably has a full stomach and techniques to avoid aspiration should be undertaken. Marked blood loss may occur during reimplantation of the digits. Blood loss and urine output should be monitored carefully.

Regional Anesthesia

Brachial plexus block can be used either as a single injection technique or alternatively with the use of a continuous catheter technique to provide prolonged anesthesia, continuous postoperative pain relief, and sympathetic blockade in the postoperative period.

Continuous regional anesthesia can also be performed in combination with general anesthesia to provide the same benefits described above (see Ch. 6).

Forearm or Arm

Considerations in reimplantation surgery at the forearm or arm level include the following:

1. It will be a very long case.
2. Multiple transfusions may be needed.
3. The patient must be protected from hypothermia.

Patient Preparation

Insert adequate lines for large volume of blood and fluid replacement.

Insert arterial line to monitor blood pressure and obtain blood gases and serial hematocrit values.

Insert Foley catheter.

Arrange for adequate blood replacement.

Monitor body temperature.

Use Bair Hugger or other warming methods to keep the patient normothermic.

Prepare for postoperative sympathetic blockade and pain relief by inserting a continuous brachial plexus block cannula.

FRACTURES

Associated Conditions

In all cases of fracture, assessment must be made of the neurologic and vascular status because such injuries can occur in association with the fracture.

Fractures of the humerus in the midshaft may involve radial nerve injury.

Fractures in the area of the elbow may involve injury to ulnar, median, or radial nerves.

Supracondylar fracture of the humerus in children is a medical emergency because Volkmann's ischemic contracture may result.

Wrist fractures may lead to carpal tunnel syndrome.

Closed Reduction

Anesthesia may be necessary if a good reduction cannot be obtained after infiltration into the hematoma and attempts at reduction.

Operation for Open Fractures

Open fractures are medical emergencies and should be treated as early as possible after injury.

Antitetanus medication was probably administered in the emergency department. It is important to check and make sure.

Antibiotics should be administered as requested by the surgeon. Remember, the antibiotic is given *before* the tourniquet is inflated.

Irrigation and débridement with stabilization of the fracture is the usual operative procedure. Use of external fixator devices has made treatment of difficult fractures easier.

Open Reduction and Internal Fixation

Regional or general anesthetic techniques are equally useful, and one is not more beneficial than the other.

The position used is determined by the surgical approach. Some situations may require the prone position with the arm placed on a hand table.

Types of Surgery

Open reduction with application of plates and screws
Open reduction with intramedullary rods
Open reduction and internal fixation with hardware plus bone graft

Bone Graft Sites

Bone grafts may be obtained from the iliac crest, which involves surgery at another operative site.

Bone grafts may be obtained from a bone bank.

Anesthetic Considerations

General Anesthesia

If there are no special problems with the patient, general anesthesia can be administered.

Regional Anesthesia

In complex reconstructions, the time element must be considered if regional anesthesia is contemplated.

If iliac bone graft harvesting is necessary, regional anesthesia of the upper extremity alone will not be sufficient. If regional anesthesia is mandatory when a bone graft is to be harvested, it is possible to administer spinal or epidural anesthesia for the harvesting of the bone graft and an upper extremity block for the surgery.

Continuous upper extremity blocks may be useful in such cases.

Innovative approaches can carry the anesthesiologist through some problems.

In some instances, multiple regional anesthetics may be indicated.

Case Study

> While in the army, one of us (RLB) attended to a military policeman who accidentally shot himself through the hand and into the thigh just after eating lunch. Spinal anesthesia was given for treatment of the thigh wound. While the extensive preparation was being performed, a brachial plexus block was given for the surgical procedure on the hand. Both operations proceeded without incident.

SHOULDER SURGERY

Frequently, shoulder surgery is performed in the sitting position. General or regional anesthetic techniques are acceptable. Special considerations include

1. If general anesthesia is used, place the endotracheal tube on the side of the mouth opposite surgery.
2. Check the blood pressure as the patient is placed into the sitting position from the supine position.
3. If intra-arterial monitoring is used, place transducers at the level of the ear to monitor pressure in the brain.

Case Study

A 62-year-old man with a history of previous stroke and hypertension came to the operating room for rotator cuff repair. Baseline blood pressure was 160/80 mmHg. An arterial line was placed in the nonsurgical hand, and the patient was induced and intubated with minimal change in blood pressure. The endotracheal tube was positioned to exit the mouth from the nonoperative side. A head rest was prepared. In elevating the head of the bed, the systolic blood pressure decreased to 100 mmHg. Neosynephrine (100 μg) was administered to return the blood pressure to baseline. The arterial line was positioned at the height of the carotid artery. Intraoperatively, the blood pressure was maintained at the patient's baseline. The nonsurgical arm was padded and supported. The patient tolerated the procedure well and had no perioperative complications.

4. Maintain the head in neutral. Avoid traction on the brachial plexus. Secure the head well.

Case Study

After shoulder repair, a patient complained of some numbness in his operative hand. The surgeon informed the patient that the anesthesiologist had the patient's head turned too far away from the site of surgery and that was the reason for the patient's problem. The anesthesiologist's record documented that the patient's head was placed midline in a head rest and taped into position.

5. Pad and support the extremity not being operated on.
6. Flex the knees and hips to avoid traction on the sciatic nerve.
7. Be aware of possible venous air embolism because the operative site is above the level of the heart.

LOWER EXTREMITY

Surgery on the lower extremity can be performed under general or regional anesthesia (see Ch. 6).

Position

Care must be taken in positioning patients who are having surgery on the lower extremity so that the chance of perioperative nerve damage is minimized.

The fracture table may be used for operative procedures on the hip (e.g., operative arthroscopy of the hip). Adequate perineal padding while avoiding direct pressure on the genitalia is important. The upper torso should be adequately strapped to avoid movement. If the nonoperated leg is rotated into abduction, the patient's upper body can rotate. Any foot that has traction applied should be adequately padded.

Case Study

An elderly patient with a hip fracture had the leg opposite the fracture rotated into abduction after the fracture side had been secured and padded. The patient was not adequately secured to the table, and the upper body rotated as the leg was abducted. The endotracheal tube, which was held in place by tape and supported by a tube support, "Christmas tree," did not rotate with the patient, and the patient was extubated.

The anesthesiologist should be aware that the surgeons will be applying traction to the patient, and this may result in inadvertent extubation.

Foot Surgery

Surgery of the forefoot, such as bunionectomies, hammertoes, tendon releases, resections of ganglia, and excision of neuromas, lends itself to management under ankle block (see Ch. 6).

Ankle fusion, triple arthrodesis, reconstructions involving bones and soft tissue, open reduction, and internal fixation of fractures can be performed under spinal anesthesia, epidural anesthesia, or general anesthesia. Care should be taken if epidural anesthesia is chosen for ankle surgery because it takes time for the lower lumbar and upper sacral roots to become adequately anesthetized. Two percent lidocaine with epinephrine 1:200,000 is used, and an appropriate time should pass before allowing the surgeon to proceed.

Tibia and Fibula Fractures

Fractures of the malleoli requiring open reduction and internal fixation are common. The fibula on the lateral aspect is usually repaired first and then the medial malleolus.

Tibia

Fractures of the tibia involve
   Insertion of intramedullary rods
   Other methods of fixation involving the use of plates and screws with possible
      bone grafts when indicated
   Use of external fixators

Warning:

   Always be aware of the possible development of a compartment syndrome
      in surgery in this area. Check neurovascular status after the procedure.
   If wires are passed for external fixation devices, beware of neurologic or
      vascular damage. Be especially alert if this is performed near the neck of
      the fibula.

Tibial Plateau

Fractures of the tibial plateau are fractures in the upper end of the tibia involving the knee joint.

Reconstruction of this type of fracture requires elevation of the depressed fragment to re-establish the continuity of the cartilaginous plate of the proximal tibia. Insertion of bone grafts and application of a plate and screws are also involved in repair of this type of fracture. Depending on the surgeon, these may be very long and involved procedures.

Anesthetic Considerations

General anesthesia or regional anesthesia is equally satisfactory, and the choice of anesthesia should be determined by the needs of the patient, surgeon, and anesthesiologist.

Knee Injury

Massive trauma in the area of the knee can lead to fractures and destruction of tendons and ligaments. Vascular and neural injury may also occur.

If a vascular injury occurs, this should be repaired first before engaging in reconstruction of bone and soft tissue. An arteriogram can be performed in the operating room if any question exists concerning the vascular status.

Combined Tibial and Femoral Fractures Resulting in a "Floating" Knee

Neurovascular status must be evaluated first.

Stabilization can be accomplished by fixation techniques involving the tibia and the femur. Major blood loss must be considered in these injuries.

Femoral Shaft Fractures

Fractures of the femoral shaft may involve massive blood loss. Measurement of the circumference of the thigh in comparison with the uninjured side can reveal the extent of blood loss, which can amount to 2,000 ml. Stabilization of the patient is performed first. Blood and fluids are administered as needed.

Associated injuries should be evaluated, and serious or life-threatening problems treated.

Early treatment of this fracture involves immobilization to decrease pain and stabilization to decrease the chance of fat embolism and to help get the patient out of bed (see Ch. 2).

A femoral nerve block (see Ch. 6) is useful in providing pain relief before the surgery and can aid in making the patient more comfortable during movement and positioning.

Femoral Neck Fractures

See Chapter 3 for a discussion of femoral neck fractures.

Bilateral Tourniquets

Simultaneous bilateral tourniquets should not be used in lower extremity surgery. The increased afterload on the heart may cause the patient to develop congestive heart failure (see Ch. 7).

Patient Evaluation

Surgery on the lower extremity can be associated with injury to nerves and vessels. The patients' neurovascular status should be evaluated carefully.

REFERENCES

1. Stoelting RK: Postoperative ulnar nerve palsy—is it a preventable complication? Anesth Analg 76:7, 1993
2. Kroll DA, Caplan RA, Posner K et al: Nerve injury associated with anesthesia. Anesthesiology 73:202, 1990
3. Wadsworth TG: The cubital tunnel and external compression syndrome. Anesth Analg 53:303, 1974
4. Smith TC: Anesthesia and orthopedic surgery. p. 1215. In Barash PG, Cullen BF, Stoelting RK (eds): Clinical Anesthesia. 2nd Ed. JB Lippincott, Philadelphia, 1992

9

Ambulatory Surgery

The number of procedures performed in an ambulatory surgery setting has grown rapidly in the past few years. At the Hospital for Joint Disease Orthopaedic Institute, 40 to 50 percent of the operating schedule is in the Ambulatory Surgery Center.

We have constructed an ambulatory center one floor above the regular operating room suite, with an internal circular staircase connecting the operating rooms. This has made more operating rooms available for inpatient surgery and has essentially separated the patients undergoing ambulatory surgery from those undergoing inpatient surgery.

PREOPERATIVE ASSESSMENT

All patients undergoing ambulatory surgery are required to undergo preoperative testing within 1 week before the scheduled date of surgery, at which time a history, physical examination, and nursing assessment are performed.

The preoperative assessment decreases the time spent on the day of surgery and provides for a smoother schedule.

Laboratory studies, chest radiograph, and electrocardiogram (ECG) are performed when indicated.

Any abnormalities detected during the preoperative assessment are treated before the scheduled date of surgery.

Medical Evaluation

When indicated, a medical evaluation by an internist is obtained before surgery. The report is forwarded to the attending surgeon and the anesthesiologist. The indication for medical evaluation is any condition or abnormality that may cause a problem (e.g., patient who is wheezing, patient with a murmur, arrhythmias, abnormal ECG, abnormal liver function tests).

Preoperative Anesthesia Assessment

When the patient comes for pretesting, the anesthesiologist also sees the patient. A complete medical history is taken, a physical examination is performed, and the patient's anesthetic history is discussed.

Anesthesiologist's Evaluation

The following items should be addressed:

Exactly which surgical procedure is to be performed

Which side will be operated on (this is very important and can help avoid errors later on)

Medications (will help indicate pre-existing conditions)

Allergies

Smoking

Alcohol

Drug abuse

Previous surgical procedures

Whether the patient or any family member has had any problems with anesthesia

History of any serious illnesses (patients do not always tell the anesthesiologist about their illnesses)

History of shortness of breath on exertion

History of cough or wheezing, asthma, pneumonia

Chest pain on exertion, murmur, myocardial infarction, angina, ankle swelling

History of hypertension

Diabetes

Gastrointestinal problems—hiatal hernia, ulcer, hepatitis, liver problems

Genitourinary problems—urinary tract infections, renal problems

History of headaches, especially migraine headaches

> If patient has headaches, the patient is questioned concerning a neurologic workup. We know of patients who had a history of migraine headaches, one treated with Fiorinal, who, after surgery, did not wake up. Workups revealed meningiomas of the brain that would have been discovered on a preoperative evaluation had the history of migraines been pursued

Last menstrual period, perform pregnancy test, when indicated

Physical Examination

Airway Assessment

The airway should be assessed at the preanesthetic visit to avoid trouble on the morning of surgery.

The ability to flex and extend the neck should be checked.

If there is a question of the status of the airway, appropriate management arrangements can be made in advance and explained to the patient. This avoids sending for a fiberoptic bronchoscope after muscle relaxant has been given and the patient cannot be intubated.

Opening the Mouth

Many patients with rheumatoid arthritis or ankylosing spondylitis may be unable to open the mouth because of temporomandibular joint problems. The following should be checked:

Status of the teeth
> Check for dentures, prosthetic devices, caps, loose teeth, necrotic teeth
> Discuss dental problems—have patient see dentist, if necessary, before surgery.

Ability to view the uvula

Status of the mandible—early fusion of the mandible seen in patients with arthritis, leading to intubation problems

Mentum to hyoid cartilage distance (should be at least three to four fingers)

Chest

The chest should be examined for breath sounds and their quality.

Cardiac Evaluation

The heart should be examined for rate, rhythm, and presence or absence of murmurs.

Carotid arteries should be auscultated for *bruits*.

Intravenous Access

The hands and arms should be examined for intravenous access.

Review of Electrocardiogram

The ECG that was taken by the ambulatory surgery testing service is reviewed. Any abnormalities are discussed with the patient. If abnormalities exist, the patient is requested to obtain old ECGs. On occasion, the ECG is faxed to the patient's cardiologist, or the patient's cardiologist is asked to fax old ECGs for comparison.

Laboratory Tests

Requests for laboratory tests should not be on a routine basis nor should a complete screening be performed on every patient.

Laboratory tests should be selected based on history and physical examination of the patient.

Hematocrit level
> Probably necessary in most female patients and in both men and women older than 60 years of age

Prothrombin time and partial thromboplastin time
> Patients with hepatic disease, bleeding disorders, anticoagulant use

Electrolytes
> Patients with renal disease, diabetes, diuretic use, steroid use, digoxin use

Creatinine and blood urea nitrogen
> Patients older than 60 years of age, those with renal disease, diabetes, diuretic use, digoxin use

Blood glucose
> Patients with diabetes, patients using steroids

Liver function tests
> Patients with hepatic disease, hepatitis exposure, drinking histories

Chest radiograph
> Patients older than 60 years of age, those with cardiovascular disease, pulmonary disease, wheezing and cough, smoking history

ECG
> Patients older than 40 years of age, those with known cardiovascular disease, pulmonary disease, diabetes, antihypertensive and/or cardiac drug use

Anesthetic Management Discussion

A discussion is held concerning the anesthetic management. At this time, the preference for regional or general anesthesia is determined.

An explanation of the anesthetic management is then carried out, starting with instructions about being on nothing-by-mouth (NPO) status.

Notes of the preoperative visit are placed in the record and can be read by the anesthesiologist on the day of surgery.

Regional or General Anesthesia

Help the patient make a proper decision as to which type of anesthesia is best for the patient.

Explain in great detail all the considerations concerning the type of anesthesia that the patient has requested including the risks and benefits.

Choosing the Patient for Ambulatory Surgery

Cases scheduled for ambulatory surgery are usually elective.

The patient should be in the best possible health. Surgery should be deferred in any patient who does not meet this criterion.

If a condition exists in which deferring the procedure would not provide any benefit, the procedure can be carried out taking the condition into consideration. However, if it is anticipated that problems may develop after surgery, plans for postoperative admission should be made.

The patient must be motivated to have the procedure performed on an ambulatory basis. The patient must understand that the postoperative care will be at home, and the patient must be able to follow the instructions provided for the postoperative care.

The patient must be accompanied home by a responsible adult.

The patient must have a responsible adult at home to help with the postoperative care.

The patient must realize that sedatives and general anesthetics may impair mental acuity on the day of surgery and into the next day. The patient must be informed that driving, operating machinery, or making very complex decisions will not be possible in the immediate postoperative period.

Both the person accompanying the patient home and the patient must be able to recognize any complications and know how to seek emergency treatment.

Warning: Under no circumstances should a patient be allowed to leave the ambulatory care unit without a responsible individual.

Case Study

A 55-year-old woman in good general health underwent an operative arthroscopy of the right knee. She made an uneventful recovery in the postanesthesia care unit (PACU) and was prepared for discharge. When the patient was dressed, she said that her son and daughter, whom she had just called, were unable to come to take her home because of business responsibilities. When the patient was instructed in crutch-walking, it was noted that she was not able to ambulate without support by the nurse. Although the patient insisted on going home by herself with a car service, the staff did not allow her to do so because she could have easily fallen when ambulating with crutches without assistance.

Pressure is on the ambulatory surgery staff to move patients out because usually no area is available where postoperative patients ready for discharge can stay and be observed. However, under no circumstances should a patient be allowed to go home unaccompanied by a responsible individual.

Small Children

Small children should be accompanied by an adult to care for them as well as another individual who will drive the car. A small child cannot be left strapped into a carseat while the responsible individual is involved in driving through traffic.

Problem Patients

It is markedly advantageous that any patient scheduled for ambulatory surgery who suffers from another illness be seen by the anesthesiologist at the preadmission testing visit. At this time, the anesthesiologist can determine whether the condition from which the patient suffers would render the patient unable to undergo surgery on an ambulatory basis.

Insulin-Dependent Diabetic Patients

Insulin-dependent diabetic patients are instructed not to take any insulin before arriving in the hospital. A blood glucose determination is made by a fingerstick, a glucose-containing intravenous fluid is administered, and insulin is given based on the blood sugar level.

Regional anesthesia is used, whenever possible, so that the patient will not suffer from nausea or vomiting and be able to start taking fluids and food orally. An assessment is made concerning whether evidence of diabetic neuropathy is present, and this is noted in the medical record.

The insulin-dependent diabetic patient who is in reasonable control may go out of control after the stress of surgery and anesthesia. Alterations in blood sugar level, electrolytes, and status of hydration after surgery may make this patient unable to be sent home to be cared for by a member of the family. This type of patient would benefit from admission to the hospital for monitoring and control of the diabetes and be sent home the following day, if stable.

Diabetic Patients on Oral Hypoglycemic Agents

Diabetic patients on oral hypoglycemic agents are instructed not to take any medication and to remain on NPO status. They are monitored by fingerstick glucose determinations, encouraged to have regional anesthesia, and to take food and fluids as soon as possible.

Patients with Multi-Organ System Diseases

The patient with hypertension, arteriosclerotic heart disease, a history of congestive heart failure, and arrhythmias requiring several medications and almost constant attention would probably not benefit from ambulatory surgery. Surgical procedures on this patient should be performed with the patient admitted to the hospital and observed until the following day so that the patient can be discharged in the best possible condition.

Elderly Patients

We frequently encounter elderly patients living at home who are scheduled for surgery on an ambulatory basis. When questioned, it is revealed that the "responsible person" living at home with the patient is in poor general health and requires the help of the patient to perform daily activities. If the patient is discharged home, no one will be at home to take care of the patient nor to take care of the dependent family member. This is a medical problem, a family problem, and a social problem. These situations must be taken into consideration and special arrangements made through other family members and the social work service representative.

Interventions by the Anesthesiologist

At the preoperative visit, the anesthesiologist can determine whether the patient is a candidate for ambulatory surgery. If not, arrangements can be made at this time for inpatient care.

If the patient requires evaluation or treatment for a medical condition, this can be arranged at this time and avoided on the morning of surgery. An example, is the patient with a murmur. If an echocardiogram is obtained after the preanesthetic visit and the results forwarded to the anesthesiologist, hassles are avoided on the morning of surgery.

What to Tell the Patient

The patient may have some soreness in the throat if general anesthesia with an endotracheal tube is to be given.

The patient will be groggy after general anesthesia or regional anesthesia with sedation.

The benefits and risks of regional anesthesia should be explained. This is the chance to sell the patient a block.

The pros and cons of epidural and spinal anesthesia should be explained, especially residual numbness, motor weakness, and backache.

The patient should be assured that if regional anesthesia is administered, sedation can be given so that the patient will not be completely awake.

In discussing epidural or spinal anesthesia, the patient should be told about the dreaded postdural puncture headache, which may develop. Also, the patient should be told about an epidural blood patch.

Some of our surgeons encourage the patient to have regional anesthesia so that they can "share" in the experience. The patients all want to see their arthroscopy on the television screen. Some patients even ask the surgeon for a copy of the tape so that they can regale their friends and family with videos of their operation.

The Surgeon

The surgeon should contact the anesthesiologist when a patient is seen who has a condition that may cause anesthetic problems during surgery. The anesthesiologist will then be alerted to pay special attention to this patient's problems so that the anesthesia and surgery can be carried out in a smooth fashion.

Medications

Any medications that may be necessary are ordered.

The patient is instructed to take cardiac and antihypertensive medications as usual in the morning with a sip of water.

We prescribe 150 mg ranitidine or 400 mg cimetidine orally before the patient goes to sleep on the night before surgery and with a sip of water on awakening in the morning before coming to the Ambulatory Surgery Center in an attempt to decrease the volume and increase the pH of gastric juice. If we desire to decrease gastric volume further, metoclopramide is administered the day of surgery. We are especially concerned about the obese patient and the patient with a history of hiatal hernia, regurgitation, peptic ulcer disease, or previous gastrointestinal surgery (see Premedication below).

Premedication in the Hospital

Anticholinergics

Routine use of anticholinergic agents should be avoided. Some anesthesiologists use glycopyrrolate in certain selected cases in which they want intense drying of secretions during the induction and maintenance of the surgical procedure in patients who have a large amount of secretions. Anticholinergics are avoided in patients scheduled for regional anesthesia, they will complain about a dry mouth the entire case.

Sedatives, Hypnotics, or Tranquilizers

If sedation is needed, it can be given intravenously in the ambulatory surgery unit.

The patient should not be given any sedatives, hypnotics, or tranquilizers to be taken at home before arriving in the ambulatory surgery center.

Patients are discouraged from taking their own medications from their "personal pharmacy."

Midazolam

Midazolam is titrated intravenously until proper sedation has been achieved.

Because of individual variation, each patient's response must be observed to determine the dose and rate of administration.

The intravenous administration of up to 2 mg midazolam can start to have its effect within a few minutes.

Up to 2 mg intramuscular midazolam administered in the holding room will provide sedation before the beginning of anesthesia.

Opioids

Opioids can be administered in combination with midazolam to patients who are experiencing pain before surgery while in the operating room. Opioids can also be given to patients while regional anesthesia is being administered.

Meperidine or morphine should not be used for premedication in the ambulatory surgery patient because they prolong recovery time.[1]

Antacids and H₂ Antagonists

It is difficult to determine which patients have a gastric pH less than 2.5 and gastric volume greater than 25 ml; these patients are considered to be those who are at risk of developing the acid aspiration syndrome.

Patients who are at increased risk of acid aspiration are those with

Hiatal hernia

Obesity

Peptic ulcer disease

Diabetes mellitus

Nervousness

Old age

Previous gastric surgery

As mentioned, at our ambulatory center we prescribe 150 mg ranitidine or 400 mg cimetidine orally before the patient retires at night and another dose with a sip of water on awakening in the morning.

Metoclopramide is frequently administered to patients at risk for aspiration.

Oral antacids are not used.

In conjunction with the H_2 blocker, the nurse re-emphasizes the importance of maintaining the NPO status.

Chewing Gum

Patients are instructed *not* to chew gum on the morning of surgery. Some anesthesiologists cancel surgery for patients who come in chewing gum or have reported that they chewed gum that morning because gastric volume is increased and acidity is decreased in these patients.

Preoperative Call by Ambulatory Surgery Center Nurse

The patient is called on the telephone the night before surgery.

The patient is reminded to remain on NPO status and to take any medications that have been ordered.

The patient is instructed that an adult must be present to accompany the patient home after surgery.

The patient is questioned whether any changes have occurred, such as the onset of a cold or cough.

ORTHOPEDIC SURGERY IN THE AMBULATORY SETTING

Orthopedic surgical procedures that may safely be conducted on an ambulatory basis should be ones that

1. Do not involve severe postoperative pain, especially in lower extremities that require the patient to have the operative extremity dependent on discharge from the unit.

2. Will not cause bleeding in the postoperative period (procedures that involve extensive dissections and undermining of tissues).

Orthopedic procedures that lend themselves to ambulatory surgery include

Arthroscopic surgery
    Shoulder
    Elbow
    Wrist
    Hip
    Knee
    Ankle

Arthroscopic surgical procedures include

Diagnostic arthroscopy

Débridement

Synovectomy

Removal of torn meniscus

Repair of torn meniscus

Repair of dislocating shoulder

Ligament repair of the knee
    This procedure may involve extensive reconstruction. Some surgeons admit these patients on an overnight basis; some surgeons discharge them home on the day of surgery. These are the patients who will probably have the highest number of unscheduled admissions and will affect the quality assurance assessment

Hand Surgery

Carpal tunnel release

Closed reduction of simple fractures

Removal of foreign bodies

Excision of ganglion

Fasciectomy (release of Dupuytren's contracture)

Release of flexor tendon sheath

Removal of hardware

Open reduction and internal fixation of fractures of the finger

DeQuervain's release

Trigger thumb release

Elbow Surgery

Arthroscopy of the elbow

Ulnar nerve transfer

Hip Surgery

Arthroscopy of the hip is a procedure that lends itself to ambulatory surgery.

Foot Surgery

Bunionectomies

Release of hammertoes

Excision of plantar neuroma

Arthroscopy of the ankle

Tendon releases

Removal of hardware

Some procedures may not lend themselves to ambulatory surgery. After procedures such as bilateral bunionectomies or bilateral hand surgery, it may be difficult for patients to care for themselves at home.

The Day of Surgery

Patients who have had preoperative testing and a preoperative anesthesia visit are assessed as to the status of their health, vital signs are taken, they are dressed in hospital attire, and they are brought to the holding room. The anesthesiologist sees the patient and performs an assessment, and the patient walks to the operating room accompanied by a nurse.

Patients who Have Slipped through the Preoperative Testing Net

Although preoperative testing of all patients is encouraged, some patients do arrive in the ambulatory surgery center who have not had preoperative testing.

Although these patients hold up and interfere with the smooth flow, they are not sent home but are taken care of. A history, physical examination, nursing assessment, and laboratory work are performed as expeditiously as possible. It is necessary to make sure these patients have maintained their NPO status.

Induction and Maintenance of Anesthesia

Early discharge is a consideration when deciding which anesthetic agents and techniques would be most beneficial for a given patient. Agents such as propofol, alfentanil, and desflurane help achieve a rapid induction and allow for quick awakening.

Propofol

Propofol is a rapid and short-acting anesthetic agent. The concentration of propofol in the blood falls rapidly after a single bolus injection because of its rapid distribution and elimination.

Pain associated with injection can be avoided if lidocaine is injected with the propofol.

Induction with propofol in a dose of 2.5 mg/kg leads to very rapid loss of consciousness. In the older age group, the induction dose is decreased to 1 to 1.5 mg/kg.

The induction dose should be decreased in patients who have been premedicated with benzodiazepines or opioids.

We have noted that after the use of propofol for induction, patients are able to respond and stand up significantly quicker than if barbiturates are used for induction.

Propofol can be used for maintenance of anesthesia as well as for induction. Maintenance of anesthesia requires an infusion rate of 0.1 to 0.2 mg/kg/min. Higher doses for infusion in the early part of the operation may be required because of the rapid redistribution of the agent.

The infusion rate is adjusted during surgery according to the response of the patient.

It is very valuable for short procedures.

Alfentanil

Small bolus doses of alfentanil (250 to 500 μg) provide analgesia when combined with nitrous oxide/oxygen and muscle relaxants. Alfentanil is also used for sedation during monitored anesthesia care.

Desflurane

This anesthetic agent, with its low solubility coefficient, has rapid onset and reversibility—important characteristics for the ambulatory surgery setting. White[2] demonstrated rapid recovery after its use.

Although desflurane has few adverse effects, its respiratory irritant properties make it unsuitable as an induction agent, and it does not possess as much of an antiemetic effect as propofol.[2]

Muscle Relaxants

Short- and immediate-acting muscle relaxants such as succinylcholine, atracurium, vecuronium, and mivacurium should be used in the ambulatory setting.

MANAGEMENT OF AMBULATORY SURGICAL PROCEDURES

Shoulder Arthroscopy

Operations performed include

Diagnostic arthroscopy

Synovectomy

Repair of dislocating shoulder

Position
Lateral Decubitus Position

The patient is placed on the operating table in the lateral decubitus position. A folded sheet is placed in the axilla of the dependent side to prevent pressure on the vessels and brachial plexus. Pulses in the dependent arm are checked.

A traction pulley device with 5 lb of weight is attached to the extremity on which the operation is to be performed. Excessive weights can cause traction injury to the brachial plexus. In our institution, somatosensory evoked potentials (SSEPs) may be used during surgery to detect any injury that may be developing.

If SSEP monitoring is used, a narcotic, nitrous oxide/oxygen, relaxant technique is recommended to avoid the effects of inhalation agents on the SSEPs.

Beach Chair Position

The patient is placed on the operating table in a sitting position after anesthesia has been induced. The table is flexed at the hips and knees. The patient is placed so that the shoulder on which the operation is to be performed is over the edge of the table.

Care must be taken to secure the patient on the table so that the patient does not fall off.

The endotracheal tube is secured to the opposite side from the surgery to prevent inadvertent kinking or dislodgment.

The head is kept in the neutral position and not turned away from the side of surgery, which can cause traction on the brachial plexus when traction is placed on the arm.

A neurosurgical head rest extension is used by some surgeons.

Arthroscopy of the shoulder is a complex procedure and may last for at least 1 hour or longer.

Choice of Anesthesia

General endotracheal anesthesia

The endotracheal tube must be properly secured. Movement of the shoulder during the procedure may lead to movement of the tube. Proper position should be checked.

Interscalene brachial plexus block is an excellent method of providing anesthesia for shoulder surgery and can be used whenever indicated.
　A superficial cervical plexus block should be performed for the posterior aspect of shoulder.

If irrigation pumps are used, the possibility of fluid dissection into the upper torso and neck with airway obstruction exists. This may be secondary to a tear in the capsule of the shoulder. The anesthesiologist should carefully monitor inflow and outflow volumes.[6]

Elbow Arthroscopy

Position

The patient may be prone or supine on the operating table.

Choice of Anesthesia

General anesthesia

Brachial plexus block
　The block must be working *100 percent* before the patient is placed in the prone position. Sedation is minimized in this position.

Hand Surgery

See Chapters 6 and 8.

Upper Extremity Brachial Plexus Blocks

For regional anesthesia for surgical procedures requiring about 1 hour, Chloro-procaine Methylparaben-free (MPF) formulation is used (see ch. 6 for choice of local anesthetic based on time consideration).

The use of long-acting local anesthetic agents for ambulatory surgery should be avoided if the anesthesiologist does not want the patient to be hanging around in the ambulatory center into the night.

Hip Arthroscopy

Arthroscopy of the hip is not a common procedure.

It is performed with the patient positioned on a fracture table with the use of a C-arm image intensifier. This setup may not be readily available in ambulatory surgery centers.

Choice of Anesthesia

General anesthesia

Spinal or epidural anesthesia

After the administration of anesthesia, the anesthesiologist should put on an x-ray apron and any other necessary protective devices such as a thyroid shield and lead glasses. A perineal post is inserted in the fracture table, traction is applied to the extremities, and the hip to be arthroscoped is abducted. The C-arm is placed. The arthroscope is inserted under guidance of the image intensifier. Adequate relaxation is required because of the need to move the hip during the procedure.

Knee Arthroscopy

This procedure is performed for diagnostic as well as operative procedures such as synovectomies, removal or repair of torn menisci, and reconstruction of torn ligaments. It is difficult to predict the length of time that will be needed for an arthroscopy because that will be determined by the findings.

Position

The patient is placed on the operating table in the supine position. The foot of the operating table is dropped, and the knees are flexed 90 degrees.

The thigh is immobilized in a leg holder, which is attached to the operating table. It consists of a soft circular foam collar held in place by rigid holders. This allows the leg to be manipulated and the thigh to be kept firmly in place above the knee.

The operated knee is controlled by the surgeon, who holds the extremity while manipulating the arthroscope and instruments.

Choice of Anesthesia

General anesthesia

Spinal anesthesia

Epidural anesthesia

Regional nerve block anesthesia consisting of femoral, sciatic, lateral femoral cutaneous, and obturator nerve blocks (a sciatic-femoral block is sufficient). Local anesthesia with sedation—an injection of 50 ml of 0.5 percent bupivacaine into the capsule of the knee joint

Local anesthesia with sedation

The surgeon infiltrates the ports with a local anesthetic agent, and the anesthesiologist provides sedation with a benzodiazepine such as midazolam and administers narcotics such as fentanyl, sufentanil, or alfentanil as needed. A propofol infusion may also be useful.

Sensory Block Only

Some surgeons want to have the patient move the leg while under sensory blockade. In such cases, use epidural anesthesia with a low concentration of anesthetic agent to provide sensory blockade but no motor blockade.

Surgical Procedure

After adequate anesthesia, the surgeon makes incisions for the arthroscopy instruments and channels for the irrigating fluid. The operation is performed with the capsule of the knee distended by irrigating fluid, which is introduced into the knee either by gravity or by a pump.

Tourniquet

A tourniquet is applied on the thigh, but it may not be inflated for the procedure. Whether a tourniquet is used depends on the procedure and the needs of the surgeon.

Pumps

On two occasions, after the use of a pump for the arthroscopy the entire lower extremity was found to be cold and swollen after the drapes were removed.

In one instance, the swelling extended into the scrotum and up the abdominal wall almost to the umbilicus.

In the other case, the swelling extended only up to the thigh.

The cause of this was extravasation of the irrigating fluid through a tear in the capsule of the knee and the dissection of the fluid along tissue planes. The concern in these situations was the possibility of the development of a compartment syndrome involving the calf. In the case in which the fluid had dissected into the scrotum, a Foley catheter was inserted to decompress the bladder and to provide a conduit for the urine if further swelling occurred. In both cases, fasciotomies did not have to be performed.

The patients were admitted to the hospital and observed. Within 12 hours the swelling had almost entirely disappeared, with the fluid being recruited back into the circulation.

Warning: If a tear in the capsule is suspected, the infusion pump should not be used. The irrigating solution should be monitored carefully as far as inflow and outflow volumes are concerned.

The anesthesiologist, the surgeon, and the nursing team should constantly be on the alert for the possibility of the development of this complication; constant observation is useful to help prevent this problem.

Special Observation after Lateral Releases

After lateral release, injury to the lateral geniculate artery may occur, leading to hematoma formation in the immediate postoperative period. This is usually avoided by placing a wound evacuation device after surgery. However, if this is not done, swelling may occur in the PACU. The surgeon should be notified if swelling occurs.

Ligament Reconstruction

Reconstruction of ligaments through the arthroscope has been developed. Reconstruction may be by the use of autologous tissue or tissue derived from a bone bank. This is a complex procedure requiring more than 1.5 hours, depending on the complexity of the problem.

This information is important when designing an anesthetic technique.

Warning: Make sure the anesthesia lasts as long as the surgery if regional anesthesia is used.

Ankle Arthroscopy

Position

The patient is placed on the operating table in the supine position.

Choice of Anesthesia

General anesthesia

Spinal anesthesia

Epidural anesthesia

Femoral-sciatic nerve blocks

Foot Surgery

After foot surgery, it is important to make sure the patient can ambulate without excessive pain.

To decrease swelling, the foot must be elevated above the level of the heart.

REDUCING THE PATIENT'S STAY IN THE RECOVERY ROOM

Narcotics such as meperidine and morphine should be avoided for premedication or intraoperative use.

If pain medication is required, short-acting narcotics should be used intravenously.

Prevention of Postoperative Nausea and Vomiting

The incidence of nausea and vomiting is higher after anesthesia with the use of narcotics as compared with an inhalation agent. If high doses of droperidol (more than 1.25 mg) are administered during anesthesia to prevent postoperative nausea, awakening may be prolonged.

Droperidol (0.625 to 1.25 mg IV) immediately after intubation is an effective antiemetic in outpatients. Those patients receiving droperidol had a lower incidence of nausea and vomiting in the PACU and a shorter length of stay than the control group.[3]

Droperidol may also cause extrapyramidal reactions consisting of restlessness, anxiety, and dystonia. Benztropine, which is a centrally acting anticholinergic, in a dose of 2 mg IM followed by 2 mg IV 15 minutes later is useful in relieving these symptoms. The dystonia can also be treated by β-blockers such as propranolol.

An induction with propofol followed by an inhalation agent will probably lessen the incidence of nausea and vomiting than if a narcotic were used.[4] Ondansetron, a new antiemetic agent, may also be useful for postoperative nausea and vomiting.

RECOVERY ROOM CARE

Make sure the tourniquet has been deflated and removed from the extremity.

Remove the underlying padding from beneath the tourniquet. This can act as a tourniquet itself.

Make certain the operated extremity is elevated properly.

> The hand should be above the level of the heart on a number of pillows or suspended from an intravenous pole. When the patient sits upright, the hand should be in a sling with the elbow lower than the hand, with the hand above the level of the heart.
>
> Elevate the foot in the recovery room above the level of the heart.
>
> Observe for adequate peripheral pulses, color, and warmth.
>
> Check the neurologic status by determining sensation and ability to move the fingers and toes.
>
> Check the forearm and the leg for swelling. Be alert for the development of a compartment syndrome.
>
> If any problems develop, alert the surgeon immediately.

Transfer from Recovery Bed to Chair

After General Anesthesia

Our PACU is divided into

Phase 1—immediate postoperative

Phase 2—lounge area where patient continues to recover until time of discharge

After an initial period in phase 1 when the patients are monitored as immediate postoperative patients, they are moved to phase 2 recovery, which is made up of lounge chairs with appropriate monitoring devices available. The patients are then placed in a sitting position and after a while are allowed to stand and then ambulate after they have received appropriate education based on their site of surgery.

After Spinal or Epidural Anesthesia

In the patient who has received spinal or epidural anesthesia, it is important to make certain that all motor strength and sensation has returned. Assuming the upright position and walking may be difficult if sensation has not returned because proprioception may be poor.

The ability of the patient to void is a good test of return of complete neurologic function. This is especially useful after spinal or epidural anesthesia.

After an Ankle Block

After an ankle block, the forefoot may remain numb for a rather long period of time even though epinephrine has not been and must not be used. If bupivacaine has been used, anesthesia may last for up to 24 hours. Such a patient may be discharged if a warning is given that sensation is not present and that the foot should be protected from injury. Lack of pain sensation may be beneficial to the patient in the immediate postoperative period at home.

Reasons for Keeping Patients in the Hospital

Pain that cannot be controlled with oral analgesics

Prolonged nausea and vomiting

Bleeding

Inability to ambulate as had been planned

PATIENT DISCHARGE

Getting the Patient Home

The patient must be motivated to go home.

The patient must be able to follow instructions.

The accompanying responsible adult should be able to care for the patient.

Role of the Surgeon

Should not undertake a major surgical procedure on an outpatient basis if the procedure will not allow the patient to be ready to be discharged in a reasonable time

Provide specific discharge instructions

Prescribe medication for control of postoperative pain

Role of the Anesthesiologist

Tailor the anesthetic management and technique so that the patient will be ready to go home in a reasonable time

Evaluate the patient in the PACU for home readiness

Role of the PACU Nurse

Encourage the patient to be motivated to go home

Review discharge instructions with the patient

Make certain the patient has proper prescriptions for pain medication

Discuss home care with the responsible person

Role of the Responsible Person

Arrive in PACU on time to take the patient home when ready

Check with the nurse and surgeon if necessary for home care instructions

Be willing to provide necessary at-home care for the patient

Postanesthesia Recovery Scoring Systems

Scoring systems can be used to determine if the patient is ready for discharge from the ambulatory center.

Early Release

Avoid premedication

Avoid postoperative pain because this is a common cause of nausea and vomiting (one of the major postanesthesia problems in ambulatory recovery areas).

Control pain in the PACU with small does of narcotics. Use rapid-acting narcotics intravenously and titrate until the desired effect is achieved.

Discharge Instructions

Patients should be provided with specific written discharge instructions.

These instructions should be read to the patient, and then the form should be given to the patient with instructions to retain the form at home on discharge.

There is a higher incidence of compliance in patients who are given written discharge instructions.[5]

Understanding the Language

In patients who do not understand and speak English, smiling and nodding of the head should not be accepted as evidence of comprehension of instructions. Everything told to the patient should be clearly understood whether the instructions are given directly to the patient or through an interpreter. On many occasions, an adult who does not speak or understand the language is accompanied by an older child or adolescent who may understand some of what is said but does not understand the significance.

Discharge Criteria

Clear sensorium

Stable vital signs

Ability to understand instructions

Ability to ambulate easily

Ability to tolerate oral fluids

Free from nausea and vomiting

Void before discharge

Specific Criteria for Orthopedic Surgical Patients

1. Dry wound with no bleeding or oozing.
2. Evidence of good circulation to the operated extremity.
3. Return of sensation, except in instances in which long-acting anesthetic agents have been used to provide postoperative pain relief.
   In this situation undue pressure should not be placed on the extremity nor should it be placed in a position where nerve damage can occur. Hot or cold items should not be allowed to touch the extremity.
4. In an extremity with a cast, no evidence of swelling, impaired circulation, or decreased sensation.

Postrelease Assistance

A mechanism must be in place for the patient to contact someone at the facility for help if a complication should arise.

Arrangements should be in place to be able to see the patient on n emergency basis if a problem arises that requires medical attention.

If the patient undergoing ambulatory surgery lives far from the ambulatory surgery facility, it is important that the patient has an emergency department close to home. If the patient must go to a close-by emergency department, the patient should also be told to inform the anesthesiologist, surgeon, or nursing personnel in the emergency department where the surgery was performed.

REFERENCES

1. Meridy HW: Criteria for selection of ambulatory surgery patients and guidelines for anesthetic management: a retrospective study of 1553 cases. Anesth Analg 61:921, 1982
2. White PF: Studies of desflurane in outpatient anesthesia. Anesth Analg 75:S47, 1992
3. Wetchler BV, Collins IS, Jacob L: Antiemetic effects of droperidol on the ambulatory surgery patient. Anesthesiol Rev 9:23, 1982
4. Gaskey NG, Ferriero L, Pournaras L et al: Use of fentanyl markedly increases nausea and vomiting in gynecological short-stay patients. Am Assoc Nurs Anesth J 54:309, 1986
5. Malens AF: Do they do as they are instructed? A review of outpatient anaesthesia. Anaesthesia 33:832, 1978
6. Hynson JM, Tung A, Guevara JE et al: Complete airway obstruction during arthroscopic shoulder surgery. Anesth Analg 76:875, 1993

10

Pediatric Orthopedics

Pediatric orthopedic surgery involves the care of patients with discrete musculoskeletal abnormalities for which operative correction is undertaken, as well as orthopedic problems associated with defects of major organ systems of the body.

We often develop a rapport with the child and parents because of their repeated return to the operating room for multiple procedures.

The anesthesiologist should become familiar with the different conditions involved in pediatric orthopedics. Consultation with the pediatrician and orthopedic surgeon will help to develop a treatment plan for those children who must undergo several orthopedic procedures.

NECK PROBLEMS

Congenital Muscular Torticollis

In congenital muscular torticollis, unilateral contraction of the sternocleidomastoid muscle occurs as a result of fibrosis. The head is tilted on the side of the shortened muscle with the chin pointed to the opposite side.[1,2]

Clinical Manifestations

Face is widened.

Position of eyes and ears changes to remain parallel to the ground although head is tilted.

Deep cervical fascia is thickened.

Anterior and medial scalene muscles are shortened.

Carotid sheath with vessels contracts.

Scoliosis may develop.

Deformity is noted at birth or very soon thereafter.[1,2]

Anesthetic Considerations

Contracture of the sternocleidomastoid muscle with altered position of the head and deformity of the facial structures may present a problem in airway management and endotracheal intubation.

Muscle relaxants should be avoided before determining the status of the upper airway.

Anesthesia is induced with an inhalation agent that can provide muscular relaxation at deeper levels of anesthesia to be able to visualize the vocal cords under spontaneous respiration.

A muscle relaxant can be administered to facilitate endotracheal intubation once it has been determined that the airway can be visualized.

Fiberoptic intubation may be necessary if visualization of the vocal cords is not possible.

Surgical Procedure

An incision is made over the sternocleidomastoid muscle parallel to the clavicle with deeper dissection and severing of the clavicular head and sternal head of the muscle.

Patients are then placed in restraints to prevent return of the head to the former position.[1,2]

Klippel-Feil Syndrome

Klippel-Feil syndrome is a congenital condition more common in females in which synostosis of the cervical vertebrae occurs, with fusion of two or more in the cervical region.[1,3,4]

Clinical Manifestations

There is shortening of the neck and limitation of lateral motion. When more than two vertebrae are fused, the neck is short and the head appears to sit directly on the thorax.

There is marked limitation of motion of the cervical spine. Flexion and extension are intact because these occur between the occiput and atlas.[1,3,4]

Associated Congenital Deformities

Torticollis

Webbing of soft tissues of neck

Congenital high scapula (Sprengel's deformity)

Cervical ribs

Scoliosis

Kyphosis

Cleft palate

Lung abnormalities

Ovarian agenesis

Patent foramen ovale

Hearing problems—deafness

Interventricular septal defect[1,3]

Kidney malformation

Anesthetic Considerations

Awareness of the possible presence of the Klippel-Feil syndrome should lead to evaluation of the neck in patients with short necks who are being considered for surgery.

Manipulation of the neck in Klippel-Feil syndrome is avoided because it may lead to neurologic changes as a result of compression of the spinal cord.[3]

Fiberoptic intubation should be used if any question arises concerning airway management.

CONGENITAL HIGH SCAPULA

Congenital high scapula (Sprengel's deformity) is caused by an upward and forward displacement of the scapula and leads to asymmetric shoulders.[1]

Associated Deformities

Scoliosis and kyphosis

Torticollis

Klippel-Feil syndrome[1]

Surgical Procedure

The surgical procedure involves release of muscles, removal of the omovertebral bone that may be present, and excision of portions of the scapula. The scapula is then displaced distally and held in position by wires.[1]

Position

The patient is anesthetized in the supine position and then placed prone on the operating table with the head and neck extending beyond the operating table, supported on a head rest. Supports are placed under the anterior part of the chest and under the ipsilateral side of the pelvis, tilting the patient to the opposite side. The patient's chin is placed on the head rest, which must be well padded.

Adequate blood must be available because the procedure may involve a fair amount of blood loss.[1]

CERVICAL SPINE PROBLEMS

Conditions associated with spinal deformities[5] include

Apert syndrome

Treacher Collins syndrome

Larsen syndrome

Klippel-Feil syndrome

Morquio syndrome

Down syndrome

Congenital scoliosis

Osteogenesis imperfecta

Neurofibromatosis

Disproportionate dwarfism

Odontoid Process

The odontoid process is the upward extension of the C2 vertebra and lies against the posterior aspect of the anterior arch of C1. It is kept in position by the transverse axial ligament and other ligaments, which ensure that the odontoid process does not move into the area of the cervical canal occupied by the spinal cord.

The odontoid process may be separated from the body of C2 because of congenital causes such as lack of fusion or trauma.

Trauma

As a result of trauma, the tip of the odontoid process may be separated and lie between the arch of the atlas and the spinal cord.

After a history of mild trauma, there may be only pain and limitation of motion of the neck or there may be signs of spinal cord compression or even quadriplegia.

The clinical picture after trauma with a fracture of the odontoid process may be similar to the picture seen with congenital separation of the odontoid, known as os odontoideum.[6]

The absence of stability between the axis and atlas will cause the anterior body of the axis and the base of the odontoid process to impinge on the spinal cord when the neck is slightly flexed. The atlas rides forward on the axis during this maneuver.

The neck must be kept in *extension* to reduce the dislocation and provide stability.

Treatment may be a plaster cast with the neck in extension. If this treatment fails, surgery involving a posterior cervical spinal fusion is carried out.[3]

Abnormalities

The following situations exist:

1. Congenital separation—os odontoideum
2. Congenital absence
3. Hypoplasia
4. Infection of the retropharyngeal space—Grisel syndrome
5. Trauma—absorption of the odontoid process after fracture[6]

The anesthesiologist involved in the care of pediatric patients should be aware of and consult with the orthopedic surgeon when patients with the foregoing syndromes are scheduled for surgery. Cervical spine radiographs in flexion and extension as well as magnetic resonance imaging may be necessary before surgery to detect an anomaly of the cervical spine.

If anomalies of the cervical spine exist, it may be necessary to stabilize these surgically before embarking on other procedures in the patient.

Clinical Manifestations

Patients with hypoplasia of the odontoid cannot maintain the alignment of the axis and the atlas. Therefore, in hyperextension the first cervical vertebrae can move anteriorly on the axis, causing a decrease in the available area for the cord with possible compression.

Patients with Morquio syndrome with odontoid hypoplasia are at risk for traumatic quadriparesis after minor trauma.[7]

Achondroplastic dwarfs may develop cervical spinal stenosis and foramen magnum stenosis. They do not have a significant incidence of odontoid abnormalities except that the odontoid process may encroach on the foramen magnum.

Traumatic Atlantoaxial Subluxation

Cervical spine injuries in children occur in the region of the atlantoaxial articulation.

Atlantoaxial subluxation as a result of tearing of the transverse axial ligament can occur, which may result in a decreased area for the spinal cord.

Diagnosis

Lateral flexion radiographs of the cervical spine are obtained in patients who complain of pain in the neck after an injury.

Cervical spine radiographs are obtained in all patients suffering from head injury or facial injury.

In adults, the normal distance between the posterior aspect of the anterior arch of the atlas and the dens in 3 mm.

There is no definite figure for normal atlas dens interval in children. Steel[8] suggests an upper limit of 4 mm in adults.

Fielding[9] suggests the upper limit of normal is 5 mm in adults.

Treatment

1. Immobilization in jackets
2. Surgical fusion

Anesthetic Considerations

If the patients are placed in halo traction before surgery with fixation to a vest, endotracheal intubation will be difficult because the halo interferes with ability to move the head.

It may be more advantageous to perform the endotracheal intubation before application of the halo, during which time the head is held in extension and then fixed after intubation.

If endotracheal intubation must be performed after application of the halo, fiberoptic intubation will be necessary.

The wrenches should always be available to release the halo immediately if fiberoptic intubation cannot be performed and direct laryngoscopy is necessary. The anesthesiologist and the surgeon should cooperate and be facile in adjusting the connections of the halo.

The patient should be kept in extension before induction of anesthesia to decrease the encroachment on the spinal cord by the odontoid process.

Somatosensory evoked potential (SSEP) monitoring may be used to monitor spinal cord function. If this is the case, a narcotic, nitrous oxide/oxygen, relaxant technique is used for maintenance of anesthesia.

Position

The head is kept in extension during positioning.

Anesthetic Management During Radiographic Evaluation

Myelography, computed tomography (CT) scanning, or magnetic resonance imaging may be necessary in patients with cervical spine injuries who may not be cooperative during a radiographic study.

Ketamine may be used if no other injuries are present. Under ketamine anesthesia, the patients remain calm and tolerate the procedure. A propofol infusion may also be used.

Trisomy 21 (Down Syndrome)

Patients with trisomy 21 may have laxity of the transverse axial ligament. Extension of the head may cause the atlas to sublux onto the axis. Before anesthesia in patients with Down syndrome, cervical spine radiographs in neutral, extension, and flexion are obtained. The compression of the cord by the odontoid process may be seen in extension in some patients and in flexion or in neutral radiographic views in other patients. If abnormalities of the cervical spine are noted, care must be exercised during intubation and positioning.

Juvenile Rheumatoid Arthritis

Abnormality of the cervical spine may be present in patients with juvenile rheumatoid arthritis. Atlantoaxial subluxation is marked by an increase in the distance between the atlas and the odontoid process. It is noted on cervical spine films with the neck flexed.

Anesthetic Management for Posterior Cervical Spine Fusion

The neck is kept in extension to prevent injury to the cervical spinal cord. The patient may be placed in a halo apparatus to maintain stability.

General anesthesia is induced in the supine position.

After induction of anesthesia, the halo may have to be loosened and the head placed in extension to intubate the patient. If this is not performed, the handle of the laryngoscope will abut against the halo and intubation may not be possible. If neck motion is not allowed, a fiberoptic intubation is necessary.

Case Study

A 4-year-old child with Morquio syndrome was placed into a halo vest for cervical spine stabilization before surgery. After general anesthesia was induced, endotracheal intubation could not be performed because the handle of the laryngoscope abutted against the halo. The halo had to be loosened before intubation.

In this case, it was acceptable to loosen the halo and extend the neck because preoperative radiographs revealed stability in extension.

Note: Do not extubate until the patient is awake and has control of the airway because management of the airway may be difficult with the halo in place.

LOWER EXTREMITY PROBLEMS

Congenital Club Foot

Congenital club foot (talipes equinovarus) may be related to neurologic, neuromuscular, teratogenic, genetic, embryonic, or environmental factors.[1]

Acquired club foot may be as a result of such conditions as poliomyelitis, intraspinal tumors, myelomeningocele, progressive muscular atrophy, or cerebral palsy.

Surgical Management

If conservative measures cannot correct the club foot, surgery will be recommended. Surgery involves soft tissue releases, tendon transfers, and in some instances, osteotomies.

Operative procedures on congenital club foot are usually performed in the first few months of life.

The Child with the "Runny" Nose

Some of the problems hindering the completion of surgery are constant colds or runny noses. It is important to try to schedule the child for operation when problems in the upper respiratory tract have been stabilized.

Premedication

Premedication usually consists of atropine.

Anesthetic Considerations

The child is brought to the holding room accompanied by the parent. The patient is then transferred to the operating room accompanied by the anesthesiologist and circulating nurse. At the discretion of the institution, parents occasionally accompany the child into the operating room.

Intravenous Access

The main problem is securing an intravenous line, which is usually reserved for the period after induction of anesthesia.

Monitoring

Monitoring devices include electrocardiogram (ECG), blood pressure cuff, pulse oximeter, end-tidal carbon dioxide monitor, precordial stethoscope, and temperature probe.

Anesthetic Induction

Induction of anesthesia is usually carried out by administering halothane, nitrous oxide, and oxygen by mask. Succinylcholine is avoided. Atracurium or vecuronium is used to facilitate endotracheal intubation.

Starting the Intravenous Line

When the patient is adequately anesthetized, an assistant is asked to insert the intravenous line. The dorsum of the hand is the site that is most useful. However, intravenous lines may have to be inserted into the external jugular vein or the scalp.

Parents do not like to see intravenous lines in the scalp, and these should be used only when absolutely necessary. The parents should be told that this route may be necessary if all other attempts fail.

Anesthetic Maintenance

Anesthesia is maintained with nitrous oxide, oxygen, and an inhalation agent after endotracheal intubation is accomplished by means of a muscle relaxant. End-tidal carbon dioxide monitoring is then instituted.

Intravenous Narcotics for Postoperative Pain Relief

Toward the end of the procedure, a small dose of a narcotic such as 5 μg/kg fentanyl or 0.5 mg/kg meperidene if the patient received narcotics preoperatively and 1 mg/kg meperidene if none had been given is administered intravenously. The child wakes up alert, calm, and pain-free.

The procedure is performed under tourniquet. Blood loss is usually 10 to 15 ml.

Body Temperature

Body temperature is monitored throughout the procedure, and efforts are made to keep the child normothermic. Body temperature may rise when tourniquets are used (see Ch. 7). Elevated body temperature may occur if the child is warmed during the procedure.[10]

Casting

At the end of the procedure, a cast is applied. The patient is kept anesthetized until the cast hardens.

The child is transferred to the recovery room and sent back to his or her room when completely recovered.

Postoperative Pain Medication

Rectal acetaminophen is given during the first 24 hours.

The parents who stay with the children postoperatively throughout the night have never indicated that the children suffer from pain.

Change of Plaster

Three weeks after the original surgery, the patient is brought back to the operating room for change of plaster.

Preoperative laboratory testing for patients undergoing change of plaster is not usually obtained. Only if the patient has shown signs or symptoms of problems in the interval between the operative procedure and the scheduled change of plaster is further laboratory work requested.

Change of plaster is usually a very quick procedure, and the anesthesia is carried out by mask using nitrous oxide, oxygen, and halothane.

Monitoring for this procedure is by means of ECG, blood pressure cuff, pulse oximeter, and precordial stethoscope.

An intravenous line is usually not placed.

Developmental Dislocation of the Hip

Normal growth and development of the hip joint will not occur unless the head of the femur and the acetabulum are in their normal anatomic relationship.

Etiology

1. Ligamentous laxity—laxity of the capsule of the hip joint and ligaments
2. Malposition in utero—breech position at birth
3. Extension of the hips during breech delivery[1]
4. Genetic
5. Occurs in females more frequently

Treatment

Closed Reduction

Closed reduction of the hip involves application of a hip spica.

It is usually performed in patients who are between 2 and 18 months old.

Closed reduction and application of a hip spica for developmental dislocation of the hip may be carried out under general endotracheal anesthesia. The child is placed on a spica table for application of the cast.

Warning:

The patient is anesthetized on the operating table in the supine position. Careful attention should be paid to the endotracheal tube during the maneuvers involved in moving the child from the operating table onto the hip spica table.

The endotracheal tube is disconnected from the breathing circuit when moving the child to avoid dislodgment and accidental extubation. The endotracheal tube is held at the mouth with one hand while supporting the head with the other.

Open Reduction

Open reduction of the hip for developmental dislocation of the hip is usually performed in children between 18 to 36 months of age.

Soft Tissue Releases

Soft tissue releases are performed in an attempt to provide contact between the femoral head and the pelvis.

Osteotomies

Osteotomies, bone grafts, and soft tissue releases may be necessary to develop a covering for the femoral head. Fixation with pins and wires may be used to stabilize the fragments.

Derotational Osteotomy of the Femur

Derotational osteotomy of the femur is performed if the femoral head is not placed concentrically in the acetabular socket.

An osteotomy is performed in the subtrochanteric area of the femur. The distal fragment is externally rotated and fixed so that the femoral head is placed in a less anteverted position.[1]

This surgery may be performed in conjunction with pelvic reconstruction.

Blood Loss

Blood loss should be determined by means of measuring the blood in the suction and weighing the sponges. Adequate replacement should be carried out as needed.

Coxa Vara

Coxa vara is a failure of the mean angle of the femoral neck and shaft to decrease to 120 degrees from 148 degrees.

A valgus osteotomy of the proximal femur is performed in this procedure.

The femoral head and neck are osteotomized and placed into the acetabulum in a horizontal position.[1]

Slipped Capital Femoral Epiphysis

In slipped capital femoral epiphysis, forces on the epiphyseal plate cause the femoral head to shift from its normal position on the femur. This condition is seen in young adolescents.[1]

Patient Characteristics

Slipped capital femoral epiphysis is an emergency and should be treated quickly.

It is seen frequently in young, large, and obese individuals.

The patient is placed in traction immediately.

Surgical Treatment

The treatment for this condition is surgical, and the operation is dependent on the extent of the displacement of the femoral head.

Hip pinning is performed with the patient on a fracture table under image intensification. A series of pins are passed through the lateral aspect of the femur into the femoral head, avoiding the hip joint.

Anesthetic Considerations

There are usually no associated illnesses or conditions with slipped capital femoral epiphysis.

The tall, obese adolescent in whom this condition frequently occurs should be managed so that aspiration of gastric contents is avoided. The patient is prepared with metoclopramide and ranitidine to help empty the stomach and to increase the pH of the gastric contents.

Congenital Pseudarthrosis of the Tibia

Congenital pseudarthrosis of the tibia is weakening of the bone in the distal half of the tibia with failure of normal bone formation. There is anterior angulation and pathologic fracture.

There appears to be a relationship between congenital pseudarthrosis of the tibia and neurofibromatosis.[1]

Management in this condition involves caring for a patient who may return for multiple surgical procedures with some failures occurring. Psychological support of the patient and good rapport with the family is of vital importance.

Anesthetic Management

After an intravenous line is obtained, the patient can be induced with intravenous barbiturates followed by endotracheal intubation with muscle relaxants and maintained with an inhalation agent.

Surgical Procedure

Many corrective procedures have been advocated; however, there is no one method that is known to be completely effective.

UPPER EXTREMITY PROBLEMS

Syndactyly

Syndactyly is an anomaly of the hand in which the skin of the fingers is not separated, leading to webbing. In some instances, the bones and joints of the fingers may be involved as well as the skin.

Syndactyly may be an isolated condition, or it may be associated with other abnormalities such as acrocephalosyndactyly.

The *acrocephalosyndactylies* are a group of conditions with abnormalities in the skull and face as well as the extremities and include such conditions as

  Apert syndrome

  Pfeiffer syndrome

  Carpenter syndrome

  Crouzon syndrome

In these conditions, there are associated cranial abnormalities, facial abnormalities, and abnormalities of the palate.

Early treatment involves surgery on the skull to avoid increased intracranial pressure.[1,11,12]

Anesthetic Considerations

Problems involve securing the airway because of the associated facial abnormalities.[11,12] Endotracheal intubation should be performed only after visualization of the vocal cords is ensured under spontaneous ventilation.

Supracondylar Fractures of the Humerus

Supracondylar fractures of the humerus in children may lead to ischemic muscle contracture because of the vascular compromise that may occur with this fracture. Reduction of supracondylar fractures is a medical emergency and should be performed as soon as possible after the injury to decrease the chances of vascular compromise.

Congenital Constrictive Bands

Constrictive bands (Streeter's dysplasia) may be present at birth, affecting either the upper or lower extremity.[3]

The constrictions associated with the bands may impair circulation of both blood and lymphatics, resulting in a swollen extremity distal to the band.[3]

These bands may form from improper embryonic development of the extremity[1,3] or from failure of development of the mesodermal masses under the skin.

Anesthetic Considerations

This condition does not require any special anesthetic considerations.

Avoidance of Hypotension

Hypotension should be avoided because the constricting bands may interfere with blood supply. Normal blood pressure aids in perfusion of the tissues during the procedure and is beneficial to the outcome.

Surgical Procedure

Deep bands are divided and excised down to normal structures by use of a Z-plasty incision. This may be performed in stages to avoid circulatory problems.

Associated Problems in Patients with Limb Abnormalities

Craniofacial abnormalities (cleft lip, cleft palate, abnormalities of the respiratory tract)

Cardiac anomalies (Holt-Oram syndrome is associated with atrial septal defect and radial aplasia; atrial and ventricular rhythm disturbances and conduction defects may be present[3])

Vater syndrome (*v*ertebra, *a*nus, *t*racheal, *e*sophageal fistula, *r*enal) (Vertebral abnormalities, scoliosis, imperforate anus, tracheal esophageal fistula, and renal abnormalities; possible congenital heart disease and absence of the radius[3])

Renal problems (Fanconi syndrome—renal acidosis, bone marrow abnormalities, hypoplasia, and pancytopenia are associated with abnormalities of the radius[3])

OTHER MEDICAL DISORDERS

Myelodysplasia, Latex Allergy, and Anaphylactic Reactions

Clinical Manifestations

Neural tube defects result in abnormalities of the spinal cord and surrounding tissues, causing disorders such as myelomeningocele and spina bifida.[1,13]

Loss of sensation and motor function is frequently related to the spinal level of the disorder.[1]

Also, many of these patients have other congenital deformities, including genitourinary and orthopedic anomalies.[1]

Patients with myelomeningocele and spina bifida frequently undergo multiple procedures during their lifetime, including repair of the meningocele, ventriculoperitoneal shunt (more than 80 percent of patients), and orthopedic surgery.[1]

Surgical Procedures

Orthopedic procedures are oriented toward correcting spinal deformities such as scoliosis as well as correcting deformities of the hip, knee, foot, and ankle that result from contractures, fibrosis, and muscle imbalance.[1]

Allergy and Anaphylactic Reactions to Latex

Anaphylatic reactions to latex characterized by marked decreases in blood pressure and elevated airway pressures requiring intravenous epinephrine and cardiopulmonary resuscitation have been reported in myelodysplasia cases.[14-20] Slater[14] reported two such cases in 1989, one case during hamstring lengthening and one during ventriculoperitoneal shunt revision. After Slater's initial report, other cases surfaced, and investigations were conducted in myelodysplasia clinics and hospitals to determine the incidence of latex allergy among the patient population.[15,16] Patients with myelodysplasia are frequently exposed to latex gloves and catheters, and complaints of rashes, urticaria, and respiratory symptoms are common.[14-20]

In a study conducted at 16 Shriners hospitals, a 22 percent incidence of allergy was reported and 22 of 2,925 children had anaphylactic reactions.[16]

Allergic reactions to latex and rubber result from exposure to these products, which are produced from the *H. brasiliensis* tree, and are probably mediated through IgE reactions. Continued exposure to latex-containing items such as rubber gloves and catheters are thought to contribute to the development of the allergy.[14–20]

An allergic interaction with materials sterilized with ethylene oxide appears to also exist in these patients.[18]

Although some authors suggest skin prick tests or radioallergosorbent test (RAST) to determine latex allergy, others do not believe this is mandatory in patients with myelodysplasia.[18,19]

Current recommendations for patients with myelodysplasia as outlined by the Shriners Hospital[16] and the *Morbidity and Mortality Weekly Review*[20] include

1. Determine whether an allergic history is present.
2. Create a latex-free environment during the hospital stay.
3. Administer prophylactic medications for allergic patients 24 hours preoperatively and 24 hours postoperatively.
   Diphenhydramine 1 mg/kg every 6 hours, maximum dose of 50 mg
   Methylprednisolene 1 mg/kg every 6 hours, maximum dose 125 mg
   Cimetidine 5 mg/kg every 6 hours, maximum dose 300 mg

Additional intraoperative considerations include

1. Put a "Latex Free Environment" sign on operating room door.
2. Do not use a rubber face mask or rubber tubing.
3. Wear nonlatex gloves.
4. Avoid using intravenous tubing with rubber injection ports—use stopcocks.
5. Filter drugs drawn up by using filtered needles—check with the pharmacy for these.
6. Pad skin areas that might come in contact with items that might contain latex or rubber (e.g., Webril padding under a blood pressure cuff).
7. Do not inject through the rubber port in the intravenous bag.
8. Use urinary catheters that are latex-free.
9. Have an epinephrine infusion ready.

Arthrogryposis

Arthrogryposis is characterized by congenital immobility of multiple joints fixed in different postures. Arthrogryposis is from the Greek word meaning "curved joints."[21]

Disease Presentation

Arthrogryposis may be noted at birth or in the first few months of life.

Disease Types

Neuropathic—results from a developmental defect in the central nervous system. A narrow spinal cord and abnormalities in the neural canal are present in 50 percent of patients with arthrogryposis.[1,3,22]

Myopathic—may represent intrauterine progressive muscular dystrophy. Site of the disease is in the muscles; the joint changes are secondary to the muscle changes. The contractures are caused by a shortening of the flexor muscles.[3,22]

Mixed—may be a mixed form of arthrogryposis in which findings of both the neuropathic and myopathic forms are present.[1,3,22]

Clinical Manifestations

Arthrogryposis usually affects all four limbs but sometimes only one or two are involved.

Joints are fixed in extension or flexion.

Skin is tense and glossy with an absence of normal skin creases.

Intelligence is usually normal, but mental retardation may be present in the severe neuropathic form.

Club feet, dislocated hips, and subluxation or dislocation of the knees may be present.

Shoulders are internally rotated.

Forearms are pronated; wrists and fingers are flexed.[1,3,22]

Associated Conditions

Mandibular hypoplasia, which may make exposure of the larynx and endotracheal intubation difficult.

Scoliosis with rib cage deformities resulting in abnormal pulmonary function (some deformities are of such a magnitude that the rib cage and iliac crest are practically touching each other)

Dislocation of the hip

Cardiac abnormalities

Abnormalities of the genitourinary tract[1,3,22]

Surgical Procedure

In the upper extremity, osteotomies, capsulotomies, and tissue releases to place the joints in positions of use are performed.

Other surgical treatments include procedures for correction of scoliosis.

Anesthetic Considerations

Intravenous Access

Intravenous access is usually very difficult because of the abnormalities of the joints and alterations in the soft tissues.

There is no definite delineation of anatomic structures because of the pronation of the forearms.

Intubation

Intubation may be difficult if mandibular hypoplasia is present.

Position

Contracture of joints and severe kyphoscoliosis make positioning the patient difficult.

Ventilatory Problems

Postoperative ventilatory problems will occur in patients with severe kyphoscoliosis.

Achondroplasia

Achondroplasia may develop as a result of a new mutation. The reduction in height may be due to shortness of the lower limbs.[23]

Clinical Manifestations

Enlarged head, possibly caused by hydrocephalus

Small foramen magnum with possible signs of spinal cord compression.

Abnormalities of the odontoid process with encroachment on the small foramen magnum

Shortness of limbs

Prominent mandible, short maxilla

Chest deformity[1,23,24]

Spinal Involvement

The spinal canal tapers from the top to the bottom.

Also, the vertebral structure is abnormal.[24]

Surgical Procedures

These patients may present for spinal surgery to relieve spinal stenosis.

Anesthetic Considerations

Cervical spine abnormalities may cause problems in flexion and extension.

The cervical spine should not be hyperextended or hyperflexed during intubation.[23,25]

Osteogenesis Imperfecta

The major error in osteogenesis imperfecta is in the synthesis of collagen. Poor bone formation results in fractures.[1,3,26]

Clinical Manifestations

Type I (osteogenesis imperfecta congenita): is the severe form of the disease. Fractures and deformities are noted at birth. Intracranial hemorrhage usually results in death.[1,3,26]

Type II (osteogenesis imperfecta tarda gravis): is a less severe form of the disease. Fractures are common because of the abnormal bones, which are osteopenic. These fractures occur during infancy. The vertebrae may fracture easily.[1,3,26]

Type III (osteogenesis imperfecta tarda levis): fractures occur later.

In the Levis form, blue sclerae may be the only manifestation, and there may not be any fractures at all.

Characteristics

The patient appears short because of deformities of the limbs caused by angulation and overriding of the fractures.[1,3,23,26]

Blue sclerae are present. This is because of the thinness of the sclera, permitting visibility of the intraocular pigment.

Laxity of ligaments leads to hypermobile joints and increased joint dislocation.

Odontoid problems or atlantoaxial instability may be present. Radiographs in flexion and extension will demonstrate whether subluxation is present.

Marked kyphoscoliosis may be present.

Chest wall appears small. There may be poor compliance.

Forehead is broad; head is enlarged.

There may be middle ear deafness.

Inguinal, umbilical, and diaphragmatic hernias are common.

Other characteristics include

Scoliosis

Brittle teeth

Abnormal platelet function

Aortic and mitral regurgitation

Medial necrosis of the aorta[1,3,23,26]

Metabolic Abnormalities

Increased sweating, heat intolerance, and increased body temperature

Tachycardia at rest

Tachypnea

These findings suggest a relationship with hyperthyroidism; however, increased serum thyroxine levels have not been noted.

Hyperthermia during anesthesia has been seen, which is part of the disease itself. However, occasionally a patient manifests true malignant hyperthermia.[27]

Hypermetabolism with increased temperature, and tachycardia must be distinguished from the onset of malignant hyperthermia. Malignant hyperthermia may occur in patients with osteogenesis imperfecta, but there is not an increased risk in these patients.

Leukocyte metabolism studies suggest an uncoupling of oxidative phosphorylation.

Platelet function studies demonstrate defects in adhesion and clot retraction.

Cardiovascular Abnormalities

Aortic and mitral regurgitation

Medial necrosis of the aorta

Surgical Procedures

Intramedullary rodding is performed to correct fractures of long bones. Sofield procedures involve segmental osteotomies of the fractured long bones with insertion of rods to correct the deformities. Further developments in rodding have taken place using elongating rods to take growth into consideration.[28]

Another surgical procedure is correction of scoliosis by spinal instrumentation.

Anesthetic Considerations

Deafness may make communication difficult.

Antibiotic prophylaxis is provided if cardiac abnormalities are present.

Any manipulation in these patients can lead to fractures.

Care is used in applying blood pressure cuffs and placing tourniquets for intravenous lines.

Application of a pneumatic tourniquet to the limbs for control of bleeding during surgery may cause fractures and may possibly have to be avoided.[23]

Securing the Airway

The oral airway is inserted carefully—teeth are easily broken. Care should be taken during endotracheal intubation.

The enlarged head may cause problems in positioning. A folded sheet is placed under the shoulders to bring the occiput in line with the rest of the body.

Cervical spine fractures may occur during positioning of the head.[1,3,23,26]

Intraoperative Considerations

Metabolic Abnormalities

Tachycardia and elevated body temperature may occur as a result of metabolic abnormalities and thyroid dysfunction.

This abnormality is apparently not related to malignant hyperthermia and can be treated with conservative measures. However, it is important to be on the alert for malignant hyperthermia.

Cardiovascular Problems

Cardiovascular problems include valvular disease.

Increases in blood pressure with forceful ejection against the wall of the aorta are avoided because medial necrosis of the aorta may be present.

Scoliosis

Ventilatory support is needed if ventilation abnormalities exist.

Postoperative Care

Tachycardia and hyperthermia may be present. Use surface cooling.

Ensure adequate ventilation.

Observe for abnormal bleeding caused by platelet dysfunction.

Case Study

A patient with osteogenesis imperfecta had a rapid heart rate in the postanesthesia care unit. The pediatric resident thought it was a result of volume overload and administered furosemide. Severe hypotension developed because of the loss of intravascular fluid following the diuresis.

The tachycardia was a manifestation of the hypermetabolic state, which did not require treatment.

Craniofacial Abnormalities

Apert Syndrome

Clinical Manifestations

1. Syndactyly of the hands and feet, which is a failure of separation of the fingers and toes leading to a fusiform mass
2. Craniosynostosis affecting the coronal suture (head peaked and vertically elongated; possible increased intracranial pressure may result)
3. Increased intracranial pressure
4. Prominent mandible (fusion defects of the maxilla and mandible seen)
5. High arched posterior palate (cleft palate present in approximately 35 percent)
6. Sphenoid, ethmoid, and maxillary hypoplasia (malocclusion)
7. Spinal deformities[1,11,12]

Treatment
Early treatment involves neurosurgical procedures to provide space for the brain to expand.[1,11,12]

Pfeiffer Syndrome

Clinical Manifestations
   Craniosynostis

   Wide towering skull

   Hypoplastic mandible and maxilla

   Possible cleft palate

   Syndactyly of the thumbs and great toes

   Depressed nasal bridge[11,12]

Carpenter Syndrome

Clinical Manifestations
   Cloverleaf-shaped skull because of the rate of fusion of the different cranial sutures

   Short neck

   Omphalocele

   Syndactyly

   Hypoplasia of the middle phalanges[11,12]

Cardiac Defects
Cardiac defects include atrial and ventricular septal defects, patent ductus arteriosis, pulmonary stenosis, and tetralogy of Fallot.[11,12]

Crouzon Syndrome

Clinical Manifestations
   Widened skull, hypoplasia of the maxilla. No special shape of the skull because closure of the sutures occurs in a variable manner.

   Hypoplastic maxilla

   High arched palate

   May be associated with increased intracranial pressure

   Spinal deformities[11,12]

Whistling Face Syndrome

Clinical Manifestations

Flat stiff face

Small mouth

Tissue band at midchin

Talipes equinovarus[11]

Anesthetic Considerations

The status of the patient's intracranial pressure and intracranial compliance must be addressed.[11]

1. Avoid medications that will cause hypoventilation.
2. Plan premedication and anesthetic management to avoid elevations in $PaCO_2$ and increased cerebral blood flow.
3. Maintain anesthesia with a narcotic, nitrous oxide/oxygen, relaxant technique rather than an inhalation agent.
4. Hyperventilate during surgery to ensure a low $PaCO_2$.

NPO Status

If patients are not able to comprehend because of mental deficiency, adequate care must be taken to make certain that patients remain on nothing-by-mouth (NPO) status.

Airway

The airway is evaluated carefully because many of these patients have attendant upper airway abnormalities, such as high arched palate or abnormality of the mandible, which may lead to problems with endotracheal intubation.

Extubation is not performed until adequate ventilation is ensured.

Postoperative hypoventilation with its attendant elevation of $PaCO_2$ should be avoided.[11]

Monitors

Monitors used are ECG, blood pressure cuff, end-tidal carbon dioxide, pulse oximeter, nerve stimulator, temperature probe, and esophageal stethoscope.

Surgical Procedure

Simple separation of the fingers is not usually performed because inadequate skin is available for closure after separation.

After separation, skin grafts are placed to provide adequate skin for closure.

Case Study

A child younger than 1 year of age with Apert syndrome presented with syndactyly of both hands for reconstruction. He had an enlarged head, a big forehead, a large mandible, and a *scar from an earlier tracheotomy*. There was no evidence of increased intracranial pressure. The main concern was to secure an airway. Induction was with halothane, nitrous oxide, and oxygen. The vocal cords were visualized, and a muscle relaxant was administered to facilitate relaxation for endotracheal intubation. The procedure progressed without any problems.

Muscular Dystrophy

Types of muscular dystrophy include

1. Becker's dystrophy
2. Facioscapulohumeral (FSH) dystrophy
3. Limb-girdle dystrophy
4. Duchenne's dystrophy

Becker's Dystrophy

Only males are affected.

It has a later onset than Duchenne's muscular dystrophy.

Patients are wheelchair bound at about 30 years of age.

Pneumonia is a major problem and is the leading cause of death.

Cardiac involvement with cardiac failure is a major cause of death.[1,29-31]

Facioscapulohumeral Dystrophy

Males and females are equally affected.

Pectoral and facial muscles are weak.

Symptoms appear at about 12 years of age.

Patient may undergo surgery for stabilizing the scapula.

Patient may have cardiac involvement with no atrial activity. Patients cannot be electrically paced from the atrium but need ventricular pacing.[1,3,29-31]

Attention should be directed to the respiratory system to avoid problems.[1,26]

Limb-girdle Dystrophy

Shoulder girdle or pelvic girdle is involved.

Onset is between the first and third decade of life.

Cardiac and ECG changes include sinus tachycardia and bundle branch block.

Diaphragmatic weakness may lead to hypoventilation.[1,3,29-31]

Duchenne's Dystrophy

Duchenne's muscular dystrophy is transmitted by a recessive gene. A positive family history is present in more than 60 percent of cases. Duchenne's dystrophy is a progressive disease. It presents between the ages of 3 to 5 years.[1,3,29–31]

Hyperkalemia and Rhabdomyolysis

Many patients with Duchenne's dystrophy have had hyperkalemia and rhabdomyolysis either intraoperatively or postoperatively. It was believed that these were variants of or occurred in association with malignant hyperthermia. One case report describes cardiac arrest after isoflurane anesthesia in a patient with Duchenne's dystrophy associated hyperkalemia and rhabdomyolysis.[32]

Diagnosis

Some patients in whom the disease has not been diagnosed may come to surgery. Care must be taken because the first sign may be malignant hyperthermia (MH). Undiagnosed muscular dystrophy must be considered if the patients have any of the following signs or symptoms:

Slow motor development

Waddling gait

Hypertrophy of calf muscles

Weakness of the hip area, causing patients to use hands to assist in standing up—known as Gowers sign[1,3,29–31]

Progression

The weakness of the muscles is first proximal and then distal.

Most boys with Duchenne's dystrophy show steady deterioration. Initially having trouble walking, by early adolescence many children are in wheelchairs that they have trouble propelling by themselves. Motorized wheelchairs may then be required.

Contractures develop in the limbs.

Kyphoscoliosis develops because of muscle weakness.[1,3,29–31]

Clinical Changes

Pharyngeal involvement leads to difficulty in swallowing and may lead to aspiration.

Respiratory Muscle Weakness

If the vital capacity falls below 35 percent of predicted value, postoperative respiratory assistance will be needed. In these patients, endotracheal intubation and assisted respirations are provided in the postoperative period.

For patients undergoing spinal fusion, a vital capacity of at least 20 ml/kg and inspiratory capacity of at least 15 ml/kg should be present.[33]

Cardiac Involvement

Cardiomyopathy is present as a result of involvement of cardiac muscle.

Obstructive cardiomyopathy with right ventricular hypertrophy can affect outflow.[34]

Electrocardiographic Changes

Characteristic ECG changes include a tall R wave in lead V_1, a deep Q wave in the lateral precordial and limb leads, and a shortened P-R interval.[35]

Sinus tachycardia is present.

Gastrointestinal Changes

Aspiration may result from impaired laryngeal and pharyngeal reflexes as well as gastric hypomotility.

Laboratory Studies

Serum creatine phosphokinase concentrations may be markedly elevated. This occurs early in the disease.

Surgical Procedures

Muscle biopsies to make the diagnosis

Fixation of fractures occurring when patients fall out of wheelchairs

Tendon lengthening procedures

Procedures for correction of scoliosis

Anesthetic Considerations

Overall muscle strength can be judged by the patient's status in a wheelchair. Those in motorized wheelchairs are more debilitated than those who are strong enough to control the wheelchair.[1,3,29-31,36]

1. Upper airway
   Be alert to the possibility of aspiration because of decreased laryngeal and pharyngeal reflexes.
2. Gastrointestinal
   Keep patient NPO for at least 8 hours because of decreased gastric motility.
   Insert a nasogastric tube if gastric dilatation present.

3. Pulmonary

Evaluate vital capacity and inspiratory capacity. If these are decreased, consider preparation for postoperative pulmonary ventilation.

4. Cardiac Changes

Obtain ECG and echocardiogram to evaluate cardiac status.

Avoid atropine during surgery because patients already have baseline tachycardia.[3]

Avoid inhalation agents to prevent cardiac depression.

Association with Malignant Hyperthermia

Patients with Duchenne's muscular dystrophy are susceptible to MH. These patients should be prepared preoperatively and managed intraoperatively as though they have MH.[37]

Take the following precautions in the perioperative period:

1. Avoid atropine because it may cause tachycardia.
2. Flush the anesthesia machine with air or oxygen.
3. Use a fresh, disposable anesthetic circuit, breathing bag, and mask.
4. Avoid potent volatile anesthetic agents.
5. Do not use succinylcholine; cardiac arrest can occur.
6. Use monitors: ECG, pulse oximeter, end-tidal carbon dioxide, temperature, nerve stimulator.
7. Alert operating room staff and have MH cart ready.[38,39]

Endotracheal intubation can be carried out with atracurium.

Narcotics, nitrous oxide/oxygen, and a muscle relaxant such as atracurium are used. Atracurium is recommended because reversal using atropine may not be necessary if atracurium is carefully titrated, because it is metabolized by Hofmann on degradation.

Succinylcholine

Smith and Bush reported[36] a group of patients with Duchenne's dystrophy who underwent surgical procedures and had apparent uneventful recovery. However, between 5 and 36 hours later, the patients had delayed respiratory insufficiency. The common medication was succinylcholine, which should not be used in these patients.[36]

Other Associated Problems

Other problems seen in patients with Duchenne's dystrophy during anesthesia include

1. *Acute hyperkalemia* can lead to cardiac arrest. This hyperkalemia may be an isolated finding or it may be due to association with malignant hyperthermia. The role of blood transfusion in increasing potassium should be considered.
2. *Heart failure* can occur as a result of cardiomyopathy and the stress of surgery.

Complications appear to be related to the use of potent inhalation agents during surgery. They should be avoided.[32,40]

It is important to be alert for rhabdomyolysis with myoglobinemia and myoglobinuria.

Postanesthetic Considerations

Maintain assisted or controlled ventilation if patient does not show evidence of adequate ventilation.

Be on the alert for the possible development of MH.

Mobilize as soon as possible to prevent pulmonary problems.

Cerebral Palsy

Cerebral palsy is not a specific disease but a group of disorders affecting neuromuscular function.[41]

The patient demonstrates abnormalities of movement and posture and possibly other evidence of central nervous system dysfunction.[41]

Upper motor neuron damage in the spinal cord or brain is present.[3]

Clinical Manifestations

There may be spasticity, athetoid movement, paralysis, hypotonia, or a mixture of these types.

Delayed motor development is common, and an abnormal crawling pattern or gait is often noted.[41]

Patients with cerebral palsy may have problems involving only one or two limbs or the entire body.[3]

In some, there may be associated developmental delay.

Surgical Procedures

Surgical procedures include tendon transfers, other soft tissue procedures, oste-otomies to reconstruct joints that have been chronically dislocated because of spasticity, and correction of scoliosis.

Anesthetic Considerations

Upper Airway

Problems with swallowing and regurgitation after feeding may be noted. Parents have learned to maintain their child in the upright position for several hours after feeding to avoid regurgitation and aspiration. This matter should be discussed during the preoperative visit.

Regurgitation and aspiration of gastric contents may be a problem.

Induction and Maintenance

If intravenous access can be obtained, the patient is induced with a barbiturate followed by a muscle relaxant for endotracheal intubation. Maintenance can be carried out in the usual fashion.

In patients in whom intravenous access cannot be obtained because of noncoop-eration, anesthesia is induced with an inhalation agent or ketamine and main-tained with nitrous oxide/oxygen, narcotics, and an inhalation agent, plus a muscle relaxant when needed.

In patients with severe spasticity or athetoid movements, there is no problem after anesthetic induction and maintenance has been established.

Spasticity

Spasticity is a motor disorder characterized by an increase in muscle tone and exaggerated tendon reflexes, which result from hyperexcitability of the stretch reflex.[42,43]

In cerebral palsy, there is a loss of inhibition of the higher centers of the cerebral cortex, leading to abnormalities in muscle tone with excessive contraction be-cause of poor control at the level of the spinal reflex arc.

Selective Posterior Rhizotomy

Patients are selected for posterior rhizotomy who have spasticity and no con-tractures and have not undergone prior spinal fusion.

Selective posterior rhizotomy involves the selective division of certain posterior roots of the second, third, fourth, and fifth lumbar and first sacral spinal nerves.

Intraoperative nerve stimulation with peripheral electromyographic recordings are carried out to determine which roots are to be cut.

Anesthetic Management

Selective posterior rhizotomy is performed under general endotracheal anesthesia. The anesthetic agents used can be either nitrous oxide/oxygen and an inhalation agent or narcotic.

Muscle relaxants should not be used because electromyographic recordings are performed.[42,43]

Mucopolysaccharidoses

Mucopolysaccharidoses are due to a deficiency of the enzymes involved in the degradation of mucopolysaccharides.

Type I—Hurler Syndrome

The patient may appear normal early in infancy.

Features of the disease include

Enlarged head

Enlarged tongue (macroglossia) with large open lips

Nasal obstruction

Short thick neck

Narrowing of the larynx and tracheobronchial tree

Hydrocephalus

Hepatosplenomegaly

Thoracolumbar kyphosis—hypoplastic vertebrae

Decreased compliance of chest wall

Coronary artery disease

Valvular disease

Sleep apnea

Cor pulmonale

Cardiomyopathy

Congestive heart failure

Mental retardation

Clouding of corneas

Flexion contractures of joints[44-46]

Anesthetic Considerations

Cervical spine involvement may be present with odontoid hypoplasia and atlantoaxial subluxation.

Thick skin and joint contractures may make intravenous access difficult.

An enlarged tongue, short neck, and cervical spine abnormalities may make endotracheal intubation difficult.[45]

Tracheobronchial Involvement

Because a narrowed tracheal lumen may be present, the tracheal diameter is assessed. CT scan is helpful to determine size of lumen.

Pulmonary involvement should be evaluated (chest radiograph, blood gas determinations).

Cardiac Involvement

ECG and echocardiogram should be performed.

The patient is evaluated for myocardial ischemia and valvular heart disease.

Hepatic Involvement

The patient should be checked for abnormalities in hepatic function.

Type II—Hunter Syndrome

Clinical manifestations include dwarfism, deafness, and hydrocephalus.

Cardiac disease involving valvular abnormalities and ischemia may be present.

Pulmonary hypertension may occur.

Airway problems may require tracheotomy.[45,46]

Type IV—Morquio Syndrome

The abnormalities in Morquio syndrome involve connective tissues, cartilage, and bone. There is also involvement of the cornea.

These patients develop severe skeletal abnormalities, including marked shortening of the neck with a head that appears enlarged compared with the body.

Pectus carinatum (pigeon breast) may develop.

Valvular disease may occur.

A hypoplastic odontoid may result in cervical instability requiring surgery. Neurologic symptoms, including paraplegia, may result.

The chest deformity and neurologic weakness lead to chronic pulmonary infections, symptoms of dyspnea on exertion, and low exercise tolerance.[44–47]

Anesthetic Considerations

1. Obtaining an airway in a patient with an unstable neck can be accomplished with a fiberoptic bronchoscope. If a transoral odontoidectomy is performed the options are a nasal fiberoptic intubation or a preoperative tracheotomy. The neck in these patients is very small and this makes a tracheotomy very difficult. Flexion can result in tracheal obstruction.
2. Pulmonary status—meticulous attention to pulmonary status is crucial in these patients because they have low tidal volumes, functional residual capacities, and vital capacities.[45,47]
3. If SSEP monitoring is to be used, a narcotic, nitrous oxide/oxygen, relaxant technique should be used.
4. In patients with pulmonary problems, postoperative observation in an intensive care unit with careful monitoring of respiratory function and blood gases should be carried out.

Case Study

A 19-year-old woman with Morquio syndrome and spinal cord narrowing presented for transoral decompression of C2 and C3, anterior vertebrectomy, and posterior spinal fusion for progressing upper and lower extremity weakness. The patient complained of muscle weakness with dyspnea on exertion and minimal exercise tolerance. Preoperative pulmonary function tests revealed severe restrictive impairment. Echocardiogram was negative. Medications included 5 mg oxybutynin chloride daily to help control bladder function. Hemoglobin was 14.9g and hematocrit value was 43.1 percent. Because the procedure was to be performed under SSEP monitoring, a narcotic, nitrous oxide/oxygen, muscle relaxant technique was planned. After adequate topicalization and sedation, a nasal fiberoptic intubation was performed, and the patient was induced with etomidate, sufentanil, and vecuronium. Maintenance agents were sufentanil, nitrous oxide/oxygen, and vecuronium. The procedure was performed uneventfully. Postoperatively, the patient was weaned from mechanical ventilation after 2 days and extubated. A few hours after extubation, the patient required reintubation for collapsed right upper lobe, low PaO_2 values, and secretions. Tracheotomy was performed with difficulty because of the large head compared with the smaller neck and trachea.

Comment

This case describes the main problems of obtaining an airway and administering an anesthetic in a patient with Morquio syndrome who has significant respiratory involvement caused by the disease. The complicated postoperative respiratory course must be considered preoperatively and appropriate perioperative plans outlined, including the possibility of elective preoperative tracheotomy.

Juvenile Rheumatoid Arthritis

Juvenile rheumatoid arthritis is a systemic disease not only involving the joints but many organ systems of the body[3,23,48] (see also Ch. 1).

Rheumatoid arthritis may begin at any age.

Rheumatoid arthritis is an autoimmune disease. There may be an increased familial incidence of this condition.

The disease may be characterized by arthritis with varying degrees of systemic involvement with polyarthritis.

Cricoarytenoid Arthritis

Cricoarytenoid joints may be involved by inflammation, with occasional hoarseness and laryngeal stridor.

Cervical Spine Involvement

Inability to extend the neck, flexion deformities, and torticollis may be present.

Atlantoaxial subluxation may be seen on radiograph examination.

Systemic Involvement

Pericarditis with effusions

Hepatosplenomegaly

Pneumonia and pleural effusions

Renal Impairment

Renal impairment may result from amyloidosis.

Ocular Manifestations

Involvement of the iris and ciliary body (iridocyclitis) may lead to chronic eye problems.

Anesthetic Considerations

Airway problems include

Temporomandibular joint ankylosis

Mandibular hypoplasia

Inability to extend neck

Cricoarytenoid arthritis

Atlantoaxial subluxation

During the preoperative visit, an assessment must be made of the upper airway because of the foregoing problems.

Evaluation must be made of the ability to open the mouth and extend the neck.

If atlantoaxial subluxation is present, extension of the neck reduces the cervical spine subluxation.

Inability to extend the neck because of flexion deformity secondary to C2 and C3 fusion may make extension impossible.[23,48]

Hoarseness, stridor, pain on swallowing, and earache may be a result of cricoarytenoid arthritis. Indirect laryngoscopy should be performed before surgery to rule out this problem.

Management of the airway may necessitate fiberoptic intubation. The patient receives topical application of local anesthetics to the oral mucosa, block of the recurrent laryngeal nerves, and transtracheal installation of local anesthetic agents.

Cardiovascular Problems
ECG should be performed to detect any abnormalities of rate or rhythm.

Echocardiogram is indicated if pericarditis or pericardial effusion is suspected.

Chest Radiograph
A chest radiograph is performed to detect any pulmonary changes or effusions.

Complete Blood Count
Anemia may be present, especially in the acute systemic form of the disease. Iron therapy is usually not effective for increasing the hemoglobin level. If the hemoglobin needs to be increased, blood transfusions are usually needed.

Abdominal Examination
Evaluation of the liver and spleen in small children should be performed because compromise of ventilation may occur due to the enlarged abdominal organs.

Bleeding Time

A bleeding time is performed to determine the extent of platelet involvement.

Patients on salicylate therapy may have problems in coagulation.

Platelet counts may be normal because the salicylates affect the quality of the platelets.

Position

Positioning of the child is important to avoid injuries to joints because flexion deformities may be present. Painful joints may need special padding and positioning.[23,48]

Cricoarytenoid Arthritis

Cricoarytenoid arthritis has not been documented frequently in children, but when it does occur, it can progress to a life-threatening airway emergency. Four well-documented cases exist in the literature. All four cases had increasing stridor, which was usually present on inspiration. When both inspiratory and expiratory stridor occurred, the situation became critical. In one recently presented case, a 4½-year-old child progressed over a short period from dyspnea to stridor, nasal flaring, substernal retractions, air hunger, and anxiety. On direct laryngoscopy, bilateral vocal cord immobility and a slit-like airway were present. The arytenoids were fixed, and a tracheotomy was performed.

Childhood cricoarytenoid arthritis appears to respond well to medical therapy. Steroids alone or together with nonsteriodal anti-inflammatory drugs or acetylsalicylic acid are useful. If the diagnosis is made early, acute airway problems can be avoided.[49]

Juvenile Ankylosing Spondylitis

Juvenile ankylosing spondylitis[48] (see also Ch. 1) is a disease involving arthritis of the axial and peripheral skeleton.

The male/female ratio is 6:1.

There is a strong familial incidence.

There is close association with HLA B-27 antigen.

Hips, ankles, and knees are usually involved.

Occasionally, the temporomandibular joint may be involved.

The sacroiliac joint and lumbodorsal spine involvement leads to low back pain and inability to move the lower spine.

Spinal involvement leads to the fixation and rigidity of the axial skeleton.

Costovertebral and costosternal joint involvement may lead to decreased expansion of the chest.

Aortic Insufficiency

Aortic insufficiency may be present in children.

If any question exists concerning the cardiac status, evaluation should be carried out with echocardiography.

Anesthetic Considerations

Anesthetic considerations involve evaluation of neck mobility for intubation.

Fiberoptic endotracheal intubation may be required if the cervical spine has been fixed.

Attempts to move the cervical spine may result in fracture.

Malignant Hyperthermia

MH is a hypermetabolic syndrome primarily involving changes in skeletal muscles with pathophysiologic intracellular hypercalcemia, which occurs after the administration of certain inciting anesthetic drugs and agents (Table 10-1).

If untreated, death can occur.

Table 10-1. Triggering and Nontriggering Agents

Safe	Unsafe	Controversial
Antibiotics	Volatile anesthetics	Curare
Antihistamines	Succinylcholine	Phenothiazines
Antipyretics	Potassium salts	
Atropine		
Barbiturates		
Benzodiazepines		
Dantrolene		
Digitalis drugs		
Droperidol		
Etomidate		
Ketamine		
Local anesthetics		
Narcotics		
Neostigmine		
Nitrous oxide		
Nondepolarizing muscle relaxants		
Propofol		
Propranolol		
Vasoactive drugs		

(Data from Rosenberg et al[50] and Gronert et al[53])

High fever is a sign of MH, but the syndrome may occur without extremely high temperatures. Fever may be a late sign in MH.[50]

Genetic Studies

The gene for MH has been tentatively localized to chromosome 19 in some humans.[51]

However, not all patients with MH have been found to have this gene.[52]

Masseter Muscle Rigidity

Masseter muscle rigidity (MMR) precedes MH in many cases. In some instances, when MMR occurred and the anesthetic was converted to a nontriggering technique, the procedure continued without any problems.

After MMR, in some instances there is an elevated creatine kinase (CK) and myoglobinuria. There is a 100 to 200 times greater incidence of MMR than MH in the population. One percent of all children anesthetized with halothane and paralyzed with succinylcholine developed MMR.[54,55]

Of patients with MMR, 50 to 55 percent are biopsy-positive for MH.

Succinylcholine may cause a transient increase in jaw muscle tone. This normal increase in muscle tone may be interpreted as MMR.

Patient Management

If trismus should develop, Gronert believes that the procedure may be continued. However, Rosenberg would opt to stop the procedure and observe the patient for the development of MH. If the anesthesiologist has dantrolene available and an end-tidal carbon dioxide monitor and is experienced in managing MH, the anesthesiologist may continue with nontriggering anesthetic agents.[56,57]

In an emergency procedure, Rosenberg recommends switching to nontriggering agents, observing for MH, and continuing the procedure.[56,57]

CK levels should be determined.

Patients are admitted to the hospital for observation.

Patients are observed for myoglobinuria, fever, hyperkalemia, and other signs of MH.

If symptoms develop, 2 mg/kg dantrolene is administered intravenously and the patient is treated for MH.

Diagnosis in the Operating Room

1. Signs of hypermetabolism
   Tachycardia
   Cyanosis
   Elevated end-tidal carbon dioxide
   Respiratory acidosis
   Temperature elevation
   Metabolic acidosis
   Arrhythmias
2. Muscle rigidity
   Masseter muscle spasm (intubation problems)
   Chest wall rigidity
   Limb rigidity
3. Rhabdomylysis
   Hyperkalemia
   Myoglobinuria
   Elevated creatine phosphokinase after anesthesia[50,53]

The onset of MH can be acute during anesthesia or may be delayed for hours and may not become apparent until the patient is in the recovery room.

Clinical Manifestations

Intense production of heat

Elevated carbon dioxide

Elevated lactate

Respiratory and metabolic acidosis

Whole body rigidity in a large percentage of cases

Elevated temperatures

Increased permeability of muscle

Increased serum potassium

Increased ionized calcium

Elevated CK

Elevated myoglobin

Elevated serum sodium

Decreased serum potassium and calcium levels later in the syndrome

Muscle edema

Sympathetic hyperactivity

Tachycardia

Sweating

Hypertension

Altered cellular permeability with accompanying edema, including acute cerebral edema

Disseminated intravascular coagulopathy

Cardiac failure

Renal failure[50,53]

MH Cart

An MH cart should be present in the operating rooms and recovery rooms (Table 10-2).

Treatment

If the diagnosis of MH is suspected, the following are performed simultaneously.

Surgeon: Stop surgery

Anesthesiologist: Discontinue anesthetic

Assistant: Mix dantrolene

The immediate administration of dantrolene is the most critical aspect of therapy in MH.

Table 10-2. Contents of MH Cart

MH Hotline Medic Alert (209) 634-4917 Index 0 (prominently displayed on cart)
1. Dantrolene sodium—supplied in 70-ml bottles containing 20 mg of drug. Keep at least 36 bottles immediately available in cart. Have access to at least 72 bottles.
2. Bottles of *sterile water* needed to reconstitute dantrolene, not normal saline
3. Emergency drugs
   a. Sodium bicarbonate: 12 ampules
   b. Furosemide: 4 100-mg ampules
   c. Regular insulin: 1 100-unit ampule
   d. Dextrose 50% in water: 1 50-ml ampule
   e. Mannitol 25%: 4 12.5-g ampules
   f. Procainamide: 1 1-g ampule
4. Refrigerated intravenous fluids—5 L
5. Ice—make certain supply readily available
6. Nasogastric tube
7. Urinary catheter
8. Syringes, needles
9. Blood gas kits

1. Have assistants dissolve vials of dantrolene in 50 ml *sterile distilled water*.

    Warning: Do not use 5 percent dextrose in water.

    Heat vial of dantrolene solution under hot tap water to aid in mixing the solution.

2. Administer 2.5 mg/kg dantrolene every 5 minutes. Use up to 10 mg/kg, more if needed, determined by clinical situation.

    Example: For initial treatment in a 70-kg patient, 175 mg (70 × 2.5) is needed to start. This is 9 vials because each vial contains 20 mg of drug.

3. Discontinue all anesthetic agents.

4. Hyperventilate with 100 percent oxygen.

5. Administer 2 to 4 mEq/kg bicarbonate. Follow heart rate, $PaCO_2$, and body temperature.

6. Lower body temperature—cool to 38 to 39°C. Avoid hypothermia.

    Surface cooling—place ice in axillae and groin, as well as over entire body.

    Infuse cold saline—keep bottles of saline in refrigerator at all times.

    Irrigate the bladder with iced solutions.

    Irrigate stomach through nasogastric tube with iced solution.

    If body cavities are open, use sterile iced fluids.

7. Monitor urinary output—maintain urinary output to 1 to 2 ml/kg/hr. Administer 0.25 g/kg mannitol intravenously.

8. Monitor blood gases.

9. Obtain laboratory studies. Follow electrolytes, blood urea nitrogen, obtain clotting profile, urine for myoglobinuria. Check muscle enzymes, CK, lactate dehydrogenase, aspartate aminotransferase.

10. Treat arrhythmias—200 mg procainamide infusion, repeat as needed.

11. Treat hyperkalemia by reversing MH with dantrolene. Do not administer calcium.[50,53]

It must be emphasized again that immediate administration of dantrolene is the most critical aspect of therapy.

Postoperative Management

Monitor patient in intensive care unit for 24 hours.

Administer 1 mg/kg dantrolene intravenously every 6 hours.

Discontinue dantrolene if there are no signs of recurrence.

When stable, administer 1 mg/kg oral dantrolene every 6 hours for 24 to 48 hours.

Anesthetic Management of Susceptible Patients

History

Previous anesthetic history should be determined. The anesthesiologist should inquire about problems with anesthesia and family members. Any deaths caused by anesthesia should be discussed. It should be determined whether MMR had ever developed.

Blood Creatine Kinase Levels
The blood CK level is elevated in about 70 percent of affected people. Blood CK levels must be drawn in a resting, fasting state without recent trauma.[53]

Anesthetic Approach for the High-Risk Patient—Pretreatment?
Some anesthesiologists prefer to pretreat with dantrolene in the MH susceptible patient. Rosenberg et al[50] recommends the administration of 2.5 mg/kg of dantrolene intravenously before anesthetic induction in the highly susceptible patient.

Some believe that if nontriggering agents and proper preparation of equipment has been carried out, dantrolene pretreatment may not be necessary and do not pretreat.

Preparation of the Anesthesia Machine
Remove the vaporizers if possible.

Replace the fresh gas outlet hose.

Use a disposable circuit.

Flush anesthesia machine with oxygen 6 L/min for 5 minutes.[58]

Anesthetic Induction
See Table 10-1 for a listing of safe agents[50,53]

Induce patients with barbiturates, opiates, or tranquilizers.

Use midazolam, diazepam, droperidol, narcotics.

Muscle Relaxants
Nondepolarizing muscle relaxants should be used.

Note:
Do not use succinylcholine.

Do not use curare.

Nitrous Oxide
Nitrous oxide may be administered with narcotics and muscle relaxants for maintenance.

Volatile Anesthetic Agents
Potent volatile anesthetic agents should not be used.

Regional Anesthesia
Regional anesthesia is safe and is preferred for procedures in susceptible patients.

Amide anesthetics and ester local anesthetics can be used.[50]

Keeping Current with MH

It is important to keep up with the latest information on MH.

Every person in the operating room should be familiar with the management of a patient with MH. Frequent inservice programs should be conducted for the operating room staff. The MH cart should be checked periodically.

The MH Hotline number should be permanently displayed on the MH cart and in the operating room.

The number is (209) 634-4917; request index 0 MH consultant.

Further information can be obtained from the Malignant Hyperthermia Association of the United States (MHAUS), Box 3231, Darien, CT 06820.

The address of MHA of Canada is Room 314, Elizabeth Wing, Toronto General Hospital, 101 College Street, Toronto, Ontario M5G1L7.

The hotline number in Canada is (416) 595-3000.

REFERENCES

1. Tachdjian MO: Congenital Deformities in Pediatric Orthopedics. 2nd Ed. WB Saunders, Philadelphia, 1990
2. Minamitani K, Inoue A, Okuno T: Results of surgical treatment of muscular torticollis for patients > 6 years of age. J Pediatr Orthop 10:754, 1990
3. Salem MR, Klowden AJ: Anesthesia for pediatric orthopedic surgery. p. 1203. In Gregory SA (ed): Pediatric Anesthesia. 2nd Ed. Churchill Livingstone, New York, 1989
4. Martz DG, Schriebman DL, Matjasko MJ: Neurologic diseases. In Katz J, Beneumof JL, Kadis LB (eds): Anesthesia and Uncommon Diseases. 3rd Ed. WB Saunders, Philadelphia, 1990
5. Crosby ET, Lui A: The adult cervical spine: implications for airway management. Can J Anaesth 37:77, 1990
6. de Beer J de V, Hoffman EB, Kieck CF: Traumatic atlanto-axial subluxation in children. J Pediatr Orthop 10:397, 1990
7. Lipson SJ: Dysplasia of the odontoid process in Morquio's syndrome causing quadriparesis. J Bone Joint Surg 59(A):340, 1977
8. Steel HH: Anatomical and mechanical considerations of the atlanto-axial articulations. J Bone Joint Surg 50(A):1481, 1968
9. Fielding JW: Fractures of the spine. p. 696. In Rockwood CA, Wilkins KE, King RE (eds): Fractures in Children. JB Lippincott, Philadelphia, 1984
10. Bloch EC, Ginsberg B, Binner RA et al: Limb tourniquet and central temperature in anesthetized children. Anesth Analg 74:486, 1992
11. Ward CF: Pediatric head and neck syndromes. In Katz J, Steward DJ (eds): Anesthesia and Uncommon Pediatric Disorders. WB Saunders, Philadelphia 1987

12. Gorlin RJ: Craniofacial defects. p. 465. In Oski FA (ed): Principles and Practice of Pediatrics. JB Lippincott, Philadelphia, 1990
13. Liptak GS: Spina bifida. p. 1487. In Hoekelman RA (ed): Primary Pediatric Care. CV Mosby, St. Louis, 1987
14. Slater JE: Rubber anaphylaxis. N Engl J Med 320:1126, 1989
15. Meeropol E, Kelleher R, Bell S, Leger R: Allergic reactions to rubber in patients with myelodysplasia. N Engl J Med 323:1072, 1990
16. Meeropol E, Frost J, Pugh L et al: Latex allergy in children with myelodysplasia: a survey of Shriners hospitals. J Pediatr Orthop 13:1, 1993
17. Calenda E, Durand JP, Petit J et al: Anaphylactic shock produced by latex. Anesth Analg 72:839, 1991
18. Moneret-Vautrin DA, Laxenaire MC, Bavoux F: Allergic shock to latex and ethylene oxide during surgery for spina bifida. Anesthesiology 73:556, 1990
19. Slater JE: Routine testing for latex allergy with spina bifida is not recommended. Anesthesiology 74:391, 1991
20. Kelly K, Setlock M, Davis JP: Anaphylactic reactions during general anesthesia among pediatric patients–United States. January 1990–January 1991 MMWR. 40: 437, 1991
21. Rosencranz E: Ueber Kongenitale Kontraturen der oberen Extremitaten. Z Orthop Chir 14:52, 1905
22. Duncan PG: Neuromuscular Diseases. p. 509. In Katz J, Steward DJ (eds): Anesthesia and Uncommon Pediatric Diseases. WB Saunders, Philadelphia, 1987
23. Holtby HM, Relton JS: Orthopedic diseases. p. 361. In Katz J, Steward DJ (eds): Anesthesia and Uncommon Pediatric Diseases. WB Saunders, Philadelphia, 1987
24. Hammerschlag W, Ziv I, Wald U et al: Cervical instability in an achondroplastic infant. J Pediatr Orthop 8:481, 1988
25. Mayhew JF, Katz J, Miner M et al: Anaesthesia for the achondroplastic dwarf. Can Anaesth Soc J 33:216, 1986
26. Hanscom DA, Bloom BA: The spine in osteogenesis imperfecta: scoliosis. Orthop Clin N Am 19:449, 1988
27. Rampton AJ, Kelly DA, Shanahan EC et al: Occurrence of malignant hyperpyrexies in a patient with osteogenesis imperfecta. Br J Anaesth 56:1143, 1984
28. Gamble JG, Strudwick WJ, Rinsky LA et al: Complications of intramedullary rods in osteogenesis imperfecta: Bailey-Dubow rods versus nonelongating rods. J Pediatr Orthop 8:645, 1988
29. Duncan PG: Neuromuscular diseases. p. 509. In Katz J, Steward DJ (eds): Anesthesia and Uncommon Pediatric Diseases. WB Saunders, Philadelphia, 1987
30. Miller JD, Lee C: Muscle diseases. p. 590. In Katz J, Beneumof JL, Kadis LB (eds): Anesthesia and Uncommon Diseases. WB Saunders, Philadelphia, 1990
31. Curran MJ: Muscular dystrophies and myotonic syndromes. p. 124. In Lui ACP, Crosby ET (eds): Problems in Anesthesia, Anesthesia and Musculoskeletal Disorders. Vol. 5. No. 1. JB Lippincott, Philadelphia, 1991
32. Chalkadis GA, Branch KG: Cardiac arrest after isoflorane anaesthesia in a patient with Duchenne's muscular dystrophy. Anaesthesia 45:22, 1990
33. Milne B, Rosales JK: Anaesthetic considerations in patients with muscular dystrophy undergoing spinal fusion and Harrington rod insertion. Can Anaesth Soc J 29: 250, 1982
34. Hunsaker RH, Fulkerson PK, Barry FJ et al: Cardiac function in Duchenne's muscular dystrophy. Am J Med 42:179, 1982
35. Sluck AC: The electrocardiogram in Duchenne progressive muscular dystrophy. Circulation 38:933, 1968

36. Smith CL, Bush GH: Anaesthesia and progressive muscular dystrophy. Br J Anaesth 57:1113, 1985
37. Wang JM, Stanley TH: Duchenne muscular dystrophy and malignant hyperthermia. Can Anaesth Soc J 33:492, 1986
38. Henderson WAV: Succinylcholine-induced cardiac arrest in unsuspected Duchenne's muscular dystrophy. Can Anaesth Soc J 31:444, 1984
39. Rosewarne FA: Anaesthesia, atracurium and Duchenne muscular dystrophy. Can Anaesth Soc J 33:250, 1986
40. Sethna NF, Rockoff MA, Worthen HM et al: Anesthesia-related complications in children with Duchenne muscular dystrophy. Anesthesiology 68:462, 1988
41. Molnar GE: Cerebral palsy. p. 420. In: Pediatric Rehabilitation. Williams & Williams, Baltimore, 1985
42. Oppenheim WL: Selective posterior rhizotomy for spastic cerebral palsy. Clin Orthop 253:20, 1990
43. Park TS, Owen JH: Surgical management of spastic diplegia in cerebral palsy. N Engl J Med 326:745, 1992
44. Tachdjian MD: Bone in Pediatric Orthopedics. 2nd ed. WB Saunders Philadelphia, 1990.
45. Stehling LC: Genetic metabolic diseases. p. 345. In Katz J, Steward DJ (eds): Anesthesia and Uncommon Pediatric Diseases. WB Saunders, Philadelphia, 1987
46. Wappner RS, Brandt IK: Inborn errors of metabolism. p. 110. In Oski FA (ed): Principles and Practice of Pediatrics. JB Lippincott, Philadelphia, 1990
47. Jones AEP, Croley TF: Morquio syndrome and anesthesia. Anesthesiology 51:261, 1979
48. Smith MF: Skin and connective tissue diseases. p. 378. In Katz J, Steward DJ (eds): Anesthesia and Uncommon Pediatric Diseases. WB Saunders, Philadelphia, 1987
49. Furtan ND, Sherris D, Norante JD: Cricoarytenoid arthritis in children. Otolaryngol Head Neck Surg 104:966, 1991
50. Rosenberg H, Fletcher J, Seitman D: Pharmacogenetics. p. 589. In Barash PG, Cullen BF, Stoelting RK (eds): Clinical Anesthesia. 2nd Ed. JB Lippincott, Philadelphia, 1992
51. McCarthy TV, Healy SJM, Heffron JJA et al: Localization of the malignant hyperthermia susceptibility locus to human chromosome 19q. 12-13.2. Nature 343:562, 1990
52. Levitt RC, Nouri N, Jedlicka AE et al: Evidence for a molecular heterogeneity in malignant hyperthermia susceptibility. Genomics 11:543, 1991
53. Gronert GA, Schulman SR, Mott J: Malignant hyperthermia. p. 935. In Miller RD (ed): Anesthesia. 3rd ed. Churchill Livingstone, New York, 1990
54. Schwartz L, Rockoff MA, Koka BV: Masseter spasm and succinylcholine: incidence and implications. Anesthesiology 61:772, 1984
55. Carroll JB: Increased incidence of masseter spasm in children with strabismus anesthetized with halothane and succinylcholine. Anesthesiology 67:559, 1987
56. Rosenberg H: Trismus is not trivial. Anesthesiology 67:453, 1987
57. Gronert GA, Rosenberg H: Management of patients in whom trismus occurs following succinylcholine. Anesthesiology 68:653, 1988
58. Beebe JJ, Sessler DI: Preparation of anesthesia machines for patients susceptible to malignant hyperthermia. Anesthesiology 69:395, 1988

11

Scoliosis*

Although scoliosis has been recognized for many years, the main advances have been made during this century in surgery for spinal deformities (Table 11-1).

Scoliosis is defined as one or more lateral rotatory curvatures in the spine. Figure 11-1 shows Cobb's method[4] for determining the degree of curvature.

The following is a classification of scoliosis[5]:

Idiopathic
    Infantile (less than 4 years old)
    Juvenile (4 to 9 years old)
    Adolescent (10 years to skeletal maturity)
Congenital
    Spinal deformity
    Abnormal spinal cord development
Neuromuscular
    Neuropathic
        Upper motor neuron (cerebral palsy)
        Lower motor neuron (poliomyelitis)
        Others (syringomyelia)
    Myopathic
        Progressive (muscular dystrophy)
        Static (myotonia)
        Others (Friedreich's ataxia)
Neurofibromatosis (von Recklinghausen's disease)
Mesenchymal disorders
    Congenital (Marfan syndrome)
    Acquired (rheumatoid arthritis)
Trauma
    Vertebral (fractures, radiation, surgery)
    Extravertebral (burns, thoracoplasty)
Tumors

---

* Portions of this chapter are from Bernstein,[5] with permission.

Table 11-1. Historical Developments in the Treatment of Scoliosis

5th century BC	Hippocrates	Forcible traction
1911	Hibbs	Spinal fusion for tuberculosis
1914	Hibbs	First fusion for scoliosis[1]
1962	Harrington	Instrumentation and fusion[2]
1969	Dwyer	Anterior disc excision
1978	Zielke	Stabilization and derotation
1982	Luque	Segmental wiring to flexible rods[3]
1986	Cotrel and Dubousset	Derotation and instrumentation
1989	Texas Scottish Rite Hospital	Derotation and instrumentation

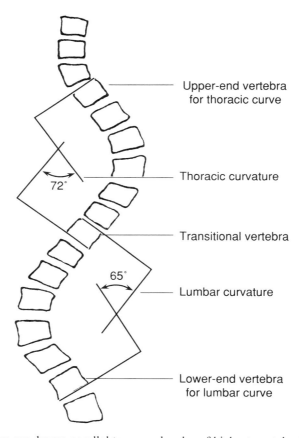

Fig. 11-1. Lines are drawn parallel to upper border of highest vertebral body and lower border of lowest vertebral body of the curve. Perpendicular lines are drawn from these lines, and the angle formed by the intersection of lines is degree of curvature. (From Cobb,[4] with permission.)

RESPIRATORY PHYSIOLOGY

Patients with idiopathic scoliosis with curves of less than 65 degrees rarely show evidence of respiratory impairment.

Patients with congenital scoliosis and weakened musculature may have significant respiratory impairment with smaller curves.

Deformities associated with muscle weakness or paralysis have the greatest impact on alterations in respiratory function.

In cerebral palsy, spasticity causes problems because of muscle imbalance.

Exercise tolerance is an important clinical determinant of the effects of the severity of the curve.

Scoliosis can be associated with neuromuscular disease.
  It is characterized by thoracic deformity, abnormalities in central respiratory control, and problems in innervation of the respiratory muscles leading to a loss of motor function.
  Patients with paralytic scoliosis are more impaired than patients with idiopathic scoliosis; those with poliomyelitis have the worst prognosis.
  Decreased respiratory muscle function leads to a reduction in inspiratory force and vital capacity.
  Poor laryngeal and pharyngeal control and ineffective cough mechanisms can further complicate respiratory function.

Effects on Pulmonary Function

Thoracic deformities lead to a restrictive lung pattern[6] with

  Decreased vital capacity

  Decreased total lung capacity

  Decreased functional residual capacity

  Decreased residual volume

  Decreased chest wall compliance

  Increased pulmonary vascular resistance

  Ventilation/perfusion imbalance

The age-associated decreased PaO_2 (resulting from the decreased mechanical properties of the lungs and the ventilation/perfusion imbalance) increases the ventilatory requirements and may ultimately lead to ventilatory failure.[6]

Vital Capacity as a Predictor of Outcome

If vital capacity is greater than 70 percent of that predicted, respiratory reserve should be adequate for the postoperative period. If the vital capacity is less than 30 percent, postoperative ventilation will be necessary.

Pathophysiology

The main defect in scoliosis is alveolar hypoventilation secondary to a ventilation/perfusion mismatch.

Rapid, shallow breathing develops because of the restrictive nature of the disease, leading to increased dead space.

Arterial blood gases indicate a reduction in PaO_2 level with a normal $PaCO_2$ level.

There is an increase in the alveolar-arterial oxygen tension difference (A-aDO$_2$)

There is an increase in the physiologic dead space ratio (dead space/tidal volume [VD/VT)]).

Hypercapnia may occur as the pulmonary disease progresses and the compensatory mechanisms begin to fail.[6]

Pulmonary Hypertension

Scoliosis that begins when a patient is very young may result in small lungs with compression of lung tissue. In areas compressed by the deformity, blood may flow through extra-alveolar vessels. Pulmonary vascular resistance may increase, leading to pulmonary hypertension.

Irreversible pulmonary hypertension may also develop from prolonged hypoxia, hypercapnia, and pulmonary artery vasoconstriction.

Polycythemia secondary to hypoxemia and cor pulmonale secondary to pulmonary hypertension may result.[6]

CARDIAC CHANGES

Hirschfeld et al[7] have found a higher than normal incidence of mitral valve prolapse in patients with scoliosis.

Primiano et al[8] reported increased pulmonary vascular resistance in asymptomatic adolescents with idiopathic scoliosis independent of the severity of the curve. Mitral valve prolapse was seen in 25 percent of these children. It is believed that cardiopulmonary abnormalities develop parallel with rather than in response to the structural changes. During the sixth week of fetal development, there is a relationship in the formation of the vertebrae, sternum, ribs, mitral valve, and breast tissue. Rosenberg et al[9] showed that there is an increased incidence of mitral valve prolapse associated with hypomastia.

Children with muscular dystrophies have myocardial abnormalities with arrhythmias as well as mitral valve prolapse.

Patients with Marfan syndrome have cardiac defects such as mitral valve prolapse, dilatation of the root of the aorta, aortic valve insufficiency, and weakening of the wall of the aorta.

SPECIAL CONSIDERATIONS

The type of scoliosis (e.g., congenital, neuromuscular), as well as defects associated with the different conditions, must be determined because this information is significant in the management.

Idiopathic Scoliosis

In patients with idiopathic scoliosis, the presence or absence of any associated pulmonary and cardiac defects, and the general condition of the patient are significant.

Congenital Deformities

Urinary tract abnormalities

Gastrointestinal tract anomalies, mediastinal cysts

Congenital bony anomalies (may be associated with Klippel-Feil syndrome and Sprengel's deformity with scapula involvement)

NEUROMUSCULAR SCOLIOSIS

The following is a classification of neuromuscular scoliosis[10]:

Neuropathic
    Upper motor neuron
        Cerebral palsy
        Spinocerebellar degeneration
            Friedreich's ataxia
            Charcot-Marie-Tooth
            Roussy-Lévy
        Syringomyelia
        Spinal cord tumor
        Spinal cord trauma
    Lower motor neuron
        Poliomyelitis
        Other viral myelitides
        Traumatic
        Spinal muscular atrophy
            Werdnig-Hoffmann
            Kugelberg-Welander
        Dysautonomia (Riley-Day)
Myopathic
    Arthrogryposis
    Muscular dystrophy
        Duchenne (pseudohypertrophic)
        Limb-girdle
        Facioscapulohumeral
    Fiber-type disproportion
    Congenital hypotonia
    Myotonia dystrophica

Characteristics

Early onset

Rapid progression

Pelvic obliquity, leading to inability to sit, dislocation of hips, and development of pressure sores[10]

Preoperative Considerations

Respiratory Factors

Patients with neuromuscular disease frequently have respiratory compromise as a result of muscle weakness and imbalance, as well as difficulty swallowing and clearing secretions. It is not unusual for patients to have a history of prior pneumonias and aspiration. A baseline chest radiograph should be obtained. It is important to check for symptoms of respiratory insufficiency such as increased respiratory rate, use of accessory muscles, and coughing.[10] In some of these patients, baseline pulmonary function tests are often impossible because of inability to understand and cooperate.[10-12]

Pulmonary Function Tests

Vital capacity is one of the most important measurements.[10]

Vital capacity less than 30 percent: postoperative respiratory assistance probably necessary

Vital capacity 35 to 70 percent: may require postoperative support

Vital capacity greater than 70 percent: probably able to tolerate surgery without postoperative respiratory support

In Duchenne's muscular dystrophy and Friedreich's ataxia, if forced vital capacity is less than 30 percent of predicted, the operation should probably not be performed.[10]

Arterial Blood Gas Determination

Patients with respiratory compromise should have a baseline arterial blood gas analysis performed. If indications exist that severe respiratory compromise is present such as a PaO_2 level less than 50 mmHg or $PaCO_2$ level more than 50 mmHg, the patient should not undergo surgery.[10,13,14]

Cardiovascular Evaluation

Cardiac dysfunction is a frequent abnormality associated with neuromuscular disease. A number of neuromuscular conditions are associated with cardiovascular abnormalities.

Duchenne's Muscular Dystrophy

See Chapter 10 for further discussion on Duchenne's muscular dystrophy.

Abnormal electrocardiogram (ECG) with tall R waves in the right precordial leads and deep Q waves in the left precordial leads[10,15,16]

Mitral valve prolapse

Conduction abnormalities

Arrhythmias

Sudden death

Dilated myocardium with abnormal contraction[10,15-17]

Friedreich's Ataxia

Cardiomyopathy with cardiac failure possible in 50 percent of patients

ECG (T wave abnormalities, sinus tachycardia, atrial flutter, atrial fibrillation, left and right ventricular hypertrophy)

Arrhythmias (may be the cause of death)

Murmurs[10,15,18,19]

Myotonic Dystrophy

Cardiac abnormalities of myotonic dystrophy include bradycardia, increased PR interval, intraventricular conduction defects, arrhythmias, mitral valve prolapse, congestive heart failure, and cardiomyopathy.[10,15,16]

Gastrointestinal Problems

Patients with neuromuscular dysfunction and developmental delay may have difficulty in swallowing and chewing their food and may have gastrointestinal reflux and hiatal hernias. This may result in development of postoperative pneumonia.[10]

Parents are knowledgeable about the child's gastrointestinal symptoms and know how to keep the child in the upright position for several hours after feeding to prevent regurgitation.

Seizure Disorders

Some patients with neuromuscular scoliosis have seizure disorders.

The levels of anticonvulsant medication should be adequate before surgery.

Anticonvulsants are maintained in the perioperative period by parenteral administration if necessary.[10]

Considerations in Different Disorders

Cerebral Palsy

See Chapter 10 for further discussion of cerebral palsy.

Compared with the general population, in patients with cerebral palsy

1. Scoliosis occurs more frequently
2. The curve progresses even after skeletal maturity has occurred[10]

Surgical Intervention

Indications for treatment include

1. Curves that progress beyond 40 degrees
2. Curves that cause pain
3. Curves that force patients to use arms to maintain stability
4. Curves that interfere with sitting[10]

Surgical Procedures

In some instances, anterior approaches to provide releases and discetomies may be needed before the posterior fixation.

In many instances, fixation may extend from T2 to include the pelvis.[10]

Friedreich's Ataxia

Patients have cardiomyopathy, muscle weakness, and ataxic gait.

Surgery should be avoided in patients with significant cardiomyopathy.[10,15,19]

Charcot-Marie-Tooth Disease

Muscle weakness and ataxia are present. The weakness is more marked in the lower extremities.[10,15,19]

Syringomyelia

The slowly progressive neuromuscular disorder of syringomyelia involves destruction of the spinal cord as a result of cavitation. These patients have muscle wasting and sympathetic disturbances with sweating disorders, Horner syndrome, and temperature changes. Deformities of the hands and feet and Charcot changes in the joints are noted.[10,15,19-22]

If syringomyelia is suspected, a preoperative computed tomographic (CT) scan or magnetic resonance imaging (MRI) should be obtained, as the findings may affect the degree of surgical correction.

Problems Associated with Surgical Correction

Postfusion paraplegia and delayed paraparesis have been reported.

Drainage of the syrinx should be performed before spinal surgery. The curve should not be corrected fully.[10,21,22]

Spinal Muscle Atrophy

Spinal muscle atrophy is a degenerative disease of the anterior horn cells of the spinal cord and motor neurons of the cranial nerves.

Clinical features include muscle weakness and pulmonary problems.

The cause of death in spinal muscle atrophy is usually due to pulmonary failure.[10,15,23–25]

Arthrogryposis

This disease is characterized by joint contractures present at birth (see Ch. 10).

Pulmonary Function

Pulmonary function may be compromised because of the severe scoliotic curves. On occasion, the lower margin of the rib cage may actually touch the pelvis.

Duchenne's Muscular Dystrophy

Weakened musculature, restrictive pulmonary disease, and cardiomyopathy are the main features and cause the most problems for the anesthesiologist[10,15,16,25,26] (see above sections on pulmonary and cardiac disease; see also Ch. 10). The possibility of malignant hyperthermia must always be kept in mind.

Surgical Treatment

Patients undergo instrumentation from the upper thoracic spine to the pelvis. It is recommended that extubation after surgery should be performed as soon as safely possible to prevent the patient from becoming dependent on the ventilator. After extubation, the anesthesiologist should stay with the patient to make sure ventilatory insufficiency does not develop.[10]

Problems Associated with Surgery

Pulmonary

Decreased pulmonary function is the main problem.

Preoperative Preparation

Preoperative pulmonary evaluation with blood gas analysis and pulmonary function studies may be necessary.

Intense pulmonary toilet and pulmonary therapy should be performed preoperatively to maximize pulmonary function and possibly minimize postoperative complications.

Postoperative Considerations

Because postoperative pulmonary complications are a main concern, early and aggressive postoperative pulmonary toilet is important.

Ventilatory support may have to be maintained in the immediate postoperative period if evidence of *inability to handle secretions* or *decreased ventilatory capability* is present.

Early Mobilization

The patient should be placed in the upright position as soon as possible to help stabilize pulmonary function.[27]

Increased Blood Loss During Surgery

There is an increase in the blood loss associated with spinal surgery in patients with neuromuscular diseases.

The anesthesiologist should be prepared for major blood loss and major transfusions.

Intraoperative Temperature Control

Hypothermia should be prevented with a warm room, warm solutions, and the Bair Hugger.

Urinary Output

Because of the secretion of antidiuretic hormone, decreased urinary output may be present.[28]

PREOPERATIVE PREPARATION AND EVALUATION FOR SCOLIOSIS SURGERY

The anesthesiologist should meet with the patient and the family to develop a rapport, to show concern for the patient, and to show confidence in the management of the case. At this time, the anesthesia plan is explained, the wake-up test is discussed, and the use of patient controlled analgesia can be suggested if indicated.

Discussion of Wake-Up Test

The anesthesiologist should explain why the wake-up test is used. The patients are told they may be awakened during surgery and asked to move their hands and then their feet, they will not feel any pain, and they will be put back to sleep as soon as they have moved their feet.

Abnormal arterial blood gas studies and pulmonary function tests and exercise tolerance determinations help identify patients in whom postoperative pulmonary insufficiency may develop. Postoperative ventilatory support should be discussed, if indicated.

An echocardiogram should be obtained if a click is heard and mitral valve prolapse is suspected. If mitral valve prolapse is present, antibiotic prophylaxis is considered. Right ventricular function abnormalities as a result of pulmonary hypertension can be detected.

Hemoglobin and hematocrit determinations may be on the low side if preoperative autologous blood donation took place.

METHODS TO DECREASE HOMOLOGOUS BLOOD TRANSFUSIONS

At the Hospital for Joint Diseases, we have a comprehensive program including predonation, intraoperative hemodilution, cell salvage, and postoperative reinfusion of blood designed to minimize the use of homologous blood (see Ch. 4).

Autologous Blood Donation

Preoperative autologous blood donation may minimize or eliminate the need for use of homologous blood. Collection should begin 3 weeks before the operation, with 4 to 7 days between collections to allow blood volume adjustments to occur. The last collection should occur 7 days before surgery. Oral iron therapy is prescribed during the autologous donation period.

Patients younger than 16 years of age can safely contribute blood for surgery.

Full units are taken from patients who weigh at least 50 kg and have hemoglobin levels of 11 mg/dl or higher.

Half units are taken from patients who weigh between 25 and 50 kg when they have hemoglobin levels of more than 11 mg/dl.[29] Others have patients predonate partial units based on body weight. The patients can continue to predonate as long as the hemoglobin level remains greater than 11 mg/dl.[30]

Newer blood preservation solutions, such as citrate, phosphate, dextrose with adenine, and adenine, dextrose, and mannitol, have allowed longer storage times than with previous solutions.

Erythropoietin

Patients undergoing orthopedic surgery were able to predonate more units of blood if they received erythropoietin while predonating. Both the amount and red blood cell mass of predonated blood was higher in erythropoietin-treated patients.[31]

Intraoperative Isovolemic Hemodilution

After the patient has been anesthetized, 1 or 2 units of blood are withdrawn into blood storage bags containing appropriate anticoagulant solution and replaced by colloid and crystalloid. The amount withdrawn is based on the estimated blood volume, starting hematocrit level, and desired final hematocrit level.

After anesthesia is induced, an arterial line is placed into the radial artery.

Then, 450 ml of blood is withdrawn through the radial artery cannula into a blood storage bag, which is placed on a scale. It is assumed that 1 ml of blood weighs 1 g. The amount of anticoagulant in the bag requires that 450 ml be withdrawn. Withdrawal of less leads to excess anticoagulant.

The blood collection bag is agitated to avoid clotting while withdrawal is in progress.

Colloid in a 1:1 ratio or crystalloid in a 3:1 ratio is administered as the blood is being withdrawn.

One or two units of blood are withdrawn.

The blood is labeled and kept in the operating room for infusion at the end of the procedure.

While surgery is progressing, the blood that is being lost has a low hematocrit level.

At the conclusion of the procedure, the withdrawn blood with normal hematocrit levels can be administered to replace the "low hematocrit" blood loss.

Case Study

A 25-kg female patient with idiopathic scoliosis presented for surgery without having predonated blood. The family requested that homologous blood transfusion not be administered.

The hemoglobin level was 12 g and the hematocrit value was 36 percent. It was believed that this patient could tolerate a hemoglobin level of 9 g and a hematocrit value of 27 percent.

It was determined that her estimated blood volume was 1,750 ml.

$$25 \text{ kg} \times 70 \text{ ml/kg} = 1,750 \text{ ml}$$

The starting hematocrit value was 36 percent, and the hematocrit value to be achieved was 27 percent. Calculations were as follows:

$$\text{Amount to be withdrawn} \quad \frac{\text{EBV} \times (\text{Ho} - \text{Hf})}{\left(\dfrac{\text{Ho} + \text{Hf}}{2}\right)}$$

Where EBV is estimated blood volume, Ho is starting hematocrit, and Hf is final hematocrit value.

$$\text{Amount to be withdrawn} \quad \frac{1750 \times (36 - 27)}{\left(\dfrac{36 + 27}{2}\right)} = 500$$

Four hundred fifty milliliters of blood was withdrawn by weight and 500 ml of hetastarch was infused as well as 100 ml of crystalloid solution.

At the conclusion of the withdrawal and hemodilution, the hemoglobin level was 8.5 g and the hematocrit value was 26.5 percent.

Also, the Cell Saver was used to salvage shed blood during surgery, and postoperative wound drainage was reinfused. There was no need to administer any homologous blood.

Isovolemic hemodilution can be carried out in patients who have already predonated autologous blood as long as the starting hemoglobin and hematocrit values are acceptable. A final hematocrit value of at least 25 to 30 percent should be achieved.

Intraoperative Scavenging of Blood

Blood loss that occurs during surgery is heparinized, collected, and processed in an apparatus such as the Haemonetics Cell Saver. The shed blood is washed, spun down, and placed into a labeled blood administration bag. This processed blood usually has a hematocrit value of 65 percent. This blood is administered during the surgical procedure or in the postanesthesia care unit (PACU).

Reinfusion of Wound Drainage Blood

At the conclusion of the surgical procedure, drains are placed into the operative site connected to a reservoir, which collects the wound drainage blood. This blood is reinfused into the patient after passage through a Pall filter.

We have noted the passage of red urine on some occasions after this procedure. This is due to free hemoglobin. When this is noted, we promote a diuresis.

Order of Blood Reinfusion

In an uncomplicated procedure, we prefer to reinfuse blood in the following order:

1. Cell Saver blood
2. Blood from the isovolemic hemodilution
3. Wound drainage blood
4. Predonated autologous blood

PREMEDICATION

Benzodiazepines are to be avoided if somatosensory evoked potential (SSEP) monitoring is contemplated.

Morphine (0.1 mg/kg) or meperidine (1 mg/kg) and hydroxyzine (25 mg) are to be administered intramuscularly approximately 1 hour before induction.

Atropine or glycopyrrolate can be administered intravenously in the operating room before induction.

EQUIPMENT

2 large-bore venous catheters

Arterial catheter

ECG

Esophageal stethescope

Pulse oximeter

End-tidal carbon dioxide monitor

Urinary catheter (placed after anesthesia is induced)

SSEP monitor

Peripheral nerve stimulator (place at wrist, not on facial nerve; facial nerve is more sensitive to stimulation and therefore more muscle relaxant than necessary will be used)

Central venous pressure line (may be used in assessment of volume status)

PROCEDURES TO AVOID HYPOTHERMIA

Warm the operating room.

Warm all intravenous fluids and blood.

Use external warming device such as a Bair Hugger on lower extremities.

Warm all irrigating solutions.

PREPARATION FOR HYPOTENSIVE ANESTHESIA

By suppressing the renin-angiotensin system, β-blockade prevents the tachycardia that results from decreased blood pressure, as well as the posthypotensive overshoot.[32] Any of the following medications are useful.

Propranolol is administered intravenously in 0.25-mg doses until pulse rate is slowed to approximately 60 beats/min.

Labetalol in 5- to 10-mg increments is administered until a pulse rate of 60 beats/min is achieved.

Alternatively, captopril (3 mg/kg by mouth preoperatively) can decrease sodium nitroprusside requirements.[33]

INDUCTION AND MAINTENANCE

Induction is accomplished with a barbiturate followed by a narcotic intravenously, nitrous oxide/oxygen by inhalation, and intubation of the trachea with the use of a muscle relaxant.

Opioids can be administered by an intermittent bolus or infusion technique. A loading dose of 10 to 15 μg/kg fentanyl or 3 μg/kg sufentanil is recommended.

If an infusion is used, 5 μg/kg/hr fentanyl or 0.5 μg/kg/hr sufentanil is used after the loading dose.

	Initial Bolus	Infusion
Sufentanil	3 μg/kg	0.5 μg/kg/hr
Fentanyl	10–15 μg/kg	5 μg/kg/hr

Opioid administration should be stopped at least 1.5 hours before the end of the procedure. An infusion of propofol can be useful to avoid awareness toward the end of the procedure after narcotics are discontinued.

High doses of opioids may necessitate prolonged postoperative intubation and ventilatory support or may require the use of a naloxone drip in the postoperative period.

Muscle relaxation can be achieved by the use of nondepolarizing agents. Curare may aid in maintaining hypotensive anesthesia. Pancuronium may cause tachycardia.

If a wake-up test is anticipated, shorter-acting nondepolarizers such as vecuronium can be used.

POSITIONING FOR POSTERIOR SPINAL SURGERY

The patient is anesthetized on a stretcher adjacent to the operating table.

The patient is then placed in the prone position on a Relton-Hall frame (Fig. 11-2). This frame supports the upper body and pelvis, leaving the chest and abdomen free.

Adequate help is needed during the positioning. The anesthesiologist controls the endotracheal tube and the lines.

Pressure in the thoracic area that may hinder respiration and pressure in the abdominal area that may be transmitted to the vertebral venous plexus and cause increased bleeding during surgery should be avoided.

Areas exposed to pressure such as the malar eminences, the tip of the nose, and the eyes are padded because perfusion may be diminished and injuries to these areas can occur. Pressure on the eye may result in blindness. There should be no interference with perfusion of the lower extremities. Pressure may cause a decreased blood flow and lead to muscle necrosis and myoglobinuria.

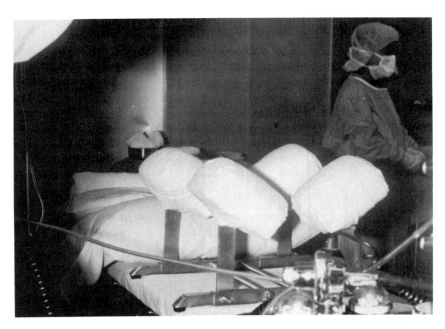

Fig. 11-2. Relton-Hall Frame. Shoulders and pelvis rest on padded bolsters. Chest and abdomen hang free.

COMBINED ANTERIOR AND POSTERIOR APPROACHES

In some situations, combinations of techniques may be indicated. Posterior instrumentation and fusion may not be adequate to treat and control certain deformities. Therefore, combined anterior and posterior approaches are now being used for treatment of these curves.

Anterior Approach

In the anterior approach, a thoracoabdominal incision is used. The anterior thoracic spine is approached through the pleural cavity, and the lumbar spine is exposed by retroperitoneal extension of the incision and detachment of the diaphragm. The intervertebral discs are removed, and appropriate soft tissue releases are performed to mobilize the spine. If necessary, bone grafts are inserted to stabilize the spine. Rib struts may be used in the fusions in this area if needed.

In most instances, after the closure of the thoracoabdominal incision and the placement of chest tubes the patient is then placed in the prone position for the posterior instrumentation and fusion.

Posterior Approach

To accomplish this, the patient is transferred from the operating table to a stretcher. All the lines are secured. The patient is then transferred to the operating table equipped with a Relton-Hall frame, onto which the patient is placed.

The incision is made so that adequate exposure of the spine is provided. Dissection is carried down to the vertebrae that are denuded, and the paraspinal muscles are retracted. Blood loss may be quite brisk at this time.

Appropriate hooks are placed on the lamina of the spines and connected to rods that can be bent to provide correction. When the instrumentation has been inserted, bone grafts from the iliac crest are placed. Muscle, subcutaneous tissues, and skin are then closed after appropriate drains are placed.

In the anterior approach, blood loss is usually not a major problem. The main blood loss occurs during the posterior portion of the procedure.

Hypothermia is noted frequently because the chest or abdomen is open, with a large surface to lose heat.

A regular endotracheal tube is used. We do not use double lumen tubes because the lung is not in the way of the surgeon. The gentle retraction used does not interfere with ventilation and usually does not result in oxygen desaturation. From time to time, the lung is inflated. After placement of the chest tube and before closure, the lung is re-inflated maximally.

CONTROL OF BLOOD LOSS AND BLOOD SALVAGE

Position the patient to avoid pressure on the abdomen, which may be transmitted to the vertebral venous plexus.

Avoid prolonged inspiratory pressure phase to minimize venous engorgement.

Provide adequate anesthesia and muscle relaxation to avoid straining and bucking.

Have the surgeon infiltrate the incision site with epinephrine 1:500,000.

Use a Cell Saver to reduce the need for transfusion.

Induced Hypotension

In young healthy normotensive patients, induced hypotension to a mean arterial pressure of 60 mmHg can materially reduce blood loss during surgery.[34,35]

In cases in which hypotensive techniques were not used, massive blood loss has been reported, and loss of one entire circulating blood volume or greater was not uncommon.[36]

In children, induced hypotension with sodium nitroprusside is more effective than use of nitroglycerin.[37] Deliberate hypotension with nitroprusside induces a reliable and rapid decrease in blood pressure. The hypotensive effect of nitroprusside is achieved more easily if adequate depth of anesthesia is maintained during administration of the hypotensive agent. Do not depend on the nitroprusside infusion alone. The patient should be kept adequately anesthetized and relaxed.

A persistent tachycardia with a high cardiac output may prevent the attainment of a dry, bloodless field. To avoid this situation, β-blockers should be administered before hypotension is induced.

Vecuronium (0.1 mg/kg) can be used to achieve relaxation for endotracheal intubation and continued during surgery.

The use of curare rather than pancuronium may be advantageous in induced hypotension because tachycardia may occur with the latter drug.

Fluid overload should be avoided. Failure to achieve and maintain the hypotensive state may be a result of excess fluid administration before induction of anesthesia.

Maintenance of Hypotensive Anesthesia

Administer β-blockers to decrease pulse rate before induction of anesthesia—propranolol in 0.25-mg IV increments or labetalol in 5- to 10-mg increments until a pulse rate of 60 beats/min is achieved.

Begin infusion of sodium nitroprusside while the patient is being prepared and draped. *Do not wait until the surgeon is holding the knife to begin preparing the solution.*

Administer nitroprusside at a rate of up to 8 to 10 µg/kg/min to achieve desired blood pressure. This dose avoids cyanide toxicity.[38]

In normotensive, healthy patients, decrease blood pressure to a mean of 60 mmHg gradually to allow autoregulation in vital organs. Accomplish the decrease in blood pressure slowly over 15 minutes to allow for autoregulation of the spinal cord blood vessels to occur. Autoregulation allows normal spinal cord function in the face of decreased arterial pressure.

Spargo et al[39] have shown that spinal cord blood flow is either unchanged or increased during hypotension induced with nitroglycerin. Fahmy et al[40] have shown that nitroprusside-induced hypotension leads to increased spinal cord blood flow at the start but the flow returned to control values when the blood pressure reached a mean arterial blood pressure of 60 to 65 mmHg. Reduction in the mean arterial blood pressure below 60 mmHg was accompanied by decreases in spinal cord blood flow.

Maintain $PaCO_2$ in the normal range to avoid vasoconstriction of spinal cord blood vessels.[41]

Make sure the patient is adequately anesthetized and relaxed.

To prevent the possibility of spinal cord ischemia during distraction, raise the blood pressure to normal levels when passing of sublaminar wires, instrumentation, or distraction is taking place.

Bring blood pressure back to normal levels before closure so bleeding points can be detected and controlled.

SPINAL CORD FUNCTION DURING OPERATIVE CORRECTION OF SCOLIOSIS

Neurologic dysfunction can occur during spinal surgery. Conditions associated with increased risk are

Kyphosis

Severe congenital scoliosis

Severe rigid deformities

Unrecognized tethering of the spinal cord

Pre-existing conditions associated with a neurologic deficit

Spinal osteotomies or surgery after preoperative skeletal traction

Stretching of the arterial supply of the spinal cord

Direct trauma

Development of hematomas

Overcorrection

Blood Supply to the Spinal Cord

The blood vessels supplying the cervical and lumbar area are increased in number and size compared with those in the thoracic cord. The thoracic cord depends on proximal and distal sources for its blood supply, and therefore the

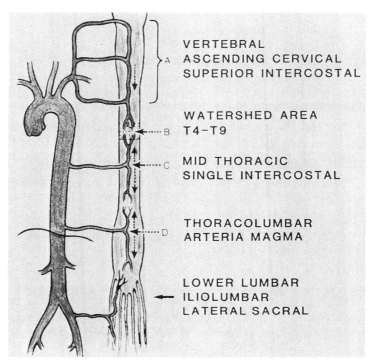

Fig. 11-3. Diagram of blood supply to spinal cord. Watershed area in midthoracic portion is supplied by a single vessel. (From Pasternak, Boyd, and Ellis,[49] with permission.)

circulation of this area has been described as a "watershed." This area of the cord that has a poorer supply of vessels extends from T4 to T9.[20] (Fig. 11-3).

ASSESSMENT OF NEUROLOGIC FUNCTION

Because of concern about neurologic damage, techniques have been developed to monitor spinal cord function during surgery.

The techniques currently in use for assessment of spinal cord function during surgery are

Wake-up test

SSEP monitoring

Neurogenic motor evoked potential (NMEP) monitoring

If these tests are to be used during surgery, *inhalation agents should not be used* because they interfere with the acquisition of accurate electrophysiologic studies, and it is difficult to reverse the effects of these agents rapidly when the wake-up test is to be performed.

Wake-up Test

In the wake-up test, motor function is evaluated during the surgical procedure by having the patient voluntarily move the legs to determine whether the spinal cord is intact.

In this test, devised by Vauzelle and Stagnara,[42] the patients are awakened momentarily during the operation, asked to move their hands and then their feet, and reanesthetized as soon as those procedures are performed. Hand movement signifies that the patient has heard the request and that there is function above the level of the surgery.

If movement does not take place in one or both lower extremities following movement of hands, it is assumed that damage has occurred to the spinal cord and actions to correct the problem are pursued. This may involve decrease in the degree of correction or removal of hardware.

A wake-up test is also performed as an adjunct to electrophysiologic monitoring of the spinal cord if responses deteriorate.

Inhalation agents are not used because their effects may take a long time to be reversed.

Procedure

When the decision is made that the wake-up test is to be performed, the effect of the relaxant is reversed.

The nitrous oxide is turned off as soon as spontaneous respiration is achieved. Small increments (20 μg) of naloxone may be administered until the patient responds by moving the hands and then the feet. After satisfactory movements, the patient is reanesthetized.

During the wake-up test, an assistant should hold the patient's head and endotracheal tube firmly.

Some complications that may occur are accidental extubation, dislodgment of the instrumentation, or air embolism on deep inspiration through open venous sinuses.[43]

Language Problems

If the patient is unable to understand the language spoken by the operating team, translators are used to speak in the patient's language. In one instance, a tape recording was made in the language spoken by the patient by the patient's sister and was played during the wake-up test with satisfactory results.

If the patient's name is Margaret but is called Peggy, or Millicent and is called Muffy, the appropriate name should be used during the test or the patient may ignore the anesthesiologist.

Somatosensory Evoked Potential Monitoring

The use of SSEP monitoring permits a moment-to-moment electrophysiologic evaluation of spinal cord function throughout the procedure. This is significant because injuries resulting from spinal surgery may be reversible if detected early. SSEP analysis indicates the integrity of the *sensory pathways*.

General Principles

SSEPs are elicited when a peripheral nerve such as the median, ulnar, or posterior tibial or pudendal nerves are stimulated.

The stimulation leads to conduction of impulses into the spinal cord by the dorsal roots through the dorsal root ganglia.

In surgical procedures involving the neck, the median and ulnar nerves are stimulated at the wrist. The ulnar nerve response may be more important in cervical spine surgery because it enters the spinal cord at a lower level than the median nerve.

The sites of stimulation for surgery in the thoracic and lumbar spine are the common peroneal and posterior tibial nerves at the ankle.

For surgery involving the lumbar and thoracic spine, both upper and lower extremities are stimulated. If changes occur in both upper stimulating site and lower stimulating sites, it is most likely that the cause of the problem is not the thoracic or lumbar spine surgery but other factors.

Sensory nerves are stimulated in the periphery, enter the spinal cord, and travel in the posterior columns to the cerebral cortex along the following path (Fig. 11-4):

1. Stimulation of peripheral nerve
2. Dorsal root ganglia
3. Posterior columns
   Funiculus gracilis (medial columns)
   Funiculus cuneatus (lateral column)
4. Nucleus gracilis (fibers from lumbar and sacral regions) and nucleus cuneatus (fibers from cervical and thoracic areas)
5. Fibers leave nuclei cross-over in medulla
6. Medial lemniscus

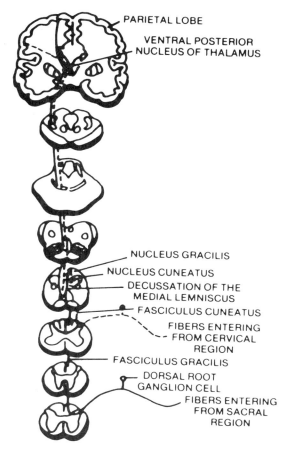

Fig. 11-4. Diagram showing pathway of conduction of impulses from periphery to cerebral cortex during SSEP monitoring.

7. Thalamus
8. Sensory area of cerebral cortex

The electrical responses occurring in the brain resulting from this stimulation denote that the pathways along the spinal cord are intact. When electrodes are placed on the scalp, spontaneous electrical activity, such as electroencephalographic and electromyographic waves, may be seen. For the purposes of the acquisition and recording of SSEPs, these waves are considered as "noise" in electrical terms and are extracted electronically.

Procedure

Sensory nerves are stimulated at the ankle by cutaneous electrodes with preamplifiers that control the amplitude, duration, and frequency of stimulation. Recording and ground electrodes are placed in the appropriate areas of the scalp

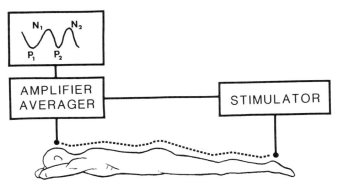

Fig. 11-5. Sensory nerves are stimulated in periphery. Impulses travel along spinal cord and are detected on scalp. They are averaged, amplified, and displayed. (From Bernstein,[5] with permission.)

according to the 10/20 International System to record the waveforms that result (Fig. 11-5).

Waveforms with specific amplitudes and latencies related to the area stimulated have been determined. These waveforms result from the computerized summation of responses to a series of repetitive stimuli that are time-locked to the stimuli. Random waveforms are rejected. The components of the wave are denoted as P1, N1, P2, and N2. The P1 component increases in latency and decreases in amplitude if spinal cord injury occurs (Fig. 11-6).

The latency and amplitude of the P1 component are observed for changes to determine if injury to the spinal cord occurs.

Factors that Affect SSEPs

A preoperative baseline response is obtained before anesthesia so that the patient's neurologic status can be assessed and pre-existing abnormalities detected. This is important in cases of pre-existing neurologic disorders, neuromuscular diseases, and trauma.

In addition to neurologic disorders, factors that affect SSEPs are

Hypoxia

Hypercarbia

Hypothermia

Hypotension

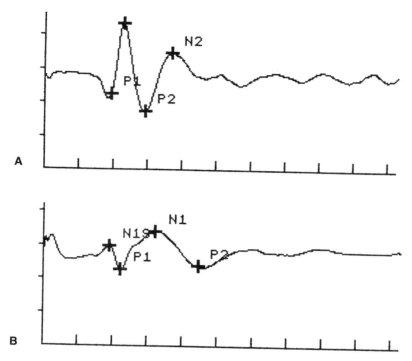

Fig. 11-6. (A) Normal SSEP waveform obtained by stimulating nerves at ankle and picking up response on scalp. Changes in latency and amplitude of P1 wave are considered evidence of spinal cord dysfunction. (B) SSEP waveform resulting from stimulation of ulnar nerve at wrist. N19 (first waveform) is normal.

Medications such as diazepam

Inhalation agents (Fig. 11-7)

Effect of Inhalation Agents

Some anesthesiologists state that low concentrations of inhalation agents are safe to use during SSEP monitoring. It must be remembered that inhalation agents cause a dose-dependent decrease in the amplitude and latency of the evoked potential, and it may be difficult to distinguish between changes that result from spinal cord dysfunction and those resulting from the effects of the inhalation agents. We have observed that waveforms caused by stimulation of the nerves of the hand and wrist may persist when those caused by ankle stimulation are diminished or absent at equipotent end-tidal concentration of inhalation agents.

To be certain that changes in SSEPs are due to spinal cord changes resulting

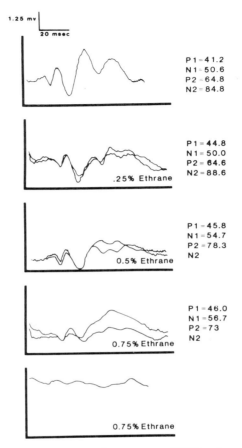

Fig. 11-7. Effect of inhalation anesthetic agents on SSEPs. As end-tidal concentration of ethrane increases, there is an increase in latency of P1 wave as well as a decrease in amplitude. **(Bottom panel)** After 15 minutes, waves disappeared.

from surgical intervention, the foregoing conditions such as hypoxia and hypercarbia must be carefully controlled.

Alterations in SSEPs

Causes
Alterations in latency or amplitude during surgery may result from direct trauma to the spinal cord, ischemia, or a combination of pressure and decreased blood flow (Fig. 11-8).

Abnormal patterns of blood supply to the spinal cord may be present in patients with congenital scoliosis or pre-existing neurologic deficits. Care must be taken

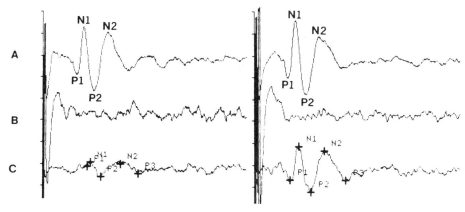

Fig. 11-8. (**A**) Normal waveform is shown. P1 wave shows an increase in latency and a decrease in amplitude if spinal cord injury occurs. (**B**) Waveform has disappeared as a result of injury to spinal cord by a bone fragment. (**C**) Waveforms return after removal of bone. Amplitude and latency of waveform on left have not recovered as much as for waveform on right because injury was on left side. (From Bernstein,[5] with permission.)

that extensive distraction and stretching of the cord not be performed in conditions in which the blood supply to the cord may be at risk.

What to Do if SSEPs Change

Although both amplitude and latency are measured during the tests, the amplitude of the response is considered to be a more valid indicator of the status of the nervous system than is the latency.

If an increase in the latency of 60 percent or a decrease in the amplitude of 10 percent of the response suddenly occurs and all other factors have been held constant,

Remain calm and do not panic; the surgeon is pretty nervous at this time.

Make certain that there is adequate ventilation and check pulse oximeter and end-tidal carbon dioxide monitor.

Make sure body temperature is within normal range.

Ask the surgeon to stop the surgical procedure.

Raise the blood pressure to above-normal levels to increase the perfusion of the cord.

Prepare to perform a wake-up test at this time.[44]

It is assumed that these parameters are being monitored closely and carefully throughout the procedure; however, check them again.

If all the foregoing conditions are normal, the surgeon must decide whether the surgery has caused any damage leading to an abnormal decrease in amplitude.

If this occurred during instrumentation, passage of sublaminar wires, or distraction, it is possible that there has been some interference with spinal cord function secondary to surgery. The surgeon can alter the instrumentation and wait to see if the amplitude returns toward normal.

Deteriorated SSEPs and the Wake-Up Test

Time Factor

It may take some time for the patient to reach a level of consciousness for determining adequacy of motor status.

If the cause of the dimunition or loss of the evoked potential is not addressed immediately, the possibility of permanent neurologic deficit increases.

It may take some time for the SSEPs to show changes after damage to the spinal cord has occurred. If it also takes time to decide whether to do the wake-up test and it also takes time to wake the patient up, there may be permanent neurologic changes by the time the test is carried out.

If the decision to do the wake-up test is made rapidly and the patient is awakened quickly, the status of the motor nerves will be determined earlier and the presence or absence of spinal cord injury will be known.

The surgeon may elect to release the instrumentation immediately and avoid all these problems.

Evoked Potential Monitoring in the Asthmatic Patient

In asthmatic patients, use of inhalation agents may be beneficial to promote bronchodilatation and prevent bronchospasm. SSEP monitoring is performed using electrodes in the epidural space. These waveforms are not altered by inhalation anesthetic agents[45] (Figs. 11-9 to 11-11).

Motor Evoked Potentials

Owen and colleagues[46] have introduced a technique of motor evoked potential monitoring through stimulation of the motor tracts of the spinal cord and recording over the sciatic nerve. There may be a sensory component of this waveform.

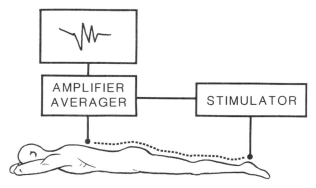

Fig. 11-9. When an epidural electrode is used, response to stimulation from peripheral nerves is detected in epidural space, averaged, amplified, and displayed. (From Bernstein,[5] with permission.)

Procedure

Stimulating electrodes are inserted by the surgeon into the spinous process at the proximal end of the incision.

Bipolar electrodes are placed over the sciatic nerve in the popliteal fossa to measure the response.

This technique does not rely on electromyographic responses but rather on the neurogenic impulse traveling along the motor nerve.

To avoid any interference by picking up recordings from muscle, the anesthesiologist should make certain that the patient is adequately paralyzed with neuromuscular blocking agents while the monitoring is being conducted.

It is important for the surgeon to make certain that fluid in the surgical site does not accumulate and shunt current away from the spinal cord.

The electrode is placed within 1 cm of the spinal cord. The anode is placed

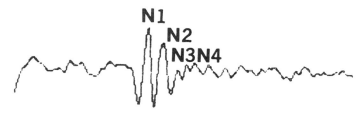

Fig. 11-10. N1–N4 demonstrate typical SSEP waveforms seen when epidural electrode is used. (From Bernstein,[5] with permission.)

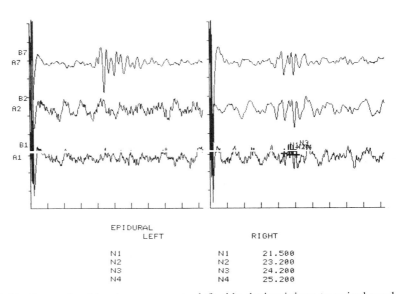

Fig. 11-11. Loss of epidural responses on left side during injury to spinal cord. (**Top**) Normal baseline; (**Middle**) normal on right, abnormal recording on left; (**Bottom**) Normal on right, abnormal recording on left.

proximal to the cathode 2.5 cm apart. This allows the placement of an electrode into two separate adjacent spinous processes.[46]

Response Characteristics

The normal NMEP consists of a sharp, biphasic component (Fig. 11-12 and 11-13).

Interpretation of Results

The interpretation is primarily based on the amplitude of the motor component and secondarily on its latency.

If the amplitude is decreased by at least 60 percent, the surgeon should be

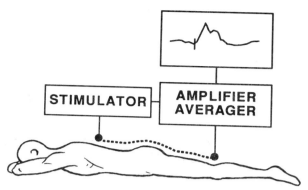

Fig. 11-12. Neurogenic motor evoked potentials. Stimulation of spinal cord above the level of surgery. Responses picked up over sciatic nerve. Latency measured at upstroke of response as shown.

notified. If the amplitude continues to diminish, the surgeon may wish to perform a wake-up test.

Case Study

A 20-year-old man with severe thoracolumbar scoliosis was undergoing correction of the condition using distraction and derotation.

Twenty minutes after the distraction and derotation were completed there was sudden disappearance of SSEPs and NMEPs (Fig. 11-14).

The surgical procedure was stopped and a wake-up test was performed. During the wake-up test, the patient was unable to move his lower extremities but was able to move the upper extremities. The patient was sufficiently awake to respond by nodding his head when asked if he understood the directions. The patient was then anesthetized, and the hardware was removed. After this, another wake-up test was performed. The patient was still unable to move the lower extremities. The patient was reanesthetized and the wound was closed. Prior to leaving the operating room the SSEP and NMEP recordings gradually improved.

In the recovery room, sensory and motor function returned to the lower extremities.

Comment

This case illustrates that the wake-up test may not always be adequate to determine whether neurologic damage had occurred after spinal instrumentation because the SSEPs and NMEPs remained normal for approximately 20 minutes after the instrumentation had been inserted. Had a wake-up test been performed immediately after the completion of the instrumentation, it may have appeared normal. Continuous monitoring of the spinal cord throughout the procedure was able to demonstrate loss of responses when they had occurred.

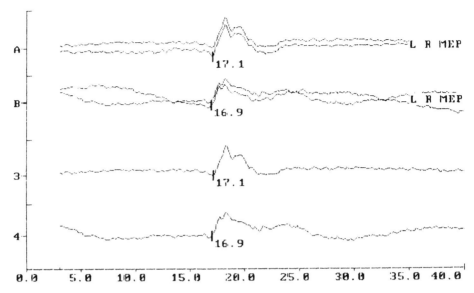

Fig. 11-13. Neurogenic motor evoked potentials. Stimulation of spinal cord above level of surgery. Responses picked up over sciatic nerve. Latency measured at upstroke of response as shown. (Courtesy of Dr. Aleksandar Beric.)

It was thought that the distraction and derotation may have been responsible for compromising the blood supply to the cord, leading to loss of sensory and motor function, which returned when the hardware was removed.

With the use of simultaneous SSEP monitoring and NMEP monitoring, it is believed that injury to the spinal cord during surgery will be detected.

STEROID USE AFTER POSSIBLE SPINAL CORD INJURY

A high-dose steroid protocol has been shown to be efficacious in patients suffering acute spinal cord trauma[47] (see Ch. 2). Although there are no documented controlled studies in patients undergoing scoliosis surgery who suffer from spinal cord trauma, we have empirically started treating such patients with the high-dose steroid protocol.

VENOUS AIR EMBOLISM

This may occur because the operative site is above the level of the heart, and open venous sinuses are present in the bone as well as in the vessels. Decreased venous pressure, decreased intra-abdominal pressure, and blood loss may pre-

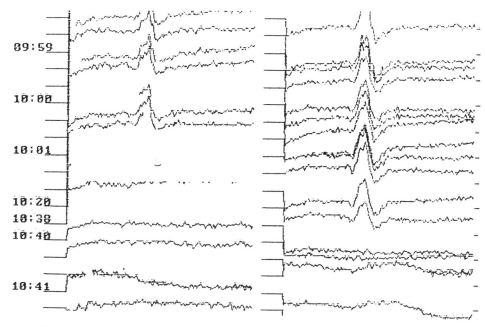

Fig. 11-14. Neurogenic motor evoked potentials. Sequential recordings at different time intervals reveal normal responses at 10:00 AM. At 10:38 AM, there is loss of response on left side followed by loss of response on right. (Courtesy of Dr. Aleksandar Beric.)

dispose to venous air embolism. A case has been reported in which the blood pressure fell, the end-tidal carbon dioxide decreased, and the end-tidal nitrogen rose.[43]

POSTOPERATIVE CARE

Neurologic Evaluation

The patient should enter the PACU awake enough to undergo a neurologic assessment. Attention must be directed to the patient's neurologic condition in the immediate postoperative period, with frequent determinations of the sensory and motor status. If any changes are observed, blood pressure should be increased to normal or even above-normal levels to improve spinal cord blood flow. If necessary, arrangements should be made for re-exploration.

Pulmonary Evaluation

At the end of surgery, a decision must be made as to the need for postoperative ventilatory support. Patients who have nonidiopathic scoliosis have a higher incidence of postoperative pulmonary complications. Patients with a paralytic scoliosis associated with neuromuscular disease may have a loss of respiratory muscle force and an ineffective cough, as well as abnormalities of the central nervous system. Airway loss because of laryngeal and pharyngeal problems may also cause difficulties in the postoperative period. Ventilatory status requires careful attention in this group of patients so that severe postoperative complications can be avoided.[48] Small amounts of respiratory depressant drugs may produce acute respiratory insufficiency or apnea in patients who have little pulmonary reserve.

Body Temperature

If the patient is hypothermic, the endotracheal tube should not be removed.

Ventilatory support should be provided and the patient rewarmed until normothermic.

The patient is assessed for extubation.

Extubation

Most patients undergoing surgery for correction of scoliosis can be extubated immediately after surgery. However, one must use extreme caution at this time because hypoventilation can occur after the stimulus of the endotracheal tube is removed, especially in patients in whom opioids and relaxants were used. Blood gas determinations and pulse oximetry are useful. In some instances, naloxone by bolus or infusion may be needed if excess opioid appears to be causing respiratory depression. The half-life of naloxone is less than that of the administered opioid, so repeat doses may be required. If a question arises as to the adequacy of ventilation, the endotracheal tube should be left in place. In patients in whom the vital capacity was less than 30 percent of normal or in patients with neuromuscular diseases, endotracheal intubation and assisted ventilation will probably be necessary for a period of time after the operation.

Volume Status

Large fluid shifts have taken place in the operating room with blood loss and fluid replacement. The patient's volume status is reassessed after arrival to the PACU.

Blood Loss

Blood may continue to be lost into drains from oozing; this must be monitored. Hemoglobin and hematocrit determinations are obtained. Complications associated with reinfusion of wound salvaged blood such as hematuria may occur.

Pneumothorax

A postoperative pneumothorax may be present, especially in patients who have had rib resections.

Ileus

Postoperative ileus is seen, and a nasogastric tube is necessary for decompression in these patients. Excessive distension of the stomach may restrict ventilation.

Cast Syndrome

A condition known as the "cast syndrome" may develop in which distension of the stomach and duodenum results from anatomic changes in the ligament of Treitz after surgical correction of the curve. This can be treated with nasogastric suction, but surgical intervention may be necessary.

Myoglobinuria

Pressure on muscles may lead to damage, and myoglobinuria may result.

Urine Output

It is necessary to observe for adequate urine output.

REFERENCES

1. Hibbs RA: An operation for progressive spinal deformity. NY Med J 93:1013, 1911
2. Harrington PR: Treatment of scoliosis. Correction and internal fixation by spine instrumentation. J Bone Joint Surg 44(A):591, 1962
3. Luque ER: Segmental spinal instrumentation for correction of scoliosis. Clin Orthop 163:192, 1982
4. Cobb JR: Outline in the study of scoliosis. Instr Course Lect 5:261, 1948
5. Bernstein RL: Anesthetic management of patients with scoliosis. p. 17. In Barash PG (ed): ASA Refresher Course Lectures. Vol. 16. JB Lippincott, Philadelphia, 1988
6. Smyth RJ, Chapman KR, Wright TA et al: Pulmonary function in adolescents with mild idiopathic scoliosis. Thorax 39:901, 1984
7. Hirschfeld SS, Rudner C, Nash CL et al: Incidence of mitral valve prolapse in adolescent scoliosis and thoracic hypokyphosis. Pediatrics 70:451, 1982
8. Primiano FP, Nussbaum E, Hirschfeld SS et al: Early echocardiographic and pulmonary function findings in idiopathic scoliosis. J Pediatr Orthop 3:475, 1983
9. Rosenberg CA, Derman GH, Grabb WC et al: Hypomastia and mitral valve prolapse: evidence of a limited embryologic and mesenchymal dysplasia. N Engl J Med 309:1230, 1983

10. Shook JE, Lubicky JP: Paralytic spinal deformity. p. 279. In Bridwell KH, Dewald RL (eds): The Textbook of Spinal Surgery. JB Lippincott, Philadelphia, 1991

11. Mackley JT, Herndon C, Inkley S et al: Pulmonary function in paralytic and non-paralytic scoliosis before and after treatment. J Bone Joint Surg 50(A):1379, 1968

12. Nickel V, Perry J, Affeldt JE et al: Elective surgery on patients with respiratory paralysis. J Bone Joint Surg 39(A):989, 1957

13. Garrett AL, Perry J, Nickel V: Stabilization of the collapsing spine. J Bone Joint Surg 43(A):474, 1961

14. Hale RA, Rash FL: Pulmonary function testing. p. 585. In Bradford DS, Lonstein JE, Moe JH et al (eds): Moe's Textbook of Scoliosis and Other Spinal Deformities. 2nd Ed. WB Saunders, Philadelphia, 1987

15. Duncan PG: Neuromuscular diseases. p. 509. In Katz J, Steward DJ (eds): Anesthesia and Uncommon Pediatric Diseases. WB Saunders, Philadelphia, 1987

16. Miller JD, Lee C: Muscle diseases. In Katz J, Benumof JL, Kadis LB (eds): Anesthesia and Uncommon Diseases. 3rd Ed. WB Saunders, Philadelphia, 1990

17. Hunsaker RH, Fulkerson PK, Barry FJ et al: Cardiac function in Duchenne's muscular dystrophy. Results of a 10 year follow-up study and non-invasive tests. Am J Med 73:235, 1982

18. Adams FH, Emmanoullides GC, Rienenschnuda TA: Heart Disease in Infants and Children. Williams & Wilkins, Baltimore, 1989

19. Martz DG, Schreibman DL, Matjasko MJ: Neurological diseases. In Katz J, Benumof JD, Kadis LB (eds): Anesthesia and Uncommon Diseases. 3rd Ed. WB Saunders, Philadelphia, 1990

20. Salem MR, Klowden AJ: Anesthesia for pediatric orthopedic surgery. p. 1203. In Gregory SA (ed): Pediatric Anesthesia. 2nd Ed. Churchill Livingstone, New York, 1989

21. Huebert HT, MacKinnon WB: Syringomyelia and scoliosis. J Bone Joint Surg 51(B): 338, 1969

22. Nordwall A, Wikkelso C: A late neurologic complication of scoliosis surgery in connection with syringomyelia. Acta Orthop Scand 50:407, 1979

23. Dubowitz V: Infantile spinal muscular atrophy: a progressive study with particular reference to a slowly progressive variety. Brain 57:767, 1974

24. Evans GA, Drennan JC: Functional classification and orthopedic management of spinal muscular atrophy. J Bone Joint Surg 63(B):516, 1981

25. Cambridge W, Drennan JC: Scoliosis associated with Duchenne's muscular dystrophy. J Pediatr Orthop 7:436, 1987

26. Milne B, Rosales JK: Anesthetic considerations in patients with muscular dystrophy undergoing spinal fusion and Harrington rod insertion. Can Anaesth Soc J 29:250, 1982

27. Aprin H, Bowen H, MacEwen GD et al: Spine fusion in patients with spinal muscular atrophy. J Bone Joint Surg 64(A):1179, 1982

28. Bell GR, Gurd AR, Orlowski JP et al: The syndrome of inappropriate antidiuretic hormone secretion following spinal fusion. J Bone Joint Surg 68(A):720, 1982

29. Silvergleid AJ: Safety and effectiveness of predeposit autologous transfusions in preteens and adolescent children. JAMA 257:3403, 1987

30. MacEwen GD, Bennett E, Guille JT: Autologous blood transfusions in children and young adults with low body weight undergoing spine surgery. J Pediatr Orthop 10: 750, 1990

31. Goodnough LT, Rudnick S, Price TH et al: Increased preoperative collection of

autologous blood with recombinant human erythropoietin therapy. N Engl J Med 321:17, 1163

32. Khambatta HJ, Stone JG, Khan E: Propranolol alters renin release during nitroprusside-induced hypotension and prevents hypertension on discontinuation of nitroprusside. Anesth Analg 60:569, 1981

33. Woodside J, Garner L, Bedfrod RF: Captopril reduces the dose requirement for sodium nitroprusside induced hypotension. Anesthesiology 60:413, 1984

34. Simpson P: Perioperative blood loss and its reduction: the role of the anaesthetist. Br J Anaesth 69:498, 1992

35. Abbott TR, Bentley G: Intraoperative awakening during scoliosis surgery. Anaesthesia 35:298, 1980

36. Bennett NR, Abbott TR: The use of sodium nitroprusside in children. Anaesthesia 32:456, 1977

37. Yaster M, Simmons RS, Tolo VT et al: A comparison of nitroglycerin and nitroprusside for inducing hypotension in children: a double blind study. Anesthesiology 65: 174, 1986

38. Tinker JH, Michenfelder JD: Sodium nitroprussive: pharmacology, toxicology, and therapeutics. Anesthesiology 45:340, 1976

39. Spargo PM, Tait AR, Knight PR, Kling TP: Effect of nitroglycerin induced hypotension on canine spinal cord blood flows. Br J Anaesth 59:640, 1987

40. Fahmy NR, Mossad B, Milad M: Spinal cord blood flow during induced hypotension: comparison of nitroprusside and trimethaphan, abstracted. Anesthesiology 53: S87, 1980

41. Jacobs HJ, Lieponis JV, Bunch WH et al: The influence of halothane and nitroprusside on canine spinal cord hemodynamics. Spine 7:35, 1982

42. Vauzelle C, Stagnara P, Jouvinroux P: Functional monitoring of spinal cord activity during spinal surgery. Clin Orthop 93:173, 1973

43. Frankel AS, Holzman RS: Air embolism during posterior spinal fusion. Can J Anaesth 35:5, 1988

44. Owen JH: Evoked potential monitoring during spinal surgery. p. 31. In Bridwell KH, DeWald RL (eds): The Textbook of Spinal Surgery. JB Lippincott, Philadelphia, 1991

45. Jones SS, Edgar MA, Ransford AO: Sensory nerve conduction in the human spinal cord: epidural recordings made during scoliosis surgery. J Neurol Neurosurg Psychiatry 45:446, 1982

46. Owen JH, Bridwell KH, Shimon SM et al: Sensitivity and specificity of somatosensory and neurogenic-motor evoked potentials in animals and humans. Spine 12: 1111, 1988

47. Bracken M, Shepard MJ, Collins WF et al: A randomized controlled trial of methylprednisolone or naloxone in the treatment of acute spine cord injury. Results of the second national acute spinal cord injury study. N Engl J Med 322:1504, 1990

48. Anderson PR, Puro MR, Lovell SL, Swayze CR: Postoperative respiratory complication in non-idiopathic scoliosis. Acta Anaesthesiol Scand 29:180, 1985

49. Pasternak BM, Boyd DP, Ellis FH: Spinal cord injury after procedures on the aorta. Surg Gynecol Obstet 135:29, 1972

12

Spinal Surgery

MYELOGRAPHY

Patients scheduled for spinal surgery may have myelography performed in the immediate preoperative period. Certain factors should be considered in caring for these patients.

Myelograms are performed with radiopaque materials that are water-soluble.

During and after myelography, it is recommended that this material not be allowed to enter the brain for fear of causing convulsions.

Therefore, after myelography it is recommended that the patients be kept in a head-up position for at least 12 hours.

Medications that lower seizure threshold should be avoided.

These drugs are

Phenothiazines

Monoamine oxidase inhibitors

Tricyclic antidepressants

Antipsychotic drugs

Droperidol

Hydroxyzine

These drugs should be discontinued 48 hours before myelography and not administered for 24 hours afterward.

Adverse Reactions

Adverse reactions that may occur after intrathecal administration of radiopaque water-soluble materials include

Headache (due either to meningeal irritation or to a leak of cerebrospinal fluid)

Stiff neck

Backache

Vomiting

Nausea

Dizziness

Neurologic symptoms
    Pain
    Hyperesthesias
    Possible urinary retention

Cerebral Symptoms
    Seizures

Generalized problems
    Fever
    Leucocytosis

After myelography, patients may be scheduled for spinal surgery in the prone position. In this position, the head may tend to be slightly lower than the back, which would allow water-soluble material to reach the brain, with the possible development of convulsions.

Renal Function

After the installation of water-soluble radiopaque material, adequate hydration should be provided to prevent renal complications.

Surgery Immediately after Myelogram

After myelography, patients may be scheduled for surgery. The postmyelogram symptoms described above are of interest to the anesthesiologist.

Dural Puncture Headache

We have encountered several patients who, after myelography, have complained of severe post-dural puncture headache. We have been called on to administer epidural blood patches for several of these patients after a day of conservative therapy. The orthopedic surgeons, neurosurgeons and radiologists should be made aware of this problem, and if the patient is suffering from a post-dural puncture headache, a blood patch should be considered.

Post-dural puncture headaches can become manifest after surgery. A patient might have a myelogram performed followed by spinal surgery. On the following day, the patient may complain of severe headache, which may be a result of the dural puncture with leaking of cerebrospinal fluid.

We have been called on to administer epidural blood patches immediately after lumbar laminectomy.

The technique used is to enter the epidural space at a lever higher than the surgical scar. As usual, meticulous attention should be paid to sterile technique.

ANESTHETIC CONSIDERATIONS FOR SPINAL SURGERY

The anesthesiologist should

1. Provide adequate anesthesia, amnesia, and muscular relaxation
2. Control blood pressure to avoid excessive bleeding
3. Provide ability to monitor spinal cord function
4. Make sure the patient is awake at the end of the procedure to assess neurologic function

ANESTHETIC MANAGEMENT

1. Balanced anesthesia with opioid administration either by continuous intravenous infusion or by intermittent bolus technique
2. Nitrous oxide/oxygen by inhalation
3. Muscle relaxation with a nondepolarizing muscle relaxant by intermittent bolus or by infusion
4. No inhalation agents if spinal cord monitoring is used

Monitoring

Electrocardiogram (ECG)

If hypotensive anesthesia is to be used, intra-arterial blood pressure monitoring

Esophageal stethescope for breath and heart sounds

Temperature

Neuromuscular blockade with a peripheral nerve stimulator

End-tidal carbon dioxide concentration

Pulse oximeter

Airway pressure

Spinal cord monitoring

Urinary catheter to monitor urinary output

Thromboembolism Prophylaxis

Some surgeons use intermittent calf compression devices to prevent thromboembolism. These must be applied before surgery to be effective. They should not be put on after surgery since clots may be dislodged and emboli may occur.

Venous Access

All intravenous catheters are inserted and secured before turning and positioning the patient.

Intravenous injection ports and stopcocks must be available at the head of the operating table after positioning and draping.

Control of Blood Pressure

Medications

If hypotensive anesthesia is necessary, consider

β-Blockers to prevent tachycardia before use of vasodilator agents
Infusion of vasodilator agents such as sodium nitroprusside or nitroglycerin
Use of agents such as labetalol alone (see Ch. 11)

Position

In the prone position, the body must be properly padded and positioned. Excess pressure on nose, ears, eyes, and face should be avoided. Acute hip flexion, which may cause occlusion of the femoral vessels, must be avoided.

Anesthesia

Provide an adequate depth of anesthesia to avoid bucking, moving, and straining
Provide muscle relaxation.
Avoid positive end-expiratory pressure with venous engorgement.
Keep mean airway pressure low.
Maintain $PaCO_2$ in normal range.

CERVICAL SPINE SURGERY

Anterior Approach

Anterior approaches are performed for

Disc excision
Disc excision and fusion
Resection of osteophytes
Anterior cervical fusion for instability

Herniated Cervical Disc

Degenerative changes in the cervical spine result in herniated discs.

Symptoms associated with acute herniated discs include

Neck pain

Occipital pain

Shoulder pain

Radicular symptoms involving a specific dermatome with sensory loss, paresthesias, hyperesthesias, or motor deficits.

Vertebral artery compression
    Symptoms of vertebral artery compression include
        Dizziness
        Vertigo
        Nausea
        Tinnitus
        Blurring of vision
        Pain behind the eye[1]

Myelopathy with complaints of pain in the upper and lower extremity

Bowel and bladder dysfunction

Role of Anesthesiologist

The degree of neck extension that is tolerable without symptoms is evaluated. If extension produces symptoms, an awake fiberoptic intubation is planned.

Somatosensory evoked potential (SSEP) monitoring may be used to detect any alterations in spinal cord function during intubation (see Ch. 11).

Position

The head and neck are maintained in a position during anesthesia that did not cause symptoms while the patient was awake.

The patient is placed supine on the operating table.

Gardner-Wells tongs for longitudinal traction may be needed.

A roll is placed under the shoulders to keep the neck in *slight* extension.

Arms are placed at the side.

All intravenous lines and monitoring devices are secured.

The patient is positioned for an intraoperative radiograph.

The surgeon must have room to work.

A pad is placed under the buttock if an iliac bone graft is to be taken.

The head is tilted 10 to 15 degrees to the opposite side of the incision to aid in the approach.

Surgical Approach

The incision in the neck is usually made on the left side to avoid injuring the recurrent laryngeal nerve. The carotid artery, internal jugular vein, and vagus nerves are retracted laterally; the trachea, larynx, and esophagus are retracted medially.[2]

Further dissection is carried out until the cervical spine is reached.

Excision of the disc is carried out.

If a bone graft is necessary, it may be obtained from the iliac crest.

SSEP monitoring is useful during the placement of the graft.

Case Study

   During a cervical spine fusion, SSEP monitoring revealed acute deterioration of spinal cord function after insertion of the graft. The graft was removed. The graft was too large and caused too much distraction of the spinal cord. After refashioning and reinsertion of the graft, the SSEPs remained normal (Fig. 12-1).

Cervical Spondylosis

Cervical spondylosis or chronic cervical disc degeneration occurs with aging and is associated with[12]

Osteophyte formation

Narrowing of the spinal canal

Narrowing of the intervertebral nerve root canals

Posterior facet arthritis

Ligamentous and capsular thickening

Instability

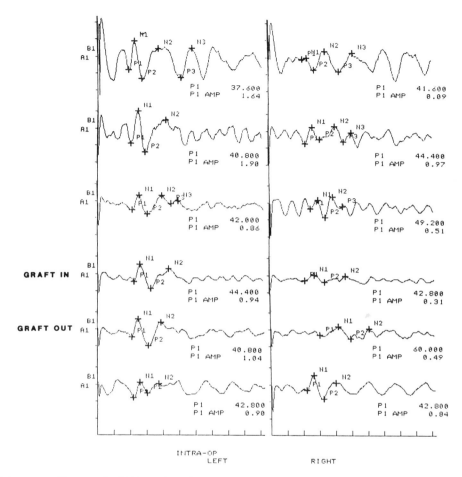

Fig. 12-1. Changes in SSEPs after placement of bone graft between two vertebrae. Note increase of latency on right side with return when graft that was too large was removed.

Subluxation

Disc protrusions

Clinical Manifestations

Neck Pain

Referred pain to the arms and shoulders

Headaches

Compression of the spinal cord with myelopathy

Compression of cervical nerve roots[13]

Surgical Procedures

1. Nerve root decompression
2. Spinal cord decompression
3. Removal of osteophytes and vertebral artery decompression
4. Vertebral fusion

The foregoing procedures may either be performed through the anterior or posterior approach. Decompression of the vertebral artery may be performed from a more lateral approach.

Position

The patient is placed on the operating table in the supine position with a sheet or towel under the shoulders and base of the neck.

The arms are placed at the sides and pulled down to allow for intraoperative lateral radiographs of the neck for identification of appropriate levels.

Skeletal traction may be applied to the head after induction of anesthesia for stabilization of the neck during surgery.

Skeletal traction also allows positioning for insertion of bone grafts. The head is placed in extension and rotated away from the site of incision.

Surgical Approach

Anterior Approach

The incision is along the anterior border of the sternocleidomastoid muscle.

The carotid sheath is retracted laterally; the trachea, esophagus, and thyroid gland are retracted medially.[2]

Complications

Temporary dysphagia, sore throat, or hoarseness
   These are related to the surgical approach and retraction. The patient should be told about these at the preoperative visit

Perforation of the trachea and esophagus
   The anesthesiologist should not tell the patient about these because it may scare them; let the surgeon do it

Perforation of the carotid and vertebral vessels

Injury to the sympathetic chain

Recurrent laryngeal nerve injury

Involvement of the recurrent laryngeal nerve is the most common neurologic complication occurring in anterior approaches. The nerve is most
exposed to injury on the right side

On the left side, thoracic duct injury

Pneumothorax and mediastinitis

Glossopharyngeal, hypoglossal, and facial nerves are at risk during exposure
of the upper cervical spines

Postoperative hematoma[2]

The dressing should always be checked for blood. This may cause tracheal
compression and may be extensive enough to cause respiratory difficulty. This
is usually avoided by adequate drainage.[2]

Conduct of Anesthesia

Adequate anesthesia and muscle relaxation should be maintained throughout
the procedure. Bucking during the procedure may lead to disastrous complications.

At the conclusion of surgery, it is essential that awakening from anesthesia be
smooth because any bucking, coughing, or movements of the head and neck
may cause disruption of graft sites.

Posterior Approach

Position

The patient is anesthetized on a stretcher adjacent to the operating table.

After endotracheal intubation, the patient is placed prone on the operating table.
The head is secured in an appropriate head holder.

The head is *slightly* flexed on the neck.

In the prone position, there should be no undue pressure on the eyes.

Contact points are padded.

The operating table is tilted foot-down so that the cervical spine is parallel to
the floor.

A lateral radiograph is taken to identify the appropriate spinous process. A 22-
gauge spinal needle is inserted through the skin as a marker.[2]

Complications

Neurologic damage to the spinal cord and nerve roots

Damage to the vertebral artery

Complications of the donor site
 Hematoma
 Injury to lateral femoral cutaneous nerve of the thigh
 Infection
 Pain over the iliac crest[2]

Sitting Position

The patient is anesthetized in the supine position on the operating table.

A central venous pressure line is inserted with the tip at the level of the junction of the superior vena cava and right atrium for aspiration of air should air embolism occur.

A Doppler monitor is placed over the precordium for detection of air embolism.

The patient is slowly placed into the sitting position while checking vital signs.

The endotracheal tube should be supported properly.

The head is fixed by the head-holding device. The pin tracts must be sealed to avoid air entrainment through these sites.

The hips and knees are flexed to decrease tension on the sciatic nerve. The buttocks are padded to avoid pressure and ischemia. The arms are supported so that they do not hang down and put tension on the neck muscles. The transducer of an arterial line is placed at the level of the head to monitor the blood pressure perfusing the brain. The blood pressure is maintained in normal range to prevent cerebral damage.

 Advantages
  Decreased venous distension and bleeding

 Disadvantages
  Air embolism
  Cerebral injury caused by severe or prolonged hypotension
  Decubiti on buttocks from pressure

Surgery for Decompression of Myelopathy

Myelopathy may be associated with compressive lesions of the spinal cord.

Anesthetic Considerations

Hyperextension of the neck should be avoided because it may produce an additional neurologic deficit.

The anterior approach is used if it is necessary to decompress three or fewer interspaces.

The posterior approach is used for three or more levels.

Surgical Technique

Anterior Approach

The patient is placed in the supine position.

The disc spaces are opened and material removed all the way to the posterior longitudinal ligament.

The vertebral bodies are then removed, leaving the posterior cortex intact.

Longitudinal traction is applied.

A bone graft is then inserted to replace the resected vertebrae.[2]

Posterior Approach

The patient is placed in the prone position with tongs applied to the skull for traction.

Warning: In positioning the patient for surgery, attention should be paid to the position of the patient's neck.

Hyperextension during posterior exposures in the prone position should be avoided. If the ligamentum flavum is hypertrophied and spinal stenosis exists, hyperextension may cause further narrowing of the spinal canal with impingement on the spinal cord.[2]

Warning: In the prone position, the eyes should always be protected from pressure. Pressure may lead to retinal artery thrombosis and blindness.

Laminectomies are performed and the spinal cord is decompressed by removing the spinous processes, the lamina, and the ligamentum flavum.

Transoral Retropharyngeal Approach

This procedure is performed through the open mouth (see Ch. 1).

Indications

Compression of the spinal cord with neurologic complications resulting from destructive changes

Involvement of the C1 and C2 vertebrae by rheumatoid arthritis because of inflammatory changes leading to instability with destruction of the dens

Upward migration of the dens toward the foramen magnum

Transoral approaches to the cervical spine have been developed to provide direct exposure.

Transoral decompression followed by posterior fusion is combined into a single two-stage operative procedure.[3–5]

Patient Assessment

There is usually cervical instability.

Neurologic deficits may be present from spinal cord compression with both upper and lower extremity weakness secondary to myelopathy.

Airway

Mouth opening usually is compromised because of temporomandibular joint ankylosis.

There is inability to move neck because of cervical spine disease. Movement of neck may cause further neurologic damage.

Airway Management

Nasotracheal intubation by means of flexible fiberoptic laryngoscopy is performed in the awake state.

Alternative Method

A tracheotomy is performed, and a cuffed tracheotomy tube is inserted. The patient is then anesthetized.

A nasogastric tube is inserted.

Anesthetic Management

A narcotic, nitrous oxide/oxygen, relaxant technique is used since spinal cord monitoring is employed.

Monitoring

ECG

Intra-arterial blood pressure monitoring

Nerve stimulator

Foley catheter

Precordial stethescope (esophageal stethoscope *not* used)

End-tidal carbon dioxide

Pulse oximetry

Surgical Procedure

Stage One

The patient is placed in the lateral position with an axillary roll to prevent pressure on the brachial artery and brachial plexus.

The head is held in position in an appropriate skull clamp.

After suitable preparation, the head is draped with the mouth exposed.

A transoral retractor is inserted into the mouth.

The retractor holds the nasotracheal tube and nasogastric tube out of the surgical field.

The operating microscope is positioned.

The mucosa of the posterior pharynx is infiltrated with epinephine 1:200,000.

A midline incision is made in the posterior pharyngeal mucosa over C1 and dissection is carried down. The anterior arch of C1 is exposed and may be removed entirely or partially.

The dens is exposed, the surrounding soft tissues are removed, and the dens is removed. This may be difficult.

Decompression is carried out until the dura is noted to pulsate freely.

Posterior Fusion—Stage Two

The patient remains in the lateral position.

The table is tilted away from the surgeon.

Posterior fusion is performed with the use of sublaminar wires or clamps.

Postoperative Management

Postoperatively, marked swelling of the posterior pharyngeal wall occurs. The endotracheal tube acts as a stent, and *its removal can result in complete airway obstruction and an airway emergency*. It is *essential* that the patient is adequately sedated and the arms restrained in the immediate postoperative period to avoid accidental dislodgement of the endotracheal tube. This should be explained to the patient during the preoperative visit.

The patient is kept in a head-up position to decrease swelling.

The nasotracheal tube remains in place for 2 to 5 days until the swelling subsides.

Ventilatory assistance is carried out as determined by blood gas analysis.

An H_2 blocker (ranitidine or cimetidine) is administered for the first 5 to 7 days.

Metoclopramide is administered to prevent regurgitation.

The patient remains on nothing-by-mouth (NPO) status for 5 days.

Intravenous fluid is administered cautiously to help reduce swelling.

Retropharyngeal Approach

Before anesthesia, the patient is asked to extend the head without help. This is the maximum extension that should be allowed during anesthesia.

The patient is placed on the operating table in the supine position with the head turned to the side. The head is stabilized by means of skull tongs.

Anesthetic Management

Fiberoptic nasotracheal intubation is performed after adequate topical anesthesia. Oral airways and esophageal stethoscopes are avoided.

A submandibular incision is used.

Use of a nerve stimulator by the surgeon to identify the facial nerve may be necessary. It must be taken into consideration that muscle relaxants have been administered. Communicate with the surgeon.

The dissection proceeds into the retropharyngeal area. The larynx and pharynx are retracted medially and the carotid sheath laterally.

Postoperative Management

The patient is maintained in skull traction.

The head is elevated to reduce edema.

The same considerations for postoperative airway management exist as after transoral surgery.

The endotracheal tube is kept in place until the swelling has diminished; its premature removal can result in an airway emergency.[6]

THORACIC SPINAL CORD SURGERY

Thoracic spinal cord surgery is performed for

Trauma

Malignancy

Scoliosis

Kyphosis

Trauma

Injuries of the thoracic spine may lead to instability of the spine with or without spinal cord compression and neurologic changes.

An unstable fracture of the thoracic spine may lead to neurologic changes if left unattended. Anterior transthoracic, anterior and posterior approaches, or a posterior approach may be indicated based on the type of fracture.

Somatosensory Evoked Potential Monitoring

SSEP monitoring should be performed before induction of anesthesia to determine baseline status.

SSEPs are repeated before and after turning the patient.

Case Study

> A patient sustained an injury to the thoracic spine without any neurologic deficit. A normal SSEP was noted before turning the patient. After placing the patient in the lateral position, the amplitude of the SSEP showed deterioration. Turning the patient affected the stability of the fracture, and compression of the spinal cord occurred because of loose fragments. After surgical stabilization, the SSEP returned to normal.

In the anterior approach, the operation is performed through a formal thoracotomy.

After stabilization by the anterior approach, the patient is turned into the prone position for posterior stabilization.

Posterior Stabilization Alone

The patient is placed in the prone position, and the procedure is carried out with decompression, stabilization, and fixation as necessary.

Anesthetic Management

A narcotic, nitrous oxide/oxygen, relaxant technique is used because SSEP monitoring is to be performed during the procedure.

Malignancy

Primary or metastatic tumors can lead to vertebral instability and neurologic changes.

Surgery involves stabilization and decompression of the spinal cord to prevent neurologic changes or reverse neurologic damage.

Anterior Approach

Certain lesions may require thoracotomy and anterior approach for decompression and stabilization.

Methylmethacrylate bone cement may be necessary in instances of vertebral body destruction in addition to the use of metallic fixation.

Posterior stabilization may be performed in combination with anterior decompression or by itself.

Posterior stabilization involves the decompression and metallic fixation to maintain correction.

These operations may need to be performed on an emergency basis because acute spinal cord compression may suddenly occur.

Factors that must be considered when operating on a patient for emergency include hemoglobin, hematocrit, full stomach, coexisting diseases, chemotherapy, and radiation therapy (see Ch. 13).

Anterior Thoracotomy

The patient is placed in the lateral decubitus position.

Care should be taken because other metastatic lesions to bone may be present that may fracture during positioning.

Anesthetic Management

General endotracheal anesthesia with a narcotic, nitrous oxide/oxygen, muscle relaxant technique is used.

SSEP monitoring may be used to follow the status of spinal cord function. Improvement may occur after decompression and stabilization of the lesion.

Posterior Decompression and Stabilization

The patient is placed on the operating table in the prone position with the shoulders and pelvis supported.

Decompression, stabilization, and fusion are carried out.

Preparation should be made to replace large volumes of blood.

LUMBAR SPINE SURGERY

Percutaneous Discectomy

The surgeon enters the disc space transcutaneously under fluoroscopic control, liquifies the contents of the disc space, and removes it by suction.

Position

The patient is placed on the operating table in the lateral position with fluoroscopic C-arm control during surgery.

Anesthetic Management

The procedure is performed under local anesthesia with sedation and monitoring provided by the anesthesiologist.

Laminectomy for Disc Removal

Laminectomy for disc removal is usually an elective procedure. However, if bowel and bladder dysfunction have occurred, emergency surgery may be necessary.

Anesthetic Management

The patient is anesthetized on a stretcher adjacent to the operating table.

No special anesthetic technique is needed unless SSEP monitoring is to be used. In this situation, a narcotic, nitrous oxide/oxygen, relaxant technique should be used.

Position

After the establishment of satisfactory general endotracheal anesthesia, the patient is carefully turned from the supine position on the stretcher to a prone position on the operating table. Adequately trained staff must be present for positioning of the patient.

The endotracheal tube must be secured before placing the patient in the prone position. Special precautions are used to make certain that the tape does not become moist and lose its grip on the endotracheal tube.

The position favored by many surgeons is the crouch position. The buttocks are placed on a board supported by upright holders attached to the table. The knees are flexed, the hips are flexed, and the shoulders are supported on rolls. The abdomen is allowed to hang freely. The head is supported on a donut. The arms are flexed at the shoulders and elbows and placed on arm boards attached to the operating table. Again, adequately trained staff must be present for positioning the patient.

Careful padding and positioning is mandatory.

Eyes
The eyes must be protected and not exposed to any pressure.

Neck
The neck should be slightly flexed; the cervical spine should be kept in the same line as the thoracic spine. Rotation and extreme lateral flexion of the head are avoided.
Note: Associated cervical spine abnormalities may also be present. If the patient complains of symptoms referable to cervical spine abnormalities with neurologic deficits in the upper extremity or vascular insufficiency when the neck is moved, the patient may need to be intubated awake. After awake intubation, the patient places his/her body in the proper position. Neuromuscular function is then tested before the induction of anesthesia.

Adequate space must exist between the mandible and the sternum when the neck is slightly flexed.

Undue flexion of the neck is avoided because venous drainage of the head may be hindered and swelling of the tongue may occur.

Arms

The arms should be positioned so that there is no traction on the brachial plexus. Any pressure on the ulna nerve is avoided by adequate padding. The wrist is supported in the neutral position, and a postoperative wristdrop due to a radial nerve palsy is avoided by making sure the upper arm is not pushed against the ether screen.

Traction on the brachial plexus should be avoided.

Chest

There should be no pressure on the chest that may hinder ventilation.

Abdomen

The abdomen must hang freely without any pressure that could be transmitted to the venous plexuses of the epidural space and spine that could cause bleeding.

Legs

Undue flexion of the hip on the abdomen should be avoided. This may interfere with circulation to the lower extremities. All surfaces around the knees are padded. The buttocks are secured to the seat so that the patient does not shift during surgery. The knees must be supported on the lateral aspects so they do not slide out from under the patient. There must be no pressure on the common peroneal nerve at the head of the fibula.

Surgical Procedure

During the removal of a disc, one of the main complications is inadvertent puncture of the anterior aspect of the annulus fibrosis by the instrument being used to remove the disc. Anterior to the annulus fibrosis is the inferior vena cava, which may be lacerated.

Case Study

A 47-year-old woman was undergoing surgery for a herniated disc in the crouch position. The anesthesiologist noted a sudden drop in blood pressure while the surgeon was removing the disc. Resuscitative measures were begun; however, it was difficult to stabilize the patient hemodynamically, although blood and crystalloid were administered.

A diagnosis of a lacerated vena cava was made. The patient was turned from the prone position to the supine position, and a laparotomy was performed. A laceration of the vena cava was noted. Attempts at controlling the bleeding were made while crystalloid and blood were administered. Bleeding was finally controlled.

If a sudden drop in blood pressure occurs during a laminectomy, laceration of the vena cava should be considered.

Anesthetic Considerations

The surgeon must be provided with proper operating conditions.

Adequate anesthesia and muscle relaxation should be ensured so that no bucking, coughing, movement, or straining occurs, which increases bleeding.

Air Embolism

Although rare, air embolism can occur because the veins in the operating field are above the level of the heart and can entrain air. Positive pressure ventilation probably results in venous bleeding rather than air entrainment. However, increased airway pressures that may cause increased right atrial pressure and possible opening of a probe-patent foramen ovale with air passage to the left side of the heart should be avoided.[7]

Lateral Position

After general anesthesia is induced, the patient is placed in the lateral position; the surgeon sits or stands adjacent to the operating table and performs the surgery in this manner.

Spinal Anesthesia

Some surgeons perform lumbar disc surgery under spinal anesthesia. Although this is possible, we do not recommend spinal anesthesia because any neurologic complication that may occur could be blamed on the spinal anesthetic.

Surgery for Spinal Stenosis

Surgery for spinal stenosis involves decompression of the spinal cord by laminectomy plus decompression of nerve roots by foraminotomy. This surgical procedure is performed in the prone position.

Patient Selection

Patients undergoing this type of surgery may be in the older age group. However, spinal stenosis can occur in young individuals as well as in patients with congenital abnormalities such as in achondroplastic dwarfs.

The patient should be properly assessed in the preoperative period and should be brought into the best possible condition before surgery.

Anesthetic Management

General endotracheal anesthesia is usually used.

The anesthetic technique that best suits the patient should be used.

Position

The head and neck are positioned carefully because there may be cervical arthritis and spondylosis. If there are any associated problems with the cervical spine, care is used in positioning. Undue flexion or extension is avoided.

SPINAL SURGERY FOR ANKYLOSING SPONDYLITIS

For discussion of ankylosing spondylitis see Chapter 1.

Indications for spinal surgery include

Correction of fixed flexion deformities of the spinal column
Stabilization of spine fractures

Fixed Flexion Deformity

Fixed flexion deformity causes the patient to be unable to look straight ahead.

In any attempt to correct a fixed flexion deformity of the spine, correction must first be carried out to fix the flexion deformities of the hips. Correction of spinal deformities without correction of hip deformities will not provide adequate extension in the upright position.

Osteotomies of the lumbar spine, thoracic spine, and cervical spine are performed at the site of the kyphosis.

Lumbar Spine Osteotomy

Patient Management

An awake fiberoptic intubation is performed before the induction of general anesthesia.

SSEP monitoring is used.

Position

These patients have severe kyphotic deformities that may result in fractures of the spine if abnormal stresses are applied. The patient is positioned so that stress is not placed on the thoracic or cervical spine. Adequate padding and care in positioning will help prevent complications.

Surgical Procedure

An osteotomy is performed at the interspace where the ankylosis is soft. This is usually at the L3–L4 interspace.

As the osteotomy is being closed manually, a snap is heard as the anterior structures are broken up, with reduction resulting.

During the closure of the osteotomy, care must be taken not to compress the cauda equina or entrap nerve roots.

Instrumentation is inserted and secured.

A wake-up test may be performed to ensure the preservation of normal neurologic function.

A bone graft is placed in the decorticated lumbar spine.

An anterior fusion is then performed to provide further stabilization.

Thoracic Osteotomy for Thoracic Kyphosis

Two groups of patients with thoracic kyphosis and ankylosing spondylitis are identified.

Group 1—Flexible Deformity

Gradual halo-gravity traction is followed by posterior fixation with instrumentation and fusion.

If posterior fusion is not satisfactory, a thoracotomy with anterior fusion with use of bone graft may need to be carried out.

Group 2—Rigid Deformity

Anterior osteotomies with resections of the discs and fusion is the first step.

The second stage consists of posterior osteotomies carried out with fixation by instrumentation and bone graft.

In this procedure, small corrections are carried out at each level, resulting in an ultimate correction.

There is a narrow spinal canal in the thoracic area. Therefore, extensive corrections may lead to problems.

The vascularity of the spinal cord in the midthoracic area is in the watershed area, and therefore the blood supply is thought to be at risk (see Fig. 11-3).[8]

Zielke's Technique

Correction of kyphosis in ankylosing spondylitis by multiple segmental osteotomies, screw fixation, and wiring between screws has been proposed by Hehne and Zielke.[9]

Position
The patient is placed on the operating table in the prone position after general anesthesia has been induced.

Anesthetic Considerations
Controlled hypotension with sodium nitroprusside may be used. Blood pressure is kept in the normal range when spinal column manipulation is carried out.

Complications
Complications include root lesions, pneumonia, and pulmonary embolism.

Cervical Osteotomy

Awake Technique

This is how it was done in the "good old days."

A halo cast is applied.

The patient is placed on the operating table in the sitting position with overhead traction applied to the halo apparatus, which is a component of the halo cast.

The operation is performed under local anesthesia. Resection of bone in the C6–T1 vertebrae is carried out.

Before straightening the neck from the flexed position after the bony resection, the patient is given 100 percent oxygen for 10 to 15 minutes. Before the fracture, halothane only is administered.

The neck is extended by the surgeon pulling the head backward, fracturing the anterior structures.

The head is stabilized while 100 percent oxygen is administered.

The neurologic status is evaluated.

The closure is completed.

The surgeon then can readjust the final position by manipulation of the halo vest.[10,11]

Warning:

This procedure is not for the faint-hearted.

Extreme caution must be exercised in managing patients for posterior osteotomy in the sitting position under local anesthesia with only an inhalation agent administered for the fracture.

General Anesthesia

This technique is much better.

A halo apparatus is applied under local anesthesia some days before the procedure.

On the day of surgery, fiberoptic endotracheal intubation is performed under topical anesthesia. A routine endotracheal intubation should not be attempted.

Local anesthetic infiltration is carried out in the area of the incision.

Sedation is provided by the infusion of propofol.

SSEP monitoring is used.

An osteotomy is performed in the appropriate area.

The patient is allowed to wake up from the infusion of propofol for a wake-up test.[8]

CERVICAL SPINE FRACTURES

For a discussion of cervical spine fractures see Chapter 2.

CHEMONUCLEOLYSIS

A technique was developed in which the enzyme chymopapain was injected into the nucleus pulposus where there was evidence of a degenerative protruded disc.

A discogram with radiopaque contrast material is first performed to delineate the pathology, after which the enzyme is injected.

Allergic reactions had been reported with the use of this agent.

Several cases of transverse myelitis have occurred.

It is recommended to precede any injections with a test for allergy to the drug.

Premedication with diphenhydramine, cimetidine, and steroids is recommended to decrease the effect of any allergic reaction.

Anesthesia

Local anesthesia is recommended because touching a nerve root with the needle will elicit a paresthesia and will alert the surgeon to change the direction.

Position

The patient is placed on the operating table in the lateral decubitus position and taped in place. An image intensifier is used to aid in finding the disc space, which is approached in laterally to avoid intrathecal injections. After a discogram is obtained, the chymopapain is injected into the disc space.

REFERENCES

1. Macnab I: Symptoms in cervical disc degeneration. p. 599. In Cervical Spine Research Society (ed): The Cervical Spine. 2nd Ed. JB Lippincott, Philadelphia, 1989
2. Transfeldt EE: Cervical spondylosis. p. 771. In Bridwell KH, DeWald RL (eds): The Textbook of Spinal Surgery. JB Lippincott, Philadelphia, 1991
3. Fang HSY, Ong GB: Direct anterior approach to the upper cervical spine. J Bone Joint Surg 44(A):1588, 1962
4. Crockard HA: Anterior approaches to lesions of the upper cervical spine. Clin Neurosurg 34:389, 1988
5. Moskovich R, Crockard HA: Post-traumatic atlanto-axial subluxation and myelopathy. Efficacy of anterior decompression. Spine 15:422, 1990
6. Moskovich R: Cervical instability (rheumatoid, dwarfism, degenerative, others). p. 813. In Bridwell KH, DeWald RL (eds): The Textbook of Spinal Surgery. JB Lippincott, Philadelphia, 1991
7. Frankel AS, Holzman RS: Air embolism during posterior spinal fusion. Can J Anaesth 35:911, 1988
8. Hammerberg KW: Ankylosing spondylitis. p. 525. In Bridwell KH, DeWald RL (eds): The Textbook of Spinal Surgery. JB Lippincott, Philadelphia, 1991
9. Hehne H, Zielke K: Correction of long curved deformities in ankylosing spondylitis. p. 547. In Bridwell KH, DeWald RL (eds): The Textbook of Spinal Surgery. JB Lippincott, Philadelphia, 1991

10. Simmons EH: Kyphotic deformity of the spine in ankylosing spondylitis. Clin Orthop 128:65, 1977
11. Simmons EH: Surgery of the spine in rheumatoid arthritis and ankylosing spondylitis. p.4. In Evarts CM (ed): Surgery of the Musculoskeletal System. Churchill Livingstone, New York, 1983
12. Friedenberg ZB, Edeiken J, Newton-Spencer H et al.: Degenerative changes in the cervical spine. J Bone Joint Surg (A) 41:61, 1959
13. Brain WB, Northfield DWC, Wilkinson M: Neurologic manifestations of cervical spondylosis. Brain 75:187, 1952

13

Orthopedic Oncology

Care of patients with cartilage, bone, and related soft tissue tumors requires knowledge and familiarity with the types of tumors, the operative procedures undertaken to treat these tumors, and the effects of chemotherapy and radiation therapy used in the management of these conditions.

INITIAL EVALUATION

Before embarking on an operative procedure, a certain protocol is followed by the surgeon.

A history, physical examination, and laboratory evaluation are performed.

Patients are also evaluated by radiographs, computed tomographic (CT) scans, magnetic resonance imaging (MRI), and angiography, when indicated. This gives the surgeon an opportunity to develop a presumptive diagnosis and plan of treatment.

BIOPSY

An initial biopsy is obtained to determine the diagnosis so that plans for definitive surgery can be made based on the results of the pathologic evaluation. There is usually a waiting period between the biopsy and the definitive surgical procedure to allow time for processing of the biopsy.

If the results of the biopsy reveal a malignancy, the patient may be scheduled for

1. Surgery
2. Further workup
3. Radiation therapy
4. Chemotherapy
5. Combination of radiation therapy and chemotherapy, followed by surgery

CHEMOTHERAPY

Chemotherapeutic agents affect both normal as well as neoplastic cells. These agents tend to be more effective against dividing cells than against resting cells. Chemotherapeutic agents are associated with several complications.[1-4]

405

Side Effects

Side effects of chemotherapy include both acute and long-term effects.[1–4]
   Acute
        Difficult intravenous access
        Alopecia
        Nausea and vomiting
        Chills and fever
        Myocarditis
        Bone marrow depression and hematologic abnormalities
        Acute respiratory distress syndrome
        Immunosuppression
        Serum calcium abnormalities
        Renal dysfunction
        Phlebitis
        Rashes
        Neuropathy

   Long-term
        Anemia
        Leukemia
        Cardiomyopathy
        Pulmonary fibrosis
        Renal dysfunction
        Hepatic dysfunction
        Neuropathy

Chemotherapeutic agents and some of their known side effects are listed in Table 13-1.

Side Effects Relevant to the Anesthesiologist

Cardiac Toxicity

Major cardiotoxic agents include

   Doxorubicin (Adriamycin)

   Daunorubicin

Cardiotoxic effects are seen in up to 20 percent of patients who receive doxorubicin.[5]

The types of toxicity include
   Nonspecific ST-T wave changes
   Sinus tachycardia
   Atrial dysrhythmias

Table 13-1. Systemic Effects of Chemotherapeutic Agents

	Myocardial	Pulmonary	Hepatic	Renal	Neurologic
Azathioprine		√	√		
1-Asparaginase			√		
Bleomycin		√			
Busulfan	√	√			
Carmustine (BCNU)		√	√	√	
Chlorambucil		√			
Cis-platinum	√			√	√
Cyclophosphamide	√	√		√	√
Cytosine arabinoside		√	√		√
Daunorubicin	√				
Doxorubicin	√				
5-Fluorouracil	√				
Lomustine (CCNU)		√	√	√	
Melphalan		√			
6-Mercaptopurine		√	√		
Methotrexate	√	√	√	√	√
Mithramycin			√	√	
Mitomycin	√	√			
Nitrogen mustards		√		√	
Procarbazine		√			
Streptozocin			√	√	
Vinblastine					√
Vincristine				√	√

(Data from Howland et al,[1] Rinder,[8] Borgeat et al,[9] Cooper,[26] and Gundlach.[27])

Ventricular dysrhythmias

Pericarditis

Low-voltage QRS complex

Cardiomyopathy
  acute congestive heart failure[1,6]
  associated with high incidence of mortality[1]

Factors affecting cardiomyopathy are

1. Dose
   While myocardial dysfunction may occur at lower doses, the incidence of congestive heart failure increases as the dose approaches 550 mg/m^2. With less than 400 mg/m^2, congestive heart failure occurred in 3 percent of patients, and the incidence was 18 percent at 700 mg/m^{2,6}
2. Previous cardiovascular disease
   Cardiac toxicity appears earlier in patients who have impaired myocardial function.[7]
3. Mediastinal radiotherapy
   Prior radiotherapy or radiation treatment in conjunction with doxorubicin therapy[1,2,8]

4. Use of other cytotoxic drugs
   Administration of other cytotoxic drugs may have a synergistic cardiomy-opathic effect[1,2,8]

Other chemotherapeutic agents associated with cardiac toxicity are listed in Table 13-1.[9]

Preoperative evaluation of patients who have received cardiotoxic doses of doxorubicin should include

1. Electrocardiogram (ECG) (may show nonspecific changes and tachy-cardia)
2. MUGA scan or echocardiogram with assessment of ejection fraction

Anesthetic Management

If perioperative cardiac evaluation reveals evidence of cardiomyopathy, these patients may require intraoperative hemodynamic monitoring with a pulmonary artery catheter. The adjustment of preload and afterload is essential.

If tachycardia is present it should not be treated with β-blockers since it is a result of the cardiomyopathy.

Cardiovascular collapse has been reported in patients undergoing general anesthesia.[9] We tend to use a narcotic, nitrous oxide/oxygen, relaxant technique.

Patients with cardiomyopathy from doxorubicin may require management in the intensive care unit postoperatively.

Pediatric Patients

In children who received at least 228 mg/m^2 doxorubicin to treat acute leukemia, 65 percent had evidence of increased afterload, decreased contractility, or both, on echocardiogram. In a follow-up study of children who had received doxorubicin, a high incidence of cardiac abnormalities was noted.[10]

Pulmonary Toxicity

Bleomycin toxicity presents as interstitial pneumonitis leading to fibrosis.

Bleomycin works by production of superoxide radicals that attack deoxyribonucleic acid.[1,11,12]

The incidence of pulmonary toxicity varies from 2 to 40 percent.[1,11,12]

Pulmonary Function Tests

Abnormalities in diffusion capacity, decreased forced vital capacity, and decreased PaO_2 may be present.[1,12]

Dosage

Bleomycin toxicity can occur at any dosage but appears to increase at 400 to 450 units; with less than 450 units, toxicity was 3 to 5 percent; at 450 to 559 units, toxicity was 13 percent; and at more than 550 units, toxicity was 17 percent.[12]

Age

Pulmonary toxicity increases with increasing age and is highest in patients older than 70 years.[13-15]

Prior Radiation Therapy

Thoracic radiation in combination with or before bleomycin therapy increases the incidence of pulmonary toxicity.[1,12]

High Oxygen Concentrations

It has been suggested that high oxygen concentrations during anesthesia result in pulmonary fibrosis in patients who have received bleomycin. The action is thought to be secondary to oxygen radicals.[12,16,17]

In one study, it has been suggested that high oxygen concentrations be avoided in patients who have received bleomycin.[16]

Other authors such as LaMantia et al[17] have found no relationship between respiratory failure, bleomycin treatment, and high oxygen concentration in the surgical patient.

As the debate is unresolved, unless hypoxia occurs, oxygen concentrations should not exceed 28 to 30 percent in patients who have been treated with bleomycin or mitomycin, which has the same effect as bleomycin.

Renal Toxicity

Nephrotoxicity may occur in 30 percent of patients who have received 50 to 75 mg/m^2 of *cis*-platinum unless the patient is adequately hydrated.[18] Patients may develop acute tubular necrosis, which may result in acute renal failure.[8,18,19]

If *cis*-platinum nephrotoxicity occurs, the patient should be hydrated and an adequate urine output must be maintained. Howland et al[1] suggest maintaining a urine output of 2 ml/kg/hr with mannitol, using a loading dose of 12.5 g followed by an infusion of 20 percent mannitol at 5 g/hr.[18]

Magnesium wasting may be associated with *cis*-platinum toxicity.[8,18]

Other renal pathologic findings with chemotherapeutic agents include azotemia, hyponatremia, hypocalcemia, and hypokalemia.[1]

Hepatic Toxicity

Because chemotherapy can affect the liver, preoperative liver function tests should be obtained.

Hematologic Effects

Most agents affect the hematologic system. Myelosuppression may result in leukopenia, anemia, and thrombocytopenia. A complete blood count, prothrombin time, partial thromboplastin time, platelet count, and bleeding time should be checked.[1,20]

Neurotoxicity

Vinblastine and vincristine are associated with neurotoxic side effects, including peripheral and autonomic neuropathies. Sensory and motor disturbances may occur.[8,18,21]

An early sign of neurotoxicity is loss of the Achilles tendon reflex.[8]

The cranial nerves may become affected and vocal cord paralysis may occur because of recurrent laryngeal nerve involvement.[1,8]

The syndrome of inappropriate antidiuretic hormone secretion may occur with vincristine.[8]

HEMOSTATIC ALTERATIONS IN MALIGNANCY

Cancer may lead to a hypercoagulable state, and patients may be at increased risk of deep vein thrombosis. There also are tumors that can release factors that result in fibrinolysis and bleeding. Prostate cancer is associated with release of urokinase and possible fibrinolysis.[8]

Because chemotherapeutic agents affect the hemostatic mechanism, abnormalities in bleeding may occur during surgery.

Metastatic tumors from sites such as thyroid, prostate, lung, colon, breast, kidney, and melanoma may bleed significantly.[1,22]

TRANSFUSION IN TUMOR SURGERY

Homologous Transfusions

Patients with some malignancies have been reported to have shorter disease-free intervals and lower survival rates when blood transfusions are administered.

It is believed that homologous blood transfusions result in immunosuppression of the recipient's defenses, making it difficult for the body to defend against the tumor cells. Irradiated blood may be used to decrease the immunologic load placed on the patient.[23]

Autologous Transfusions

Patients with malignancy are not considered candidates for autologous predonation.

Cell Saver

The Cell Saver is contraindicated in patients undergoing tumor surgery for fear of metastatic hematogenous spread.

Wound Drainage Reinfusion Devices

Wound drainage reinfusion devices are not used in cancer surgery for the same reason.

SURGICAL TREATMENT

Orthopedic oncology involves the management of patients with tumors of bone and the related extraskeletal connective tissues of the body.

Sarcomas

Soft tissue malignant tumors that arise from connective tissues are known as sarcomas, derived from the Greek *sarkoma,* which means "fleshy growth."[24]

Classification of surgical procedures includes

1. Intracapsular excision
2. Marginal excision
3. Wide excision
4. Radical resection (the tumor is removed with all soft tissue in the anatomic compartment occupied by the tumor; the resected specimen includes the muscles, bones, and joints that are contained within the compartment of resection)[24]

Lower Extremity Amputations

Amputation may be used to treat soft tissue sarcomas.

Soft tissue sarcoma of the foot: below-knee amputation

Tumors of the leg: above-knee amputation through the thigh

Lesions of the middle and distal thigh: hip disarticulation

Lesions of the proximal thigh and buttock: hemipelvectomy[24]

Hemipelvectomy

Hemipelvectomy involves removal of the entire lower extremity and hemipelvis with disarticulation of the sacroiliac joint and pubic symphysis.

Extended Hemipelvectomy

Used to treat lesions of the iliac wing, the extended hemipelvectomy includes excision of the sacral ala at the level of the vertebral bodies.

Upper Extremity Amputations

Tumors of the hand and wrist: below-elbow amputation

Tumors of the forearm: above-elbow amputation

Distal arm and elbow lesions–disarticulation of the shoulder joint

Lesions of the shoulder girdle or proximal arm–forequarter amputation[24] (involves removal of the entire upper extremity, including the scapula and clavicle)

Wide Excision

Wide excision in the treatment of sarcomas includes wide excision of all normal tissue in the tumor area for several centimeters of normal tissue in all directions. Wide excision must be combined with radiation therapy because wide excision will only result in local control 50 percent of the time if used alone.[24]

Muscle Compartment Excision

In some tumors situated in muscle compartments, excision of that compartment of the leg and thigh that is bounded by fascia may be carried out.

Bone Tumors

Surgical procedures for bone tumors as described by Enneking et al[25] are similar to those for soft tissue sarcomas.

These are intralesional, marginal, wide intracompartmental, and radical extra-compartmental techniques.

The preceding techniques can be applied as either an amputation with a marginal, wide, or radical excision or as a limb-sparing procedure.

Biopsy

Tumor biopsy may occasionally be associated with large blood loss (e.g., from thyroid, renal). Before incision, the surgeon should be asked what type of tumor it is believed the patient has and whether large blood loss is anticipated.

Biopsy and Curettage

Biopsy and curettage can be bloody procedures, such as occur with aneurysmal bone cysts. Blood loss of 1,000 to 1,500 ml in 5 minutes has occurred while the curettage was being performed. The empty space may then be filled with bone chips or methylmethacrylate cement.

More Definitive Surgical Procedures

Surgical procedures in orthopedic oncology involve resection of musculoskeletal tumors. The tumors may be either benign or malignant or may be benign with a tendency to recur continually after local excision but not considered malignant.

Excision of the entire lesion with a wide margin around the tumor may be performed. This may involve removal of the tumor, bone, adjacent soft tissue, muscle, and possibly overlying skin, requiring skin grafting. The skin grafting can be either a full-thickness skin graft or a pedicle flap. In some instances, a free flap may be necessary with the attachment of blood vessels from the donor site to the recipient site.

Amputation

Lower Extremity

Below-knee amputation

Above-knee amputation

Midthigh amputation

Disarticulation of lower extremity

Hemipelvectomy[24]

Upper Extremity

Amputation of the proximal humerus and associated soft tissues, with remainder of the distal arm left intact

Upper extremity disarticulation

Forequarter amputation (involves removal of upper extremity, scapula, clavicle, and associated soft tissues)

Limb-Sparing Procedures

Limb-sparing surgery involves the resection of the tumor in an adequate fashion, using all the principles of tumor resection.

The surgical procedures involved in limb-sparing are the following:

1. Resection of the tumor
2. Skeletal reconstruction
   This involves the resection of bone with use of prostheses that are specifically fabricated for tumor reconstruction. Prostheses are made for proximal femoral replacement, distal femur replacement with a total knee component, and total femoral replacement. For the upper extremity, proximal humeral replacements are used.
3. Soft tissue and muscle transfers
   Muscle transfers are used to cover the resection site and to restore muscle power.
4. Adequate skin coverage

Anesthetic Management

Preoperative Preparation

Patients presenting for musculoskeletal oncological surgery should have preoperative evaluations consisting of a history, physical examination, complete blood count, liver function tests, neurologic examination, evaluation of blood clotting, if indicated, and chest radiograph or CT scan of chest or head, if indicated.

The first procedure is usually the biopsy if malignancy is suspected or resectional surgery if the lesion is considered benign from preoperative radiographic, CT, and MRI evaluations.

A history of chemotherapy should be obtained as well as an examination for side effects of chemotherapy.

Psychological Preparation

The anesthesiologist should spend time with the patient and, if the patient is a child or adolescent, with the family. Every effort should be made to allay the fears and apprehensions of all concerned and to answer all questions directly and honestly.

It is wise for the anesthesiologist not to become involved with questions concerning surgery, chemotherapy, or outcomes because this is the province of the surgeon. If the anesthesiologist gets involved in this aspect, there may be small discrepancies between what the surgeon says and what the anesthesiologist says, which may lead to problems with the patient and family.

Sedation

Sedation should be provided so that the patient can get a good night's sleep before the surgery and come to the operating room in a calm, relaxed state.

Conduct of Anesthesia

General or regional anesthesia with sedation can be provided as indicated by the procedure and the needs of the surgeon.

Major Resections and Limb Salvage

Major resections and limb salvage are major surgical procedures characterized by

    Large blood loss
    Major fluid shifts
    Hemodynamic swings
    Potential for coagulopathy

The patient should have

    2 14-gauge intravenous lines
    Foley catheter
    Central venous lines for procedures with large volume shifts or a pulmonary
        artery catheter if cardiac disease is present

Arterial line

Blood available in the operating room

Component factors available (blood bank notified in advance and material needed available)—work with the hematologist.

Upper Extremity

If surgery is to be performed on an upper extremity, intravenous and arterial lines and monitoring devices must be placed on the contralateral extremity. In major resectional surgery of the upper extremity, the patient is placed in a lateral or modified lateral position to gain access to the back.

Lower Extremity

General or general with regional anesthesia can be used in lower limb tumor resectional surgery. After both general and regional anesthesia, postoperative pain relief can be provided by epidural narcotics or local anesthetics. An epidural catheter may be inserted before general anesthesia or after induction. If the epidural catheter will be in the surgical field, it can be inserted at the end of surgery.

The surgeon should be asked how long the procedure is and how much blood loss is expected.

Blood Loss

During these procedures, bleeding may get out of control at times. Ongoing evaluation of blood loss is essential. It is possible to fall behind rapidly if sudden blood loss occurs after a slow, steady loss that had not been noted.

A running calculation of blood loss is kept.

Measure volume in suction bottles.

Weigh sponges and lap pads (1 ml = 1 g).

Observe drapes, surgeons' gowns, and floor.

Hypovolemia may be manifested by hypotension and tachycardia and a decrease in central venous pressure. Serial hematocrit values are performed and are valid if fluid replacement has been adequate during blood loss.

The 14-gauge intravenous lines placed before or just after induction have been very valuable. When the patient has bled out and is in shock is *not* the time to start looking for intravenous sites.

Coagulopathy

Coagulopathy may develop perioperatively. In the operating room, this may become evident by a continuous ooze. A platelet count, prothrombin time, and partial thromboplastin time is ordered, and preparation is made to administer large amounts of blood and blood products. Sometimes the coagulopathy may not develop until the postoperative period, as raw surface areas continue to bleed.

Platelets are administered based on platelet count. After large volume blood replacement, there is usually a thrombocytopenia.

Fresh frozen plasma is administered as indicated by evaluating clotting parameters.

Postoperative Care

The patient is transferred to the recovery room and evaluated. If the procedure is long and the patient is cold, the patient should not be extubated until stable. The patient should be observed carefully for postoperative bleeding, which may manifest itself as

1. Large amount of bleeding into drains
2. Decreased urine output despite what appears to be adequate fluid administration
3. Tension on the wound
4. Tachycardia, which may be perceived as caused by pain
5. Hypotension

Case Study

A 65-year-old man underwent a major resection of a midthigh tumor involving the femur and adjacent soft tissue. The procedure was uncomplicated. Postoperatively, the patient was noted to have a low urine output despite receiving ''adequate'' fluid therapy. Twelve hours postoperatively, the patient was noted to have no movement or sensation of his toes. Examination revealed a tense, distended thigh. Studies revealed an elevated prothrombin time and partial thromboplastin time. The patient was brought to the operating room where approximately 1 L of blood was drained from the wound. The resection site was noted to be oozing without any obvious main bleeding source. Small areas were coagulated, and once the surgical site was dry and fresh frozen plasma was administered to correct the coagulation abnormality, the wound was closed. The patient had return of normal motor and sensory function.

Postoperative Pain Management

Extremely effective postoperative pain relief has been provided in patients with disarticulations and hemipelvectomies by the use of epidural narcotics after surgery.

Case Study

A 56-year-old man presented for limb salvage because of a soft tissue tumor of the left thigh, which required complete resection of his quadriceps muscle. Six weeks before, the patient had had a biopsy at a different hospital, which was complicated by severe postoperative bleeding that lead to a myocardial infarction. The high-grade nature of the tumor necessitated not waiting the usual 6 months after myocardial infarction. In the operating room, two large-bore intravenous lines, a pulmonary artery catheter, and an arterial line were placed. Resection was performed under epidural anesthesia. Postoperatively, the patient received Duramorph, which completely relieved his pain for more than 48 hours. No untoward effects were noted, and the patient had an uncomplicated postoperative course.

Patient controlled analgesia is very useful in those patients in whom epidural narcotics are not used.

Management of Metastatic Disease Involving Bone

Some primary malignancies may metastasize to bone, such as those of thyroid, breast, lung, kidney, and prostate. The surgical approach to these problems may require prophylactic fixation by means of nails and plates or intramedullary rods in the metastatic areas, which may be in danger of fracturing. Fixation with methylmethacrylate cement may be necessary.

Patients with metastatic disease must be evaluated carefully to determine the status of pulmonary, cardiac, renal, hepatic, and central nervous system function.

A history of chemotherapy should be obtained and proper evaluations performed.

The aim of surgery is to prevent a fracture. This may constitute an emergency or relatively urgent case.

Lesions in the femoral head or humeral head may require prosthetic replacement with the use of cement.

Prophylactic nailing of lesions of long bones in general tends to

Have higher blood loss than normal

Be longer in duration than usual cases

Be associated with difficulty obtaining intravenous access

Have potential for hemodynamic alterations

REFERENCES

1. Howland WS, Rooney SM, Goldiner PL: Manual of Anesthesia in Cancer Care. Churchill Livingstone, New York, 1986
2. von Hoff DD, Rosencweiz M, Piccart M: The cardiotoxicity of anti-cancer drugs. Semin Oncol 9:23, 1982
3. Ginsberg SJ, Comis RL: The pulmonary toxicity of anti-neoplastic agents. Semin Oncol 9:34, 1982
4. Schilsky RL: Renal and metabolic toxicities of cancer chemotherapy. Semin Oncol 9:75, 1982
5. Kantrowitz NE, Bristow MR: Cardiotoxicity of anti-tumor agents. Prog Cardiovasc Dis 27:195, 1984
6. Editorial: Doxorubicin-induced cardiac toxicity. N Engl J Med 324:843, 1991
7. Selvin BL: Cancer chemotherapy: implications for the anesthesiologist. Anesth Analg 60:425, 1981
8. Rinder CS: Cancer therapy and its anesthetic complications. p. 1447. In Barash PG, Cullen BF, Stoelting RK (eds): Clinical Anesthesia. 2nd Ed. JB Lippincott, Philadelphia, 1992
9. Borgeat A, Chiolero R, Baylon P et al: Perioperative cardiovascular collapse in patients previously treated with doxorubicin. Anesth Analg 67:1189, 1988
10. Lipshultz SE, Colin SD, Gelber RD et al: Late cardiac effects of doxorubicin therapy for acute lymphoblastic leukemia in childhood. N Engl J Med 324:808, 1991
11. Gilson AJ, Sahn SA: Reactivation of bleomycin lung toxicity following oxygen administration. Chest 88:304, 1985
12. Jules-Elyseek K, White DA: Bleomycin induced pulmonary toxicity. p. 1. In Cooper JAD (ed): Clinics in Chest Medicine. Vol. 11. WB Saunders, Philadelphia, 1990
13. Blum RH, Carter SK, Agre K: A clinical review of bleomycin—a new antineoplastic agent. Cancer 31:903, 1973
14. Einhorn L, Krause M, Hornback N et al: Enhanced pulmonary toxicity with bleomycin and radiotherapy in oat cell cancer. Cancer 37:2414, 1976
15. Samuels ML, Johnson DE, Holloye PY et al: Large dose bleomycin pulmonary toxicity. A possible role of prior radiotherapy. JAMA 235:117, 1976
16. Goldiner PL, Carlon GC, Cvitkovic E et al: Factors influencing postoperative morbidity and mortality in patients treated with bleomycin. Br Med J 1:1664, 1978
17. LaMantia KR, Glick JH, Marshall BM: Supplemental oxygen does not cause respiratory failure in bleomycin treated surgical patients. Anesthesiology 60:65, 1984
18. Chabner BA: Principles of cancer therapy. p. 1113. In Wyngaarden JB, Smith LH (eds): Cecil Textbook of Medicine. WB Saunders, Philadelphia, 1988
19. Schilsky RL: Renal and metabolic toxicities of cancer chemotherapy. Semin Oncol 9:75, 1982
20. Hoagland HC: Hematological complications of cancer chemotherapy. Semin Oncol 9:95, 1982
21. Kaplan RS, Wiernik PH: Neurotoxicity of anti-neoplastic drugs. Semin Oncol 9:103, 1982
22. Gralnick HR, Abrell E: Studies of the procoagulant and fibrinolytic activity of promyelocytes in acute promyelocitic leukemia. Br J Haemotol 52:167, 1952
23. Schriemer PA, Longnecker DE, Mintz PD: The possible immunosuppressive effects of perioperative blood transfusion in cancer patients. Anesthesiology 68:422, 1988
24. Enneking WF: Staging of Musculoskeletal Neoplasms in Current Concepts of Diag-

nosis and Treatment of Bone and Soft Tissue Tumors. Springer-Verlag, Heidelberg, 1984
25. Enneking WF, Spannier SS, Goodman MA: A system for the surgical staging of musculoskeletal sarcoma. Clin Orthop 153:106, 1980
26. Cooper JAD: Drug induced pulmonary disease. In: Clinics in Chest Medicine. Vol. 11. WB Saunders, Philadelphia, 1990
27. Gundlach TE: The oncology patient. Anesthesiol News 18:9, 1992

14

Postoperative Pain

Recent advances in pain management have enabled postoperative orthopedic patients to achieve significant pain relief, ambulate sooner after surgery, and be discharged from the hospital earlier than in the past. To manage postoperative pain, the anesthesiologist must understand the severity and duration of pain after particular orthopedic procedures, the specific postoperative rehabilitation, physical therapy, and ambulation plan of the orthopedic surgeon, and the capabilities and goals of the patient.

Do not let the following happen. The statement "If I knew you were going to be placed on a continuous passive motion (CPM) machine after your surgery I would not have removed the epidural catheter" demonstrates both a lack of communication and failure to plan postoperative pain management. The "pain plan" is developed preoperatively so the patient understands what to do and expect, and the surgeon's cooperation can be anticipated.

INTRAMUSCULAR NARCOTIC ADMINISTRATION

Although traditional intramuscular narcotic administration does provide pain relief, this technique may be associated with periods of oversedation and respiratory depression alternating with periods of severe pain while the patient waits for an injection.

Newer techniques for pain relief include

Patient controlled analgesia (PCA)

Spinal narcotics (intrathecal and epidural)

Spinal narcotics plus local anesthetic infusions

Regional nerve blocks

Indwelling catheter technique

Transdermal narcotics

Non-narcotic analgesics

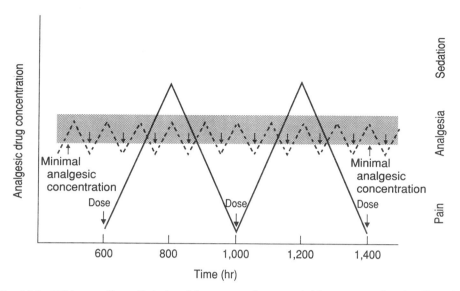

Fig. 14-1. PCA paradigm. Relationship among plasma opioid concentration *(ordinate)*, dosing interval *(abscissa)*, and analgesic effect *(z axis)* defining therapeutic effectiveness. (From Ferrante et al,[31] with permission.)

PATIENT CONTROLLED ANALGESIA

Development

The disadvantages and failure of intramuscular injections to provide good pain relief is because this method of administration results in varying plasma opioid levels. This variation in plasma levels results in the patient alternating between levels of pain, analgesia, and sedation[1] (Fig. 14-1 [solid line]).

According to Ferrante et al,[1] there is an optimal zone of analgesia, obtained at a certain systemic opioid level, that affords the patient adequate pain relief without oversedation. If the opioid level remains in this zone, the patient has optimal pain control. Pain occurs once the analgesic drug concentration falls below the minimal analgesic concentration[1] (Fig. 14-1 [dotted line]). This theory developed from research on intermittent intravenous dosing.

Intermittent Intravenous Doses

Sechzer[2,3] searching for a more satisfactory method of obtaining the optimal analgesia zone without oversedation noted that administration of smaller doses intravenously over shorter time intervals could help maintain

A more constant analgesic drug concentration

More constant pain relief

Less oversedation

A higher degree of patient satisfaction

If pain occurs while a patient is on this pain-relief regimen, as a result of the drug concentration falling below the minimal analgesic concentration or because a dressing change or physical therapy require an increase in the minimal plasma drug concentration necessary to obtain pain relief, additional intravenous doses could be administered. Because each additional dose is not very large, the chances of each dose causing oversedation is small.

The technique proved successful with nurses providing intravenous pain medication on demand.[2,3]

The intervention of machines to provide pain medication in this manner has significantly altered the postoperative pain management of many patients.

Method

PCA is a method of obtaining pain relief by which the patient controls the administration of intravenous medications on demand by pressing a button, by constant infusion, or by a combination of the two. The technique is designed to

1. Place the patient in an important role in determining when medication is needed by pushing a button that can allow for the administration of medication
2. Deliver a defined dose of pain medication on demand
3. Allow the physician to program the delivery of pain medication to meet the needs of the patient
4. Allow the patient to administer medication before an anticipated painful situation—physical therapy, log rolling, dressing change

The success of the technique requires patient understanding and cooperation. Advantages include

1. Satisfied patients
2. Patients who will "live" with some discomfort because they know they are in control and can receive more medication if necessary
3. Better pain control without increased demand on nursing staff
4. Earlier hospital discharge in some patient populations

PCA is a team effort:

1. Time must be taken to ensure nursing knowledge of PCA and create a desire for it to work.
2. Enough pumps and supplies must be present for patients who desire PCA.

3. Staff must be available to modify doses.
4. PCA should be explained so patients understand what they will need to do to obtain adequate pain relief.

Terminology

Initial bolus or loading dose

Demand dose

Lockout interval

Basal infusion

Total hourly dose[1]

Bolus or Loading Dose

The bolus or loading dose is administered to the patient by the physician when the patient is initially placed on PCA. By loading the patient with a narcotic, the drug concentration is rapidly raised into the analgesic range.

Doses of 3 to 5 mg of morphine can be administered at 10-minute intervals until adequate relief is obtained. If the patient has just undergone surgery, the effect of residual narcotics should be considered.

Demand Dose

The demand dose is the dose the patient will receive when the demand button is pushed.

The usual range is 0.5 to 1.0 mg morphine for most patients. In patients with severe pain, the demand dose can be increased. When considering the demand dose, such factors as weight, age, narcotic history, and any history of being very ''sensitive'' to narcotics must be taken into account. Young patients who have undergone extensive surgery will require higher demand doses than older patients.

Lockout or Dosage Interval

The lockout or dosage interval is the time during which a patient will not receive a dose even if the demand button is pushed. The lockout interval should be long enough to allow a demand dose to achieve its effect but not so long that the patient suffers with pain while awaiting the next dose.

The lockout interval for morphine should be 6 to 15 minutes, depending on the patient. If small demand doses are used, the lockout interval can be on the lower side.

Basal Infusion

The basal infusion is a constant infusion of pain medication that the patient receives whether or not the demand button is pressed. The basal infusion helps maintain a serum concentration in the analgesic zone.

We start at an infusion rate of 1 mg/hr and increase as necessary up to 2 mg/hr.

While infusions are frequently used at the start of PCA, after 24 hours they may only be required at night to help the patient sleep. Because constant infusions are administered regardless of the patient's level of consciousness or pain, it is important that the rate of infusion not be too high.

Total Hourly Dose

Limit: The maximal amount that can be administered in 1 hour can be calculated by adding the basal infusion rate and the demand doses that would be administered should all the doses be demanded.

Example: If the demand dose is 1 mg and the lockout time is 10 minutes with a basal infusion of 1 mg/hr, the total hourly dose would be 7 mg.

Drugs and concentration: We use morphine in a concentration of 1 mg/ml. Meperidine (10 mg/ml), hydromorphone (0.2 mg/ml), or fentanyl (5 to 50 μg/ml) are alternatives.

Order Sheet

The order sheet (Fig. 14-2) provides space for the anesthesiologist to order doses, lockout times, and basal infusion rates for the individual patient. It also instructs the nursing staff about the potential side effects and their treatment.

When ordering PCA, the following should be considered:

1. Patient's general medical condition (decreased dose in frail patients)
2. Age (lower dose in very old)
3. History of use of narcotics preoperatively (possible tolerance)

We have found that patients younger than 50 years old undergoing surgery will generally need more than the intramuscular dose given every 3 hours that would ordinarily be ordered for them. In elderly patients, the medication should be lowered to avoid oversedation. When PCA is started, morphine should be ordered cautiously and side effects such as respiratory depression must be watched for. However, if insufficient amounts are ordered, the method may

Patient Controlled Analgesia (IV-PCA) Order:

1. Give no other analgesic/sedative while patient on PCA
2. Meds: Morphine 1 mg/ml in 60-ml Luer-Lock syringe
3. Mode: PCA with basal rate
   a. Bolus dose: _____ mg (loading dose)
   b. PCA dose: _____ mg/injection
   c. Delay interval: _____ min (lock-out interval)
   d. Basal rate: _____ mg/hr (continuous rate)
   e. 1-Hour limit: _____ mg
4. Tylenol: 2 325-mg tablets q4h PRN for the duration of treatment. If unable to take PO, give Tylenol 650-mg suppository per rectum
5. Narcan 0.4 mg available on unit for Rx side effects
6. For nausea and vomiting, give Compazine 25-mg suppository per rectum or Compazine 10 mg IM
7. Call MD if patient is difficult to arouse, is confused, or if respiratory rate is <10 breaths/min
8. Monitor vital signs (blood pressure, pulse, respiratory rate) and assess level of pain, level of consciousness, and level of anxiety q15min the 1st hr, q1h for 4 hr, then q2h for 4 hr, and then q4h while patient is on PCA
9. Continous IV LR 50 ml/hr infusion (unless otherwise specified) for the duration of treatment
10. PCA may run in an IV line containing blood, Kefzol, vancomycin, or dextran
11. Discontinue PCA at patient's or orthopedist's request, maximum 72 hr

Fig. 14-2. Example of patient controlled analgesia order sheet. LR, lactated Ringer's solution.

be deemed inadequate. Patients are closely evaluated to observe the doses required.

Starting PCA

After the patient arrives in the postanesthesia care unit (PACU), PCA is instituted when the patient starts to complain of pain.

1. Bolus dose
    If pain is significant, a 3- to 5-mg intravenous bolus dose is administered,

depending on age, weight, and level of pain. If the initial bolus is inadequate, more medication is administered until pain relief is achieved.
2. Basal infusion

   In general, for the "average" 70-kg patient, a PCA basal infusion of 1 mg/hr is started. It should be remembered that the patients receive their basal infusion whether or not they request medication.
3. Demand dose

   The demand dose is started at 1 mg, with a lockout of 6 to 10 minutes. The lockout can be decreased to 6 minutes if there is significant pain. Alternatively, the dose given for each demand can be increased. We prefer to increase demand doses in 0.5-mg increments. A lockout interval of 10 minutes and an increase of 0.5 mg per demand allows the patient to request an additional 3 mg/hr.

PCA Flow Sheet

The PCA flow sheet is used to assess and manage postoperative pain (Fig. 14-3).

It records

Levels of pain, consciousness, and anxiety

Amount of medication a patient received in a given hour

Number of attempts made

The flow sheet can help determine whether a patient who is complaining of pain is using PCA correctly.

1. Are the doses ordered being used? If the patient has complaints of pain but is using only 3 mg/hr of a possible 7 mg, the patient needs to be educated about pressing the button more frequently to receive pain medication. Re-educating the patient about the demand dose and lockout interval will help achieve adequate pain relief without increasing the medication.
2. If maximal doses are being used, the orders are increased to allow the patient to receive more medication. If maximum doses are being used, acetaminophen, hydroxyzine, or ketorolac can be added to the pain regimen if further increases in narcotic doses are undesirable.
3. The patient may actually be sleeping much of the time and have more than adequate pain relief but may have the perception of constant pain. It is necessary to explain to the patient that adequate pain relief is being received. Some patients will not admit they are receiving adequate analgesia until they are comatose.

PATIENT CONTROLLED ANALGESIA FLOW SHEET

PCA Dose: _____

Basal Rate: _____

1-Hour Limit _____

Level of Pain
1 = None
2 = Slight
3 = Tolerable
4 = Moderate
5 = Severe

Level of Consciousness (LOC)
1 = Awake/Alert
2 = Awakes w. Stimulus
3 = Disoriented
4 = Sleeping
5 = Stupor

Level of Anxiety (LOA)
1 = Calm/Relaxed
2 = Mild Anxiety
3 = Moderate Anxiety
4 = Restless
5 · Agitated

DATE	TIME	PCA DOSE/ INTERVAL	TOTAL MG DELIVERED	TOTAL # INJECTIONS	TOTAL # ATTEMPTS	RESP. RATE	PULSE	BP	PAIN RATING 1-5	LOC 1-5	LOA 1-5	COMMENTS	INITIAL

VITAL SIGNS columns: RESP. RATE, PULSE, BP

ASSESSMENT columns: PAIN RATING 1-5, LOC 1-5, LOA 1-5

Fig. 14-3. Patient controlled analgesia flow sheet.

Disadvantages

1. PCA is not for all patients.

    There are patients who do not understand and will never understand how to use the equipment or do not want to be involved in their pain management. The elderly patient who is slightly disoriented after a hip fracture is not a good candidate for PCA.
2. Undermedicating can leave a patient in pain.
3. Oversedation is a possibility, especially if a high basal rate is ordered or family members "help" control pain by pushing the demand button.
4. Nausea may cause patients to be unhappy. This is no different from nausea seen with narcotic administration in any form.

Pain Despite PCA

If postoperative orthopedic patients have pain out of proportion to that expected, causes other than postoperative pain must be considered.

1. Significant pain can be caused by

    Compartment syndrome (with or without a cast present)

    Vascular problem (intraoperative damage to a vessel resulting in postoperative ischemic pain)

    Urinary retention

    Improperly adjusted CPM machine
2. The narcotic-tolerant patient may not have adequate pain relief with normally prescribed dosages.
3. Very anxious patients also will complain of "pain" and request increased medication.

Case Study

   A 48-year-old man underwent anterior and posterior spinal fusion. After surgery, he was placed on PCA, which, although used correctly, did not provide adequate pain relief. The patient complained of pain in the left lower extremity. Investigation revealed a thrombosis of the iliac artery as a result of an aneurysm. An emergency by-pass procedure was performed.

INTRATHECAL AND EPIDURAL NARCOTICS

The discovery of opiate receptors in the spinal cord has led to the use of epidural and intrathecal narcotics for control of pain.[4,5]

When undertaking a program involving epidural and spinal narcotics, specific orders must be written for managing these patients and the potential side effects. We use a special set of orders for patients receiving narcotics by the epidural

Epidural/Spinal Narcotics Order:

1. Patient received epidural/spinal _____ mg DURAMORPH
2. Place sign "EPIDURAL/SPINAL NARCOTICS" over patient's bed x 24 hr
3. Additional narcotics may only be administered by order of an anesthesiologist
4. Check respiratory rate from time of injection: q15min for the 1st hr; q30min for 11 hr, then q1h for 12 hr
5. If respiratory rate <9 breaths/min and patient somnolent, give Narcan 0.2 mg IV immediately, and page MD STAT. If MD orders Narcan drip: 5 ampules/250 ml saline, 50 ml/hr IV
6. Have Ambu bag, mask, and oral airway readily available. VENTILATE IF NECESSARY!!
7. Tylenol 2 325-mg tablets q4h PRN pain for the duration of treatment. If unable to take PO, give Tylenol 650-mg suppository per rectum
8. For nausea and vomiting, give Compazine 10 mg IM. If no relief after 30 min, give Narcan 0.2 mg IM
9. For pruritus, give Benadryl 50 mg IM q4–6h PRN. If no relief after 2 hr, give Narcan 0.2 mg IM
10. If patient has not voided within 6 hr after arriving in PACU, straight cath. If after additional 6 hr patient has not voided, straight cath again
11. Patient to remain in PACU/SCU/MONITORED BED for 24 hr after injection, or as per anesthesia
12. Only anesthesiologist may reinject in epidural catheter

Fig. 14-4. Example of epidural/spinal narcotics order sheet. PACU, postanesthesia care unit; SCU, special care unit.

or spinal route, with emphasis on assessment of respiratory status and treatment of side effects (Fig. 14-4).

Also, we use a simple hourly flow sheet to note level of pain relief, respiratory rate, patient complaints, and complications.

Role of Lipid Solubility

The onset, spread, and duration of analgesia associated with a given opioid are related to its degree of lipid solubility.

Highly lipid-soluble narcotics such as fentanyl, sufentanil, and buprenorphine have a faster onset of action, less segmental spread, and a shorter duration of action than hydrophilic narcotics.

Hydrophilic narcotics with low lipid solubility (e.g., morphine) do not cross the dura quickly, do not bind with as high an affinity to opiate receptors, have a higher segmental distribution, have a higher tendency toward rostral spread, and have a longer duration of action.

Low Lipid Solubility Opioid

Preservative-Free Morphine

Intrathecal and epidural preservative-free morphine has been used extensively for managing postoperative pain, especially after knee and hip replacements. Its characteristics[6] include

Slow onset
> The time to onset is delayed as compared with highly lipid-soluble narcotics.
> Its low lipid solubility results in slow absorption from the epidural space and therefore longer time for onset (30 to 60 minutes)

Long-lasting analgesia
> It is not uncommon to obtain 18 to 24 hours of excellent pain relief after a single intrathecal injection of 0.3 to 0.5 mg or epidural injection of 3 to 5 mg.
> Doses greater than 3 to 5 mg epidurally or 0.5 mg intrathecally are not associated with greater analgesia but with higher incidence of complications.

Potential side effects
> Because it has low lipid solubility, morphine will remain in the cerebrospinal fluid in the unbound form, enabling rostral spread and the potential central side effects of respiratory depression, pruritis, and nausea and vomiting.[6]
> Respiratory depression
>> Incidence is noted to be less than 1 percent in cases, with higher incidence in the elderly.
>> Initial respiratory depression occurring in less than 1 hour may be due to systemic absorption. Second peak of possible respiratory depression at about 8 hours can be due to rostral spread.[6,7]
> Nausea and vomiting—30 to 40 percent[6,8]
> Urinary obstruction secondary to effect on detrusor muscle—5 to 40 percent[6,9]
> Pruritis—10 to 50 percent[6,10]
> Side effects reversible with naloxone
> Not as ideal for infusions as short-acting narcotics

Lipophilic Narcotics

Examples are fentanyl, sufentanil, buprenorphine.

In general, lipophilic narcotics have the following characteristics:

Rapid onset of action

Highly segmental effect

Shorter duration of action than morphine

Ideal for infusions

Can be diluted to increase segmental spread

Epidural Fentanyl

Dose: 50 to 100 μg

Onset of action: 2 to 10 minutes

Duration of action: 2 to 4 hours

Limited segmental spread with minimal rostral spread in doses in the 50- to 100-μg range (acts best if placed at segmental area involved in pain)

When administered in a 50- to 100-μg dose with epidural morphine, provides rapid onset of pain relief while waiting for morphine to take effect

Synergistic effect when added to bupivacaine

Works well for infusions and intermittent bolus techniques

Spread achieved by diluting medication

Side effect of respiratory depression associated with concurrent systemic narcotic use

Pruritis in 30 to 50 percent of cases[6]

Nausea and vomiting less frequent than with morphine[6,11-13]

Epidural Sufentanil

Greater lipid solubility than fentanyl (two times)

Short duration of action

Short time to onset

Increased incidence of respiratory depression in elderly as compared with fentanyl[6,14]

Good medication to initiate pain relief until morphine can take effect[15]

Buprenorphine

0.15 mg equivalent to 5 mg morphine epidurally

Fewer side effects than morphine

Use in Orthopedic Surgery

Intrathecal and epidural narcotics are useful in providing pain relief in patients undergoing repairs of fractures of the hip, total hip and total knee replacement, acetabular fracture repairs, and other lower extremity trauma surgery.

We have had excellent results with the use of both spinal and epidural narcotics in patients who have undergone total hip and total knee surgery. Preservative-free morphine in doses of 5 mg epidurally and 0.3 to 0.5 mg intrathecally have been very successful in decreasing postoperative pain.

Patients with fractured hips suffering from multiple medical problems have done well with spinal anesthesia with 0.3 mg morphine added to the local anesthetic. Avoiding pain in these patients has helped their postoperative course.

If epidural anesthesia is used for the surgical procedure, the epidural morphine is administered about 1 to 1.5 hours before the end of the surgical procedure so that the onset of the analgesic effect can coincide with the cessation of the local anesthetic effect, thus sparing the patient any pain. It is simpler to prevent pain than it is to treat it once it begins.

If the analgesic effect of the morphine has not as yet become effective, a solution of 7 to 10 ml of 0.25 percent bupivacaine can be administered in the PACU. This will provide pain relief until the morphine takes effect. The patient is observed for hypotension after the administration of the local anesthetic.

Pelvic and Acetabular Fracture Repair

Pelvic and acetabular fracture repair is associated with a painful postoperative course, CPM, and radiation therapy to avoid heterotropic bone formation. Epidural narcotics are very helpful for these patients.

Resectional Surgery for Lower Extremity Tumors

Patients who have had major resectional surgery for bone and soft tissue tumors also do well with postoperative epidural narcotics.

Case Study

A 63-year-old man who required resection of a malignant tumor of the lower extremity had suffered a myocardial infarction 6 weeks before surgery secondary to postoperative bleeding. The malignant nature of the tumor precluded waiting the usual post-myocardial infarction convalescence period. The resection was performed under epidural anesthesia. The patient received epidural morphine for the first few days postoperatively and did well without any complaints of pain.

Continuous Passive Motion Machine

Patients who require a CPM machine derive a great benefit from immediate postoperative pain relief because motion can be initiated early. This early motion hastens recovery and rehabilitation. Surgical candidates include patients undergoing ligament repair of the knee and manipulation of the knee.

Tourniquet Pain

Patients undergoing lower limb procedures under epidural anesthesia who complain of tourniquet pain obtain relief with the epidural administration of 50 to 100 μg of fentanyl.

Epidural Narcotic Infusions With and Without Local Anesthetics

Fentanyl Infusions

Fentanyl infusions are used in postoperative orthopedic patients after lower extremity surgery.

Concentrations of 10 μg/ml of fentanyl are frequently used.

An infusion rate of 5 to 10 ml/hr is given.

Patients must be watched carefully for side effects, especially somnolence and respiratory depression.

While some physicians add bupivacaine (0.1 percent) to fentanyl infusions, others have not found that this improves analgesia.[6,16]

Patient Controlled Analgesia with Epidural Infusion

At one institution, epidural narcotic PCA has been used to manage postoperative pain patients undergoing total hip replacements and total knee replacements. Emphasis is placed on close observation of patients for potential side effects (K. Sanborn, M.D. personal communication).

Total Hip Replacement

Infusions containing 5 μg/ml of fentanyl are administered in the following manner:

Basal rate: 10 ml/hr, 50 μg/hr

PCA demand dose: 5 ml, 25 μg per demand

Lockout: 15 minutes

Total allowable dose: 150 μg/hr

The basal rate is decreased in elderly and may be increased in very large patients.

These patients ambulate 2 days postoperatively after the infusion is discontinued (K. Sanborn, M.D. personal communication).

Total Knee Replacement

These patients suffer from more pain than those having total hip replacement.

Infusions containing 5 μg/ml fentanyl and 0.125 percent bupivacaine are administered in the following manner:

Basal rate: 10 ml/hr, 50 μg/hr fentanyl

PCA demand dose: 5 ml

Lockout: 15 minutes

Total narcotic dose: 150 μg/hr

There is some decreased sensation associated with this technique. Patients are not allowed to ambulate until the third postoperative day, at which time the catheter has been removed.

Adjustments to the basal rate should be considered, such as a decrease in basal rate in the elderly (K. Sanborn, M.D. personal communication).

Another anesthesiologist prefers infusions of 3 μg/ml fentanyl, 0.01 percent bupivacaine, and 0.5 μg/ml epinephrine with infusion rates of 10 to 15 ml/hr and 3-ml demand doses allowed every 15 minutes (S. Cohen, M.D. personal communication).

Patients who receive epidural bupivacaine infusions appear to be at risk for development of heel ulcers secondary to diminished sensation.[17]

Summary

Anesthesiologists at different institutions vary the concentration of epidural fentanyl and bupivacaine that they infuse into patients. Whether 3, 5, or 10 μg/ml of fentanyl or 0.01, 0.03, 0.1, or 0.125 percent of bupivacaine is used also varies by institution.

It is important that whatever technique or concentration is used, the patient be closely observed for side effects of somnolence, respiratory depression, hypotension, and motor and sensory blockade.

Problems with epidural local anesthetics for postoperative pain management include the following:

Blockade of sympathetic fibers can cause hypotension.

Blockade of motor fibers can lead to muscle weakness.

If sympathetic blockade or motor blockade occur, ambulation is not possible.[6,17]

All complications associated with epidural and spinal narcotics and local anesthetics can occur in patients receiving infusions. Special consideration should be given to possible catheter migration into the intrathecal space.

Complications of Intrathecal and Epidural Narcotics

Respiratory Depression

Narcotics administered into the epidural or intrathecal area can result in respiratory depression. An acute apneic event is uncommon, but respiratory depression may present as a progressive slowing of respiratory rate.

A bimodal respiratory depression pattern is associated with epidural narcotic administration.

Early respiratory depression results from systemic vascular absorption and a narcotic effect on the respiratory center. If this occurs, it usually happens in the first hour after narcotic administration.[18]

Late respiratory depression can occur from 4 to 12 hours or even as late as 24 hours after an epidural or spinal dose. It results from rostral spread of narcotics in the cerebrospinal fluid and suppression of respiratory centers. Respiratory depression occurs less frequently after epidural than after spinal narcotics.

The incidence of clinically significant respiratory depression from epidural narcotics is actually very low (less than 1 percent). Highly lipid-soluble narcotics have a lower incidence of respiratory depression.

Associated Factors

1. Concurrent administration of parenteral narcotics—avoid
2. Dural puncture—inadvertent administration of an epidural narcotic dose intrathecally
3. Migration of catheter into a blood vessel
4. Concurrent administration of central nervous system depressant medications
5. Too high a dose of intrathecal or epidural narcotic
6. Elderly patients
7. Patients in a generalized debilitated state
8. Respiratory disease
9. Low tolerance for narcotics

Treatment

If ventilatory assistance is required, initiate immediately.

If there is slowing of respiration, administer small doses of naloxone in 0.04-mg increments to see whether an effect occurs. Repeat if necessary.

Initiate an infusion of 5 to 10 μg/kg/hr. Place 5 ampules of naloxone in 250 ml of normal saline.

Administer at 50 ml/hr, so the patient receives 1 ampule per hour. The infusion may be necessary because the half-life of naloxone is less than that of the epidural morphine.

Pruritis

Occurs frequently

Not histamine-related but responds to antihistamines and propofol

Treatment included as part of "standing orders"[19] (Fig. 14-4)

Nausea and Vomiting

Results from rostral spread to chemoreceptor trigger zone

Treated with naloxone or antiemetics (Compazine [prochlorperazine])

Treatment included as part of "standing orders"

Urinary Retention

Effect on detrusor muscle

Can last for the duration of pain relief

Urinary catheter possibly necessary

Helped by naloxone

Migration of Catheters

Epidural catheters can migrate intravascularly or intrathecally. The anesthesiologist should aspirate before injection.

Sedation

Sedation can occur as a result of systemic absorption or with large doses.

Bleeding

The use of anticoagulation in the presence of an epidural catheter should arouse concern about the possible risk of an epidural hematoma.

Infection

Infection is a major concern for indwelling catheters. Catheters must be placed and maintained in a sterile fashion.

Masking of Perioperative Complications

Vascular compromise, compartment syndrome, neurological dysfunction, deep vein thrombosis may be masked by the pain relief afforded by narcotics.

LOCAL ANESTHETICS BY BOLUS METHOD

Local anesthetics can be administered for postoperative pain relief by the bolus technique. Motor and sensory block do occur with this method. The use of this technique requires the presence of a physician to manage inadvertent intrathecal or intravenous injections. Doses of 5 to 10 ml in concentrations of 0.125 to 0.25 percent bupivacaine provide good postoperative pain relief.

When using bolus injections, there may be intermittent episodes of sympathetic blockade with hypotension occurring.

Tachyphylaxis can occur with intermittent dosages.[25]

SPECIAL TECHNIQUES AFTER KNEE SURGERY

Intra-articular Narcotics after Arthroscopic Surgery

The installation of 1 mg of morphine in 40 ml of saline was effective in providing postoperative pain relief after arthroscopic surgery.

At the end of the surgical procedure, the morphine plus saline was introduced into the knee joint through the arthroscope.

Patients treated in this manner had less pain as measured by the visual analog scale than control patients. It is believed that there are specific opioid receptors in such peripheral tissues as the knee joint with which the narcotic interacts.

When intra-articular naloxone was instilled with the morphine, there was a significant decrease in the postoperative analgesia.[20]

In an accompanying editorial, the reviewers are puzzled by the delayed onset and prolonged duration of analgesia after the intra-articular injection of morphine. They are also concerned because the patients in the naloxone group who had higher pain scores did not use more supplementary pain medication.[21]

Intra-articular Bupivacaine

Comparison was made between the intra-articular injections of 0.25 percent and 0.5 percent bupivacaine or 0.9 percent saline injected into the knee joint after arthroscopy. There was no significant analgesic effect after the use of 0.25 or 0.5 percent bupivacaine as compared with control patients.

Femoral Nerve Block or Lumbar Plexus Block

Anker-Miller et al[22] have shown that femoral nerve block or femoral nerve blockade that includes lumbar plexus block with lateral femoral cutaneous nerve and obturator nerve block provides adequate postoperative analgesia after open knee surgery.

Patients receive approximately 20 ml of 0.25 percent bupivacaine by single injection or by means of a catheter. When the catheter technique was used, a bolus of 2 mg/kg body weight of 0.5 percent bupivacaine was followed by a constant infusion of 0.25 percent bupivacaine at a rate of 0.35 mg/kg/hr.

These techniques may be satisfactory after open knee surgery where the patient remains in the hospital and requires immediate postoperative physical therapy with CPM machines. However, such treatment may not be satisfactory in patients who have arthroscopic surgery of the knee and are to be discharged home on the day of surgery. It must be emphasized that any motor blockade will decrease the ability of the patient to ambulate and will cause a major problem in the immediate postoperative period.[29]

WOUND INFILTRATION

At the termination of surgery, local anesthetics such as bupivacaine can be infiltrated in the wound before closure.

CATHETER PLACEMENT

Catheters can be left in wounds at the end of the procedure and infiltration with local anesthetics such as 5 ml of 0.5 percent bupivacaine can be carried out at intervals to prevent pain.

Iliac Crest Graft Sites

Pain in the area of harvested iliac bone grafts is a major complaint after surgical procedures, especially spinal fusions. A catheter placed in the wound with twice-daily infiltration of 5 ml of 0.5 percent bupivacaine can give prolonged relief.

Nerve Sheaths

Catheters for postoperative pain relief can be placed into nerve sheaths during the operative procedure.

Patients undergoing amputations or limb salvage procedures for malignancies had Silastic catheters placed in the nerve sheaths at the time of surgery. Catheters were placed into the axillary sheath, the lumbosacral trunk, the femoral nerve sheaths, and the sciatic nerve sheath. The Silastic tubes were attached to an infusion pump, and 0.5 percent bupivacaine at 2 ml/hr was used in adults. In children, a 0.25 percent solution of bupivacaine was used. Some patients received the bupivacaine as intermittent boluses.[23]

TRANSDERMAL ADMINISTRATION OF ANALGESICS

A transdermal formulation of fentanyl is used to provide pain relief in the postoperative period. Transdermal preparations of fentanyl are applied to the chest wall. A mean of 9.6 hours is required before minimum effective blood fentanyl concentrations are obtained. When the fentanyl patch is removed, there is a delay until the blood fentanyl concentrations decrease to less than the minimum effective concentration for the control of postoperative pain. Some patients develop slowing of the respiratory rate. Since narcotic effect persists after removal of the patch, repeated doses of naloxone may be necessary if the patch is removed because of respiratory depression. Nausea is noted in 85 percent of patients. Also, drowsiness, unpleasant dreams, and headache are reported.

Although transdermal administration of medications is useful in certain areas, the exact role of transdermal administration of narcotics has not as yet been fully developed.[24,30]

PROSTAGLANDIN INHIBITORS

Trauma and tissue damage may cause the release of mediators, which results in the lowering of the threshold of pain receptors to painful stimuli. Nociceptors are sensitized by the prostaglandins and the products of arachidonic acid that result from the activity of the enzyme cyclo-oxygenase.

Nonsteroidal anti-inflammatory drugs (NSAIDs) produce analgesia by their ability to prevent the production of prostaglandins and prevent the sensitization of pain receptors.

The analgesic effect of a NSAID has its greatest benefit if given before the traumatic event that releases the prostaglandins. Administration of these agents should be in the preoperative period before the release of inflammatory agents occurs.

Adverse effects of NSAIDs should be taken into consideration before their use.

Effects on platelet function may lead to a problem with hemostasis.

NSAIDs may mask the febrile response to infection.

Analgesic nephropathy may occur after the administration of these agents.

NSAIDs may affect the gastric mucosa and may cause upper gastrointestinal problems as well as bleeding in some patients.

Ketorolac is a newer NSAID. Like other NSAIDs, it can increase bleeding time and has other side effects including duodenal and gastric ulcer formation and nephropathy. High doses can be associated with nausea, vomiting, somnolence, sweating, and palpation. We have used ketorolac in situations in which epidural and intrathecal narcotics have been inadequate to provide pain relief, when large doses of PCA are inadequate, and when we desire to avoid any respiratory depression.

In doses of 10 to 90 mg, ketorolac had no effect on end-tidal carbon dioxide or on the carbon dioxide response curve.[32] Ketorolac administration does not alter hemodynamics. We have had much better success with the parenteral form than the oral form.

A study using a NSAID, piroxicam, was compared with a placebo to determine the dose of morphine needed in the postoperative period for pain relief after total hip replacement. The piroxicam was given on the evening before surgery, on the evening of the day of surgery, and on the evening of the first day after operation. There was a significant decrease in the total dose of morphine needed.

It is possible that the use of NSAIDs combined with narcotic techniques can decrease the use of narcotics. It is also possible that the use of these agents before the onset of pain may act to decrease the inflammatory response and be more effective than if given after the pain has occurred.[26]

A study of NSAIDs used before and after surgery to decrease prostaglandin synthesis revealed that there was a decrease in postoperative pain score in patients undergoing laminectomy. Indomethacin (100 mg) was given by intravenous injection at induction of anesthesia, followed by rectal suppositories of 100 mg indomethicin 6 and 12 hours after surgery and three times per day on the day after surgery. The indomethacin-treated group had a lower pain score and required fewer analgesics. There was no increase in bleeding.[27]

MANAGEMENT IN CHILDREN

Infants and children do indeed perceive pain after surgery. However, it is difficult to evaluate this painful experience. Visual analog scales are a technique used in adults to determine the level of pain. This is a 10-cm line with the words "no pain" on one end and the words "worse pain possible" on the other end. The patient is asked to place a mark on the line indicating the intensity of the pain. Another technique is to ask the patients to rate pain on a scale from 0 to 10, with 0 indicating no pain. If these scales are to be used in infants and children, they must understand numbers and quantities. In children older than 7 years of age, pain assessment scales may be of use.

In children younger than 6 years of age, evaluation of the pain must be based on what the child says as well as the interpretation of the child's behavior.

Preparation for Surgery

Management of postoperative pain is intimately related to the preparation of the child for the entire perioperative period.

An adequate explanation of the admission to the hospital, the surgical procedure, and the postoperative period should be explained to the child.

A preoperative visit to the hospital when the child can meet members of the nursing staff and the anesthesiology team can provide an opportunity to discuss the surgical procedure and the postoperative management with the child.

Treatment

Infants

1. Unless the babies are going to be mechanically ventilated, narcotics should be avoided.
2. Respiratory complications are frequent in infants after narcotics.
3. Narcotic clearance is prolonged in infants compared with older children, and the prolongation of clearance leads to high levels of narcotic agents in the blood, with a greater risk of respiratory depression.[28]

If an infant is to be mechanically ventilated after surgery, opiates may be used to abolish the pain, and after the effect of the narcotic has worn off, the patient can be weaned from the ventilator.

1. The medication is limited to non-narcotic agents.
2. Acetaminophen (5 to 10 mg/kg every 4 to 6 hours) is useful in infants.
3. Infants undergoing club foot repair in our institution do not receive any pain medication in the postoperative period other than acetaminophen. They do receive intravenous narcotics during their surgical procedure and usually awaken calm and pain-free.

Children Older than 6 Months

Intravenous morphine in a starting dose of 0.05 mg/kg can be used. It is imperative that children receiving intravenous narcotics be observed constantly.

Intramuscular morphine (0.1 mg/kg) can be used.

Acetaminophen can be used for mild to moderate pain.

Aspirin has side effects that make it undesirable. Aspirin can inhibit platelet aggregation and may lead to bleeding. Aspirin may be associated with Reye syndrome.

NSAIDs have not been recommended for pediatric use.

Patient Controlled Analgesia

We have had great success with PCA for the management of postoperative pain in children who have had spinal instrumentation and fusion for scoliosis. Most children older than the age of 12 years who can understand the concept of PCA and who are adequately prepared can benefit from this technique. The patient can treat the pain when it occurs and is not dependent on a preset hospital schedule.

It is of utmost importance that the child be made aware that the PCA will not completely abolish the pain but will diminish it so that it is manageable. Many children constantly press the button and keep complaining of pain even though apparently adequate doses of morphine are being administered.

An anxious family hovering around the bedside usually makes adequate pain relief inadequate because their own anxiety is transmitted to the child.

Epidural Narcotics

In children, epidural narcotics can easily be administered through a catheter placed in the caudal canal. It is more easily placed in this area than in the lumbar epidural space. The patient can receive local anesthetic agent into the epidural catheter during surgery with light general anesthesia, or the patient can receive regular general anesthesia for the surgical procedure followed by epidural narcotics for postoperative pain relief.

Morphine can be administered through the catheter at least 1.5 hours before the end of the surgical procedure.

A dose of 0.033 to 0.050 mg/kg of morphine can be used.

When the patient starts to perceive pain, the same dose of morphine can be administered. If the pain relief is inadequate, an increased dose can be administered at the time of reinjection.

Nausea, vomiting, and urinary retention as well as delayed respiratory depression are the side effects seen in children. Itching may also be present. Diphenhydramine can be used to treat the itching. Naloxone (0.005 mg/kg) can also be used to abolish the itching. Naloxone can be used if nausea and vomiting occur. Urinary retention may be a problem necessitating catheterization. Respiratory depression can occur, and it can be delayed as in adults. Naloxone (0.01 mg/kg) can be used to treat respiratory depression. It must be emphasized that delayed respiratory depression can occur up to 12 hours after the administration of the morphine. Careful observation of the patient is mandatory because apnea monitors and pulse oximeters are of no use in detecting respiratory depression.[29,30]

REFERENCES

1. Ferrante FM, Ostheimer G, Covino B: Patient Controlled Analgesia. Blackwell Scientific Publications, Boston, 1990
2. Sechzer PH: Objective measurement of pain. Anesthesiology 29:205, 1968
3. Sechzer PH: Studies in pain with the analgesic-demand system. Anesth Analg 50: 1, 1971
4. Willer JC: Studies on pain. Effects of morphine on spinal nociceptive flexion reflex and related pain sensations in man. Brain Res 331:105, 1985
5. Willer JC, Bergeret S, Gaudy JH: Epidural morphine strongly depresses nociceptive flexion reflexes in patients with postoperative pain. Anesthesiology 63:675, 1985
6. Badner NH: Epidural agents for postoperative analgesia in current concepts of pain control. Anesth Clin North Am 10:321, 1992
7. Stenseth R, Sellevold O, Breivik H: Epidural morphine for postoperative pain. Experiences with 1085 patients. Acta Anaesthesiol Scand 29:148, 1985
8. Cousins MJ, Mather LE: Intrathecal and epidural administration of opioids. Anesthesiology 61:276, 1984
9. Gregg R: Spinal analgesia: management of postoperative pain. Anesth Clin North Am 7:79, 1989
10. Morgan M: The rational use of intrathecal and extradural opioids. Br J Anaesth 63: 165, 1989
11. Ackerman WE, Juneja MM, Colclough GW: A comparison of epidural fentanyl, buprenophone, and butorphanol for the management of post cesarian section pain. Anesthesiology 39:A401, 1988
12. Madej TH, Strunin L: Comparison of epidural fentanyl with sufentanil. Anaesthesia 42:1156, 1987
13. Naulty JS, Datta S, Ostheimer GW et al: Epidural fentanyl for post cesarian delivery pain management. Anesthesiology 63:694, 1985
14. Cheng E, Koebert RF, Hopwood M et al: Continuous epidural sufentanil for postoperative analgesia. Anesthesiology 67:A233, 1987
15. Naulty JS, Parmet J, Pate A et al: Epidural sufentanil and morphine for post cesarian delivery analgesia. Anesthesiology 73:A965, 1990
16. Fischer RL, Lubenow TR, Liceago A et al: Comparison of continuous epidural infusion of fentanyl–bupivicaine and morphine–bupivicaine in management of postoperative pain. Anesth Analg 67:559, 1988
17. Cohen S, Amar D, Pantuck CB et al: Adverse effects of epidural 0.03% bupivicaine during analgesia after cesarian section. Anesth Analg 75:753, 1992
18. Kafer ER, Brown JT, Scott D et al: Biphasic depression of ventilatory response to CO_2 following epidural morphine. Anesthesiology 58:418, 1983
19. Borgeat A, Wilder-Smith OHG, Saiah M et al: Subhypnotic doses of propofol relieve pruritis induced by epidural and intrathecal morphine. Anaesthesia 76:5110, 1992
20. Stein C, Comisel K, Haimerl E et al: Analgesic effect of intraarticular morphine after arthroscopic knee surgery. N Engl J Med 325:1123, 1991
21. Basbaum AI, Levine JD: Opiate analgesia—how central is a peripheral target? (Editorial.) N Engl J Med 325:1168, 1991

22. Anker-Miller E, Spangsberg N, Dahl JB et al: Continuous blockade of the lumbar plexus after knee surgery: a comparison of the plasma concentrations and analgesic effect of bupivacaine 0.250% and 0.125%. Acta Anaesethesiol Scand 34:468, 1990
23. Malawer MM, Buch R, Khurana JS et al: Postoperative infusional continuous regional analgesia. Clin Orthop 266:227, 1991
24. Gourlay GK, Kowalski SR, Plummer JL: The transdermal administration of fentanyl in the treatment of postoperative pain: pharmacokinetics and pharmacodynamic effects. Pain 37:193, 1989
25. Bromage PR, Peltigrew RT, Crowell DE: Tachyphylaxis in epidural analgesia. I. Augmentation and decay of local anesthetics. J Clin Pharmacol 9:30, 1969
26. Serpell MG, Thomson MF: Comparison of piroxicam with placebo in the management of pain after total hip replacement. Br J Anaesth 63:354, 1989
27. Nissen I, Jense KA, Ohrstrom JK: Indomethacin in the management of postoperative pain. Br J Anaesth 69:304, 1992
28. Lynn AM, Slattery J: Morphine kinetics in early infancy. Anesthesiology 66:136, 1987
29. Tierney E, Lewis G, Hurtig JB et al: Femoral nerve block with bupivicaine 0.25% for postoperative analgaesia after open knee surgery. Can J Anaesth 34:455, 1987
30. Plexia PM, Linford J, Kramer TH et al: Transdermal therapeutic system (fentanyl) for postoperative pain: an efficacy, toxicity and pharmacokinetic trial. Anesthesiology 65:A-210, 1986
31. Ferrante FMN, Orau EJ, Rocco AG, Gallo J: A statistical model for pain in patient-controlled analgesia and conventional intramuscular opioid regimes. Anesth Analg 67:457, 1988
32. Brandon BLJC, Mattie H, Spierdijk J et al: The effects on ventilation of ketorolacin comparison with morphine. Eur J Clin Pharmacol 35:491, 1988

15

Common Pain Syndromes

Anesthesiologists who are interested in pain management should become familiar with those conditions that are likely to respond to nerve blocks as well as with the other therapeutic modalities used in the treatment of pain.

The following are conditions that the anesthesiologist may be called on to manage:

1. Reflex sympathetic dystrophy—sympathetic mediated pain
2. Back pain
3. Facet arthropathy
4. Myofascial pain (trigger points)
5. Meralgia paresthetica
6. Occipital neuralgia
7. Phantom limb pain
8. Herpes zoster
9. Painful shoulder
10. Neuropathic pain
11. Factitious pain (Münchausen syndrome)

APPROACH TO THE PATIENT WITH PAIN

Patients suffering from acute and chronic pain have to be managed with an understanding of the emotional, social, and psychological factors that may be contributing to the main process. Patients injured on the job and those who may be seeking compensation for personal injury may find the continuation of disability an important factor.

In many instances, a series of nerve blocks or epidural steroid injections combined with physical therapy may be sufficient to provide pain relief.

Some individuals, who receive secondary gain from their families who respond to every complaint, may be using pain as a controlling mechanism.

To manage patients with chronic pain such operant mechanisms must be understood and addressed. The activities that must be recognized and rewarded are

447

increased mobility, involvement in social activities, and interpersonal relationships.

Psychological, social, and rehabilitative services must be provided in conjunction with nerve block therapy for these patients.

COMPREHENSIVE PAIN MANAGEMENT

In some instances, patients may need the services of a Comprehensive Pain Treatment Center such as the one at our institution. In such a center, patients are given a battery of tests to evaluate their emotional, social, and psychological status as related to pain. Also, family members are integrated into the program. Group therapy sessions, private sessions, biofeedback, hypnosis, Amytal interviews, and time management sessions combined with physical, occupational, and recreational therapy are used.

Patients are given an insight into their pain problems and how they can cope with them while being directed to return to occupational and family relationships.

Many patients suffering from chronic pain take large amounts of narcotics and sedatives. Also, an element of depression may be associated with the painful state. Another role of the comprehensive pain program, therefore, is to detoxify patients from their drug dependence, provide antidepressants, when indicated or before bedtime to provide sleep, and substitute non-narcotic agents such as acetaminophen.

Patients in the comprehensive pain program who may benefit from nerve block therapy are referred to the anesthesiologist for treatments, thus providing the patient with the facilities of the comprehensive pain program as well as nerve block therapy when necessary.

TERMINOLOGY

Pain: unpleasant sensory and emotional experience associated with actual or potential tissue damage

Allodynia: pain caused by a non-noxious stimulus to normal skin

Analgesia: lack of pain or noxious stimulation

Central pain: pain associated with a lesion of the central nervous system

Dysesthesia: unpleasant abnormal sensation

Hyperalgesia: increased sensitivity to noxious stimulation (a lower threshold to noxious stimulation)

Hyperesthesia: increased sensitivity to stimulation (an increased response to noxious stimulation and pain after non-noxious stimulation)

Hyperpathia: painful condition characterized by overreaction to a stimulus (there may be delay and a after-sensation to a stimulus, especially if it is repetitive; there may be faulty identification and localization of the stimulus; the pain may be explosive in character)[1]

REFLEX SYMPATHETIC DYSTROPHY SYNDROME

In 1864 during the American Civil War, Silas Weir Mitchell described a syndrome of persistent burning pain and progressive trophic changes occurring in soldiers who had received gunshot wounds in their extremities. This syndrome was named *causalgia*, which means "burning pain" in Greek. Causalgias became a subclassification of a pain syndrome known as reflex sympathetic dystrophy (RSD), which has now been termed *sympathetic mediated pain.*[2]

RSD is a syndrome of pain, hyperesthesia, vasomotor disturbances, and dystrophic changes that usually improves with sympathetic denervation.

The three cardinal features of the disease are

Pain
  The patient often complains of pain that appears to be out of proportion to the injury suffered. A constant burning pain is frequently present, which may be exacerbated by movement, touch, or even a gentle breeze over the affected extremity. Patients may shield their extremity for fear of banging it or someone touching it. The pain and guarding of the extremity can result in loss of motion and eventually cause contractures and immobilization of joints.

Vasomotor disturbances
  Vasomotor disturbances vary depending on the degree of sympathetic tone and duration of RSD. A vasoconstricted or a warm vasodilated extremity may be present. In either situation, the extremity or affected part has a significantly different appearance from the opposite side.

Trophic changes
  Hair loss, shiny skin, and poor nail growth may be present. Swelling may or may not exist. Occasionally, very long fingernails are noted because the patient has too much pain to cut them.

Precipitating Factors

The syndrome of RSD may be triggered by trauma, surgical procedures, neurologic disorders, medical conditions, and immobilization after trauma. Other conditions known to precipitate RSD are listed below:

Soft tissue injury

Arthritis

Infection

Bursitis

Trauma

Fractures, sprains, dislocations

Surgical procedures

Malignancy

Aortic injury

Venous or arterial thrombosis

Myelography

Postherpetic

Brachial plexus injury

Scalenus anticus syndrome

Radiculopathy

Immobilization with cast

Vasculitis

Myocardial infarction

Polymyalgia rheumatica

Brain tumor

Severe head injury

Cerebral infarction

Subarachnoid hemorrhage

Cervical spinal cord injury

Poliomyelitis

Trauma is the most common precipitating factor in the etiology of RSD. Wrist and hand fractures are frequent causes, as well as crushing injuries, lacerations, sprains, burns, bruises, or penetrating wounds.

RSD may be associated with injuries to the spinal cord, neck, shoulder, arm, or lower extremity.

It can follow surgical procedures such as carpal tunnel release, Dupuytren's contracture repair, or excision of a ganglion.

Strokes, subarachnoid hemorrhage, head injury, spinal cord lesions, entrapment syndromes, and herpes zoster infections have been known to be associated with the development of RSD.

Reflex Sympathetic Dystrophy Variants

Causalgia
> Peripheral nerve injury

Sudeck's atrophy of bone
> Soft tissue injury, with bony atrophy predominating

Algodystrophy
> Occurs after minor trauma

Shoulder-hand syndrome
> RSD with "frozen shoulder" that occurs after myocardial infarction, cardiovascular accident, or cervical radiculopathy

Causalgia

Causalgia is a form of sympathetic dystrophy that is the result of a severe but incomplete nerve injury, which is usually caused by a high-velocity projectile or by a blast. Causalgia may also result from crushing injuries to an extremity. In our opinion, causalgia is a variant of RSD that is very difficult to treat because the underlying cause, the nerve damage, does not resolve.

Causalgia is a syndrome of persistent burning pain, allodynia, and hyperpathia in limbs in which injury to a nerve has occurred, with development of trophic changes.

The median and sciatic nerves are most commonly involved.

Less commonly affected sites include the ulnar, radial, trigeminal, greater occipital, and intercostal nerves.

Superficial burning pain in the distal area of the affected limb is the main presenting complaint of causalgia.

The pain is first limited to the distribution of the affected nerve but, if left untreated, quickly spreads to the entire limb and becomes more diffuse.

The pain may be exacerbated by a breeze blowing over the affected area, slight movement or touch, or anxiety or emotional stress. As the disease progresses, muscle atrophy and joint capsule fibrosis may lead to contractures. Osteoporosis in the bones on the affected extremity may be seen.

Physical Examination

The physical examination may reveal vasomotor and trophic changes. The patient may exhibit erythema with patches of pallor and warmth in the effected extremity. Cyanosis and rubor may be present. Sweating may or may not be present.

The trophic changes that appear as causalgia progresses reveal a shiny skin with atrophic changes, hair loss, and coarseness of the nails.

Theoretical Considerations in RSD Development

Pathophysiology

Devor[3] thought that any form of injury damages Schwann cells or the axons of nerves with local demyelination.

Excessive numbers of sodium and calcium channels and α-adrenergic receptors are incorporated into the demyelinated segment. This may lead to formation of ectopic pacemakers, which discharge spontaneously as well as in response to stimuli. Circulating catecholamines as well as those released from sympathetic efferent sprouts activate the ectopic pacemaker. RSD may result from abnormal firing of peripheral nerves because of increased sensitivity. This would account for the pain, allodynia, and hyperesthesia. The abnormal firing may cause altered responses in the spinal cord, which then respond abnormally to brain stem and cortical influences.[4]

These mechanisms are likely responsible for the "centralization" of pain in patients with RSD, ultimately rendering the pain untreatable.

Trauma in an extremity results in C-fiber hyperactivity sensitizing large-diameter fibers in the dorsal horn, resulting in sympathetic fiber stimulation of peripheral nerve A-mechanoreceptors. This leads to spontaneous pain, hyperesthesia, and allodynia. Normal tissue that may have abnormal innervation gives rise to pain on stimulation by non-noxious means.

Extension of stimulation to the autonomic nuclei in a dorsal horn results in uninhibited sympathetic motor activity sufficient to sustain the abnormal sensitization of A-mechanoreceptors, resulting in persistent pain and physical changes.[3,5]

Stages

Stage 1: acute stage
   Stage 1 may last for several weeks to 6 months.
   Pain is described as burning or aching.

Pain is exacerbated by touch, emotional upset, or active or passive
movement.
Diffuse swelling is present, with pain and stiffness in the affected parts.
Pain is intense and burning and is not limited to a specific dermatome.
Pain is much greater than expected in relation to the original injury.
Involved limb may be either cool or warm to the touch.
Hair or nail growth may be accelerated.
Extremity is diffusely tender, edematous, and dusky, red, or pale in
color or it may have a mottled appearance.
Skin is smooth and sweaty.
Extremity is held in a guarded and flexed position.

Stage 2: dystrophic stage
Stage 2 usually lasts between 3 and 6 months.
Pain becomes constant.
Pain is exacerbated by any type of stimulation.
Skin *shows edema;* it *becomes cool and hyperhidrotic* and *may be indu-
rated, cyanotic,* or *mottled.*
Nails become brittle and ridged.
Periarticular tenderness at the wrist or metacarpophalangeal joints is
frequently present.
There may be wasting of the intrinsic hand muscles and subcutaneous
tissues.
Flexion deformities of the fingers may start to develop.
Loss of hair may begin.

Stage 3: atrophic stage
Pain may be decreased at stage 3, but it may spread proximally in the
affected extremity.
Irreversible tissue damage occurs with limitation of motion in the small
joints of the hand.
Pronounced wasting of intrinsic muscles and subcutaneous tissues
occurs.
Contractures may begin to develop.
Skin is atrophic and smooth.
Distal part of the extremity is cool and pale.
Shoulder may become immobile.
Radiograph studies disclose marked demineralization.[6]

Diagnosis

The diagnosis of RSD is primarily based on
Clinical grounds
Radiographic findings
Scintigraphy

Thermography

Diagnostic differential neural blockade

Clinical Manifestations

Pain, vasomotor disturbances, trophic changes after an injury, application of a cast, or any of the other etiologic factors mentioned previously should lead one to suspect RSD.

The injury can be a major one or inconsequential.

The symptoms may begin gradually over a period of days or weeks or may manifest themselves within a few hours of the injury.

Many physicians may not readily interpret the findings and may be concerned that the pain is stated to be much more severe than it should be from the apparent etiology of the problem. Patients become emotionally unstable, anxious, and socially withdrawn. Anxiety may increase sympathetic discharge, which may in turn exacerbate the pain.

This syndrome of pain, hyperesthesia, vasomotor disturbances, and dystrophic changes is usually diagnosed by its response to sympathetic denervation.

Radiographic Findings

The most common radiographic abnormality is osteopenia, which is the result of continuous hyperemia. Osteopenia rarely occurs before the sixth week of symptoms.

Radiographic findings include

Patchy, local or diffuse demineralization in the affected extremity

Erosions of subchondral or juxta-articular bone in the small joints of the hands and feet or wrist and ankle

Patchy demineralization of the epiphyses and short bones of the hands or feet

Subperiosteal bone resorption, striation, and tunneling in the cortices, as well as large excavations and tunneling of the endosteal surface

Swollen tissues, reticulated in appearance

These changes, which may suggest RSD, may also be seen in hyperparathyroidism, thyrotoxicosis, and other conditions associated with increased bone turnover.[7]

Scintigraphy

Bone scans using methylene diphosphonate labeled with technetium-99m show increased blood flow and regional pooling. The delayed phase of the three-phase bone scan shows diffusely increased juxta-articular uptake in multiple joints in the effected extremity. This most likely represents increased periarticular blood flow and bone turnover.[8]

Thermography

A thermogram is considered positive if there is a temperature increase or decrease of at least 1°C in the painful area as compared with the opposite side.[9]

Differential Neural Blockade

Upper Extremity

Stellate ganglion block of the upper extremity is performed using 8 ml of normal saline.

If no pain relief occurs after several minutes, a stellate ganglion block with local anesthetic is performed. If pain relief occurs, the diagnosis may be RSD.

If pain is not relieved after a stellate ganglion block, a brachial plexus block is performed. If pain is relieved, the diagnosis of RSD is suspected.

If the pain persists, it must be of central origin.

Lower Extremity

Epidural blocks in the following sequence are used:

1. 10 ml normal saline
2. 10 ml 0.375 percent lidocaine, which will block sympathetic nerves
3. 10 ml 1.0 percent lidocaine, which will block sensory nerves
4. 10 ml 1.5 percent lidocaine, which will block motor nerves[10]

Case Study

A 37-year-old woman with pain in her knee underwent an arthroscopy. After this, she had persistent pain, discoloration, and swelling. A series of lumbar sympathetic blocks were performed without long-term relief. Intravenous regional bretylium blockade of the extremity provided some relief. She was referred by a neurosurgeon who was planning to insert a dorsal column stimulator but wanted to establish whether the patient was suffering from RSD or another, more complex pain syndrome. An epidural catheter was inserted at the L2 and L3 interspace. Injection of 10 ml of normal saline did not provide any relief, nor did an injection of 0.25 percent lidocaine. After an injection of 10 ml of 0.375 percent lidocaine, the patient said she had warmth in her lower extremity, with complete relief of pain. She was able to flex and extend her knee easily. There was no decrease in sensation. It was concluded that the patient was indeed suffering from RSD. The patient reported that there was decreased pain 1 week after the epidural block. She was referred for repeat epidural blocks with 0.375 percent lidocaine.

The lowest concentration of lidocaine that relieves the patient's pain will determine whether the pain is sympathetic, peripheral, somatic, or central in origin.

Differential Diagnosis

When there is pain, swelling, and tenderness in an extremity, with signs of vasomotor changes such as vasoconstriction or vasodilatation as well as dystrophic skin and nail changes, the diagnosis of RSD may be obvious, especially when a preceding triggering event has occurred.

Other conditions may be considered in the differential diagnosis if the signs and symptoms of RSD are not clear cut.

Entrapment syndrome such as carpal tunnel syndrome

Thoracic outlet syndrome, with neurologic or neurovascular entrapment

Raynaud's disease

Mixed connective tissue disease

Vascular insufficiency

Treatment

Early recognition and aggressive treatment are essential for a successful outcome. As the disease progresses and becomes long-standing, the chance for recovery is less likely. A series of sympathetic blocks in conjunction with physical therapy should be started as soon as the diagnosis is made. The response to sympathetic blockade and physical therapy will aid in the diagnosis. Physical therapy facilitates recovery from the disability and plays a role in providing a prolonged response to other modes of therapy.

Sympathetic Ganglion Blockade

Homan[11] was the first to describe the use of paravertebral sympathetic ganglion blockade to treat RSD.

Paravertebral sympathetic ganglion blockade is now the most widely recommended treatment for RSD.

Treatment Plan

Therapeutic Block Series

The diagnosis of RSD may not be clear cut. When it is suspected, a series of nerve blocks should be instituted as a diagnostic tool. If relief is obtained after a series of blocks of the stellate ganglion or lumbar sympathetic chain, the diagnosis of RSD is probably correct.

Sympathetic block each day for 3 to 5 days in combination with physical therapy after the block should provide a decrease in signs and symptoms if treatment is instituted early in the disease (stage 1). If commenced toward the end of stage 2 (the dystrophic stage) or during the third stage (atrophic stage), beneficial effects are less likely to result because fixation of soft tissues and joints may have already progressed to the point of irreversibility. Therefore, vigorous treatment early in the disease, as soon as it is suspected, is the best approach for a chance at recovery.

If pain relief occurs as a result of these blocks but the symptoms recur, another series of blocks should be performed.

Stellate Ganglion Block for the Upper Extremity

Anatomy

The stellate ganglion is formed by the fusion of the inferior cervical and first thoracic sympathetic ganglia. It measures approximately 2.5 cm × 1 cm × 0.5 cm.

It lies between the base of the transverse process of the last cervical vertebra and the first thoracic vertebra.

It is situated behind the carotid sheath and anterior to the longus colli muscle.

Equipment
   1 3-ml syringe

   1 5-ml syringe

   1 10-ml syringe

   1 25-gauge 0.5-in. needle

   1 22-gauge 3.5-in. needle

Drugs

Lidocaine, 1 percent, 5 ml

Bupivacaine, 0.25 percent, 10 ml

Note: Emergency resuscitation equipment should always be readily available.

Position

The patient is placed on an operating table in the supine position with a folded sheet under the shoulders to extend the neck (Fig. 15-1).

The head is tilted backward so the neck is in maximum extension. This straightens the esophagus and places it directly behind the trachea.

Landmark

Sternoclavicular junction and sternocleidomastoid muscle

Transverse process of C6 (Chassaignac's tubercle)

Level of cricoid cartilage

Procedure

Prepare and drape the neck in the usual manner.

Insert two fingers above the sternoclavicular junction in the immediate paratracheal area.

Feel pulsations of the carotid artery by the fingers retracting the sternocleidomastoid muscle.

Retract the sternocleidomastoid muscle and carotid sheath laterally.

Separate the two fingers and raise a skin wheal between them at the level of the transverse process of C7 *in the immediate paratracheal area.*

Through this wheal, pass a 22-gauge 3.5-in needle perpendicularly until the transverse process is encountered.

If the transverse process is not encountered, the needle is passing between vertebrae. Reinsert the needle superiorly or inferiorly.

If paresthesias to the brachial plexus are elicited during the placement of the needle, withdraw the needle and place it more medially.

Withdraw the needle 1 mm from the longus colli fascia.

Grasp the hub of the needle with the thumb and forefinger and steady the hand against the body of the patient.

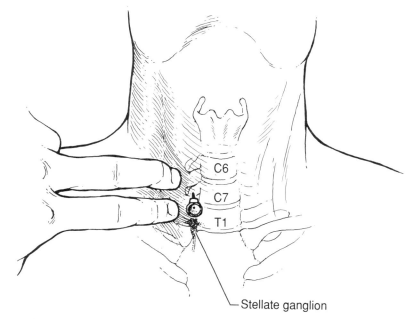

Fig. 15-1. Stellate ganglion block. Index and middle fingers are inserted at site of insertion of sternal head of sternocleidomastoid muscle and trachea. Muscle is retracted laterally. Needle is inserted perpendicularly between fingers until transverse process of C7 is encountered.

Aspirate for blood or cerebrospinal fluid.

Inject 5 ml of 1 percent lidocaine slowly, with aspiration after each 2.5 ml followed by 10 ml of 0.25 percent bupivacaine with the same technique of aspiration.

As soon as the drug is injected, withdraw the needle and elevate the head of the bed so the patient is in the sitting position.

Effects of Block

A successful block will be followed by Horner syndrome, which is

Ptosis of the eyelid

Miosis of the pupil

Enophthalmos

Absence of sweating on the side of the face

Increased temperature of the arm and face

Stuffiness of the nose

Side Effects

The patient may develop some hoarseness as well as a lump in the throat. The patient should be assured that this is not serious and will disappear.

Complications

1. Pneumothorax
2. Injection into the vertebral artery
3. Subarachnoid injection
4. Paralysis of the recurrent laryngeal nerve
5. Paralysis of all or part of the brachial plexus

If Horner syndrome develops, this means that the sympathetic chain has been blocked; however, the extremity should be checked for increased temperature, vasodilatation of the peripheral veins, and dryness. If these are not present, the block should be repeated after rechecking the landmarks. At least 15 to 30 minutes should pass before a decision is made to repeat the block because it is possible for the facial signs of Horner syndrome to appear within 2 to 5 minutes but it may take 15 to 30 minutes for the arm to show signs of an adequate block.

After observation of the patient for approximately 15 minutes, the patient is sent to physical therapy.

Paravertebral Lumbar Sympathetic Ganglion Block for the Lower Extremity

Anatomy

The lumbar portion of the sympathetic trunk lies along the anterolateral aspect of the bodies of the lumbar vertebrae. The depth from the transverse processes of the lumbar vertebrae to the sympathetic ganglia is approximately 1.5 to 2 in. The distance from the skin to the transverse process varies, depending on the size of the patient.

The sympathetic outflow to the lower extremity goes through the second lumbar sympathetic ganglion. Therefore, block of L2 is sufficient for sympathetic denervation of the lower extremity.

Premedication

In apprehensive individuals, 2 mg of midazolam (adjusted for age) can be given intramuscularly before the procedure.

Equipment

1 3-ml syringe
1 5-ml syringe
1 10-ml syringe

1 25-gauge 0.5-in. needle

1 22-gauge 3.5-in. needle

1 22-gauge 5-in. needle for heavy individuals

Drugs

Lidocaine 1 percent, 5 ml

Bupivacaine 0.25 percent, 10 ml

Position

The patient is placed on the operating table in a prone position. A pillow is placed under the abdomen between the ribs and the iliac crest to flatten the lumbar curvature of the spine and make the spinous processes more prominent.

Landmark

The iliac crests are palpated.

A line is drawn between the iliac crests. This line usually crosses the interspace between the fourth and fifth lumbar spinous processes. The fourth, third, and second lumbar spinous processes are identified.

The L2 spinous process is marked. The upper limit of the L2 spinous process identifies the level of the transverse process of the L2 vertebra.

Procedure

Prepare and drape the back in the usual manner (Fig. 15-2).

Identify the midpoint of the spinous process of L2, which corresponds to the lower border of the L2 transverse process.

Raise a skin wheal 4 cm lateral to the midpoint of the spinous process of L2.

Through this wheal, pass a needle in a perpendicular direction until the transverse process is encountered. The depth at which the transverse process is encountered will vary with the size of the patient.

Withdraw the needle to the skin and redirect it inferiorly to pass caudad to the inferior border of the transverse process and direct it to the anterolateral aspect of the vertebral body where the needle should just graze this area. When this occurs, the needle is at the level of the sympathetic ganglion. (Occasionally, the first pass of the needle may be between the transverse processes. To identify the transverse process, move the site of the skin insertion slightly cephalad.)

After advancing beyond the transverse process and the needle hits bone, the tip of the needle may have been directed too far medially and is hitting the body of the vertebra. Withdraw and redirect the needle in a more

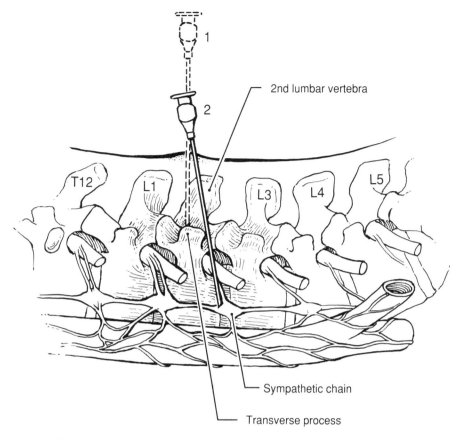

Fig. 15-2. Paravertebral lumbar sympathetic block. Needle is inserted two fingerbreaths lateral to spinous process of L2 until transverse process is encountered (1). Needle is directed to anterolateral aspect of body of vertebra at level of sympathetic ganglia (2).

perpendicular direction with the midline to avoid hitting the body in order to just graze the body of the vertebra.

Inject 5 ml of 1 percent lidocaine and 10 ml 0.25 percent bupivacaine after careful aspiration for blood and spinal fluid.

During the passage of the needle, paresthesias to the hip or thigh region may be obtained if the needle is touching somatic nerves that exit through the intervertebral foramen. This somatic nerve is located more dorsal than the sympathetic ganglia.

The paresthesias appear less commonly when inserting the needle midway between the transverse processes than when just caudad to the transverse process.

A successful block will show

1. Increase in skin temperature
2. Absence of sweating of the skin
3. Redness of the skin
4. Vascular dilatation
5. Decrease in pain

From time to time, sensory or motor anesthesia may occur as a result of the lumbar somatic nerves having been anesthetized. If this occurs, the patient should be warned not to attempt to walk because adequate motor power may not be present and falls can occur. Although rarely, postdural puncture headaches can occur possibly as a result of penetrating a dural sleeve.

Regional Sympathetic Blockade Using Bier Blocks

Guanethidine

Hannington-Kiff[12-15] describes regional sympathetic blockade with 10 to 20 mg of guanethidine. Guanethidine displaces norepinephrine in presynaptic vesicles and prevents its reuptake. Guanethidine is not commercially available in the United States for intravenous regional use.

Reserpine

Treatment of RSD with intravenous regional reserpine is recommended by Benzon et al.[16]

Reserpine is also not available in the United States for intravenous regional use.

The use of both reserpine and guanethidine results in significant systemic side effects such as hypotension, abdominal pain, and flushing after tourniquet release.

Bretylium

The treatment of RSD with intravenous regional bretylium Bier block has been recommended.[17]

It does not appear to have the serious side effects of the other drugs. However, some gastrointestinal complaints have been noted after tourniquet release.

We have had some good results with intravenous bretylium.

Patients may not allow the anesthesiologist to touch or move the painful limb to perform intravenous regional anesthesia.

The intravenous regional block may be more acceptable to the patient if sedatives and analgesics such as midazolam and alfentanil are given to decrease the pain and to make the patient more comfortable.

Monitors
Electrocardiogram (ECG)

Blood pressure

Pulse oximeter

Upper Extremity

Equipment
Tourniquet cuff

Tourniquet control apparatus, which has been checked

1 50-ml syringe

Connecting tubing

1 20-gauge cannula with stylet

Drugs
Bretylium, 1.5 mg/kg

Lidocaine, 3 mg/kg of 0.5 percent *preservative-free, epinephrine-free* solution (total dose not to exceed 40 ml)

Position
The patient is placed on the operating table in the supine position.

Procedure
Start an intravenous line in the contralateral arm.

Supply oxygen through a nasal cannula.

Apply ECG, blood pressure cuff, and pulse oximeter.

Titrate intravenous midazolam and narcotics to effect.

Place Webril padding as high in the axilla as possible on the arm to be blocked. Avoid folds or creases.

Apply a tourniquet snugly over the Webril.

Check the patient's blood pressure.

Select a suitable vein on the dorsum of the hand to be blocked.

Venous access may be difficult because of swelling and vasoconstriction. If necessary, inflate arm tourniquet for 5 minutes to obtain venous dilatation after deflation. Place a small drop of nitroglycerin ointment over a vein to cause vasodilatation. Wear gloves so you do not get a headache.

If the extremity is too painful to allow intravenous regional block, an interscalene block can be performed to decrease sensation so that tourniquet application and venous access can be obtained. We have had to resort to this on several occasions.

Place an intravenous cannula into this vein.

Place a stylet into the cannula.

Important: *Securely* tape the cannula.

Raise the arm and completely exsanguinate by tightly wrapping an Esmarch's bandage from the tip of the finger to the tourniquet. Sedation may be required to wrap the tender and sensitive extremity.

Inflate the tourniquet to 50 mmHg above the patient's systolic blood pressure.

Check for the presence of a radial pulse. It should not be felt.

Carefully remove the Esmarch's bandage. Do not dislodge the cannula from the vein.

Carefully remove the stylet from the cannula.

Attach the connecting tubing to the cannula.

Inject very, very slowly so that the pressure of the injection does not force the drug underneath the tourniquet into the general circulation.

Start an interval clock as soon as the injection is completed.

Keep the tourniquet inflated for a period of 30 minutes.

If the patient complains of discomfort, administer sedation.

At the end of 30 minutes, release the tourniquet in a cyclical fashion to allow the drugs in the arm to be released into the circulation slowly. Remove the tourniquet and observe the patient.

Observations after Block

The area distal to the tourniquet usually becomes warm and red.

The pain from which the patient suffers may be gone initially and may be diminished or absent. We have a few cases in which the patients remain pain-free for 3 months and return for blocks when the pain returns.

Repeat Block

The block can be repeated if necessary. During this period of pain relief between blocks, the patient should have physical therapy to stretch the muscles and increase the range of motion of the extremity.

Lower Extremity

Equipment

34-in. thigh tourniquet

Tourniquet control apparatus that has been checked

2 50-ml syringes

Connecting tubing

1 three-way stopcock

1 20-gauge cannula

1 20-gauge stylet

Monitors

Blood pressure

ECG

Pulse oximeter

Drugs

Epinephrine-free and preservative-free solution only

Bretylium, 1.5 mg/kg

Lidocaine, 100 ml 0.375 percent (add 25 ml preservative-free saline to 75 ml of 0.5 percent lidocaine)
    In thin individuals the total lidocaine dose is decreased.

Position

The patient is placed on the operating table in the supine position.

Procedure

Start an intravenous line in an arm vein.

Apply monitors.

Check the blood pressure.

Titrate midazolam and narcotics intravenously for sedation.

Wrap Webril padding around the upper thigh. Avoid folds and creases.

Apply tourniquet over Webril padding.

Place cannula into suitable vein in the foot. This may be the most difficult part of the procedure because of swelling and pain.

We have inflated the lower limb tourniquet for a period of 5 minutes, which provides vasodilatation after release of the tourniquet. We also have used a dab of nitroglycerin ointment on a vein to promote vasodilatation. Use gloves.

To help obtain venous access, we have performed a lumbar sympathetic block to provide venous dilatation.

Elevate lower extremity.

Exsanguinate blood by wrapping an Esmarch's bandage from the tips of the toes to the tourniquet. This may be very painful to the patient. Titrate sedation.

Inflate the tourniquet to 50 mmHg above the patient's systolic blood pressure.

Remove the Esmarch's bandage, taking care not to dislodge the cannula from the vein.

Attach connecting tubing.

Inject drugs very, very slowly to not exceed tourniquet pressure.

Administer sedation as needed.

Keep tourniquet inflated for 30 minutes.

Deflate tourniquet in a cyclical fashion.

Other Approaches to Treatment

Therapies that have proved to be effective involve blocking the effects of sympathetic hyperactivity.

Continuous Epidural Blockade

RSD of the knee has been treated by Cooper et al[18] with continuous epidural anesthesia for 4 days, combined with manipulation and continuous passive motion. The syndrome of RSD that affects the knee usually involves problems with the patellofemoral joint. In all the patients, the symptoms were relieved by a sympathetic block as an aid in the diagnosis of RSD.

A continuous epidural block through an indwelling lumbar catheter was instituted using local anesthesia followed by narcotics.

A dose of 1 mg/kg of 0.5 percent bupivacaine at a rate of 0.25 to 0.5 mg/kg/hr was titrated to give complete epidural anesthesia.[18]

Narcotics were given 2 to 3 days after the bupivacaine was started.

Morphine, 0.7 mg/kg body weight every 10 to 18 hours by bolus

or

Meperidine (Demerol), 1 mg/kg body weight by bolus followed by continuous infusion of 0.1 mg/kg body weight/hr

or

Fentanyl, 1 μg/kg body weight as a bolus followed by an infusion of 0.3 μg/kg body weight/hr.

Morphine was not infused continuously because of the possibility of respiratory depression. The continuous infusion of Demerol or fentanyl provided consistent analgesia.

Corticosteroids

The mechanism of action of corticosteroids is unknown, but they have been used systemically in patients with RSD.

Physical Therapy

Physical therapy alone or in conjunction with sympathetic blockade should be used. Passive and active motion, when adequate pain relief has been obtained from sympathetic blockade, should be directed toward improving the mobility of the affected extremity.

The anesthesiologist should arrange for physical therapy treatment to be provided immediately after the block.

RSD in Children

RSD in children is more common in girls.

A history of trauma is not as frequently noted as in adults.

The lower extremity is more frequently involved.

Knee involvement alone is present in a significant number of cases. This knee involvement may be misdiagnosed as chondromalacia of the patella.

Radiographic diagnosis is *not* helpful as it is in adults.

Deitz et al[19] have found a sign of autonomic dysfunction known as *tache cérébrale*. This is elicited by stroking the skin in the affected area with a blunt object, using the contralateral limb as control. Autonomic dysfunction is demonstrated by the appearance of an erythematous line lasting up to 30 seconds after the stimulus. This line may persist for as long as 15 minutes. All the patients described by the authors had this sign.[19]

Dietz et al[19] treated their cases with weightbearing and massage. They point out after review of the literature that a large component in the etiology is related to stress in the child or the family. They recommend that inpatient therapy or sympathetic blockade is indicated for those who fail to respond to massage. The outcome in childhood RSD is generally favorable in contrast to the adult experience.[19]

The major problem in childhood RSD is the failure to make an early diagnosis.[20]

Case Reports

Case Study

A 47-year-old police detective was shot in the left brachial plexus while pursuing an alleged perpetrator. Although emergency surgery was performed, significant median and ulnar nerve damage resulted in a nonfunctioning hand.

Postoperatively, severe, persistent burning pain with trophic changes was present. A diagnosis of causalgia was made because of the nerve injury.

A series of left stellate ganglion blocks was performed with immediate pain relief, but the pain recurred after 2 days.

A Bier block with bretylium was performed, with complete pain relief lasting 4 days. A second Bier block was performed 1 week later with similar results.

Comment

Causalgia is a result of direct nerve injury. The lack of prolonged success in this case despite early complete relief may be due to the possible irreversible effects of the nerve injury. True causalgia appears to be the most difficult variant of RSD to treat.

Case Study

A 25-year-old female model presented with pain in her right foot 2 months after a minor injury and immobilization.

Examination revealed that the patient could not move her foot or ankle because of pain. The foot was swollen and red and extremely tender to touch. A diagnosis of RSD (stage 1) was made.

After the first right lumbar sympathetic block, there was marked pain relief and improved ability to move the foot. A series of three blocks on subsequent days followed by physical therapy each day resulted in complete pain relief. The patient was discharged on the fourth hospital day.

Comment

In this case, the diagnosis was made early in the disease; treatment was instituted quickly and resulted in complete pain relief and return to work.

Case Study

A 22-year-old college student had a minor injury to the left foot, resulting in pain and inability to place the foot on the ground. She did not allow bedclothes to cover her foot.

Examination revealed a severely tender, swollen foot and ankle with mottling when left dependent.

Radiographic examination revealed patchy demineralization in the area of the cuboid bone.

Technetium-99m bone scan revealed increased uptake in the foot.

A series of five lumbar sympathetic blocks with 1 percent lidocaine and 0.25 percent bupivacaine were performed with some slight pain relief. Warmth of the lower extremity followed each block; however, permanent pain relief was not obtained.

Comment

Although evidence of sympathetic blockade was noted after blocks, partial but not complete relief was obtained.

Case Study

A 27-year-old male cyclist was struck by an automobile while riding his bicycle and was thrown 15 ft.

Examination revealed pain in the area of the right knee. The skin was mottled. The hair in the area of the knee was kept shaved, because, according to the patient, its presence exacerbated the pain.

A series of lumbar sympathetic blocks gave relief, which lasted 6 months, during which time he was able to ride on a stationary exercise bicycle.

The pain recurred, and the patient returned for another series of five sympathetic blocks, which resulted in moderate pain relief.

One year later, the patient returned with an increase in pain. He was given a Bier block with 150 mg of bretylium. Excellent pain relief lasted for about 1 month. He returns intermittently for Bier blocks with bretylium when the pain becomes severe.

Comment

This is a classic case of RSD after an injury. The patient obtains excellent relief while receiving blocks, but pain tends to recur over time.

In this patient, Bier blocks have been more successful than lumbar sympathetic blocks in controlling the pain.

RSD with an Underlying Surgically Correctable Disease

Case Study

A 33-year-old female patient complained of burning pain in the foot, for which she received a series of sympathetic blocks without significant relief.

Consultation with an orthopedic surgeon revealed a tarsal tunnel entrapment syndrome as well as RSD.

On referral to us, a management plan was developed in conjunction with the orthopedic surgeon.

A series of lumbar sympathetic blocks was performed before surgery for decompression of the tarsal tunnel. The pain did not recur.

The tarsal tunnel decompression was performed under epidural anesthesia to provide analgesia and sympathetic blockade. The epidural catheter was left in place for postoperative sympathetic blockade. Pain relief resulted.

Comment

This is an example of a patient with a remediable surgical condition and RSD. The RSD must be treated before surgery. Surgery performed in the face of untreated RSD will only serve to exacerbate the RSD.

LOW BACK PAIN

Anesthesiologists are frequently called on to provide consultations and treatment for patients with low back pain. Epidural steroid injections and nerve blocks have been found useful in treating patients with radicular pain, sacroiliitis, and facet joint problems.

Before embarking on treatment of patients with back pain, it is essential that all systemic diseases that may be involved in causing back pain be ruled out and a precise diagnosis obtained.

A careful history, physical examination, neurologic evaluation, computed tomography (CT) scan, magnetic resonance imaging (MRI), electromyography, and laboratory tests may be indicated to rule out systemic diseases and to arrive at a precise diagnosis.

Low Back Pain and Radiculopathy

Differential Diagnoses

Systemic diseases
    Dissecting aortic aneurysm
    Ruptured duodenal or gastric ulcer
    Pancreatitis
    Endometriosis
    Sickle cell disease

Organic back problems
    Arthritis
    Tumor
    Infection

Mechanical problems
    Trauma
    Scoliosis: osteoarthritis of facet joints, narrowing of disc space
    Spondylolisthesis: disc degeneration, facet joint arthrosis, narrowing intervertebral foramina, nerve root entrapment, shifting of vertebral body pulling nerve root with radiculopathy
    Spondylolysis: defect of pars interarticularis (fibrocartilage grows and impinges on nerve root exiting through foramen)
    Facet joint abnormalities: narrowing of joint, osteophyte formation, nerve root entrapment
Intervertebral disc problems
    Disc degeneration
        Narrowing of disc space
        Osteophyte formation
        Herniation
        Osteoarthritis of facet joints
    Disk bulging
        Distends posterior longitudinal ligament, resulting in localized back pain
        Increased bulging of disc: pressure on nerve roots, radicular pain
    Herniation
        Extrusion: may lead to relief if no pressure on nerve roots; radiculopathy caused by increased pressure on nerve roots

Herniated Discs

Low back pain with lumbar radiculopathy is a common pain problem seen by anesthesiologists. Herniated or bulging discs lead to mechanical compression and irritation of nerve roots.

Nerve root irritation may result from

Leakage of substances from a herniated disc, causing chemical irritation[21]

Compression of a nerve root by a herniated disc

Pressure on nerves from alterations in the bony architecture of the spinal column

Inflammatory Effect of Nucleus Pulposus

Tears in the annulus allow leakage of material from the nucleus pulposus that can act as an irritant to nerve roots and lead to back pain. In a canine model, material from the nucleus pulposus when homogenated and placed onto spinal nerves caused a chemical or immunologic inflammation of the neurosac.[22]

Pathophysiology of Nerve Root Compression

Mechanical pressure exerted by a herniated disc on a nerve root results in pain in the distribution of the nerve supplied by the irritated root (e.g., sciatic symptoms from a compressed L5 nerve root).

Compression of the nerve root may lead to alterations in the vascular dynamics involving arterial supply and venous drainage of the nerve.

Swelling and hypertrophy of the nerve root may occur, leading to sciatic symptoms.

If long-standing compression of the root occurs, inflammatory change leading to fibrosis may develop.

Prolonged irritation may lead to irreversible nerve root damage with persistent pain.

Early treatment aimed at decreasing the swelling is of benefit.

Site of Involvement

The L5 and S1 nerve roots are most commonly affected by disc disease, probably because those roots pass through a narrow lateral bony recess as they exit the spinal canal. This narrow recess increases the likelihood of root compression and irritation.[23]

Surgery

Surgical intervention for removal of herniated disks causing sciatica was introduced by Mixter and Barr.[24]

Nonsurgical Approaches

Saline Injections

Before the use of epidural steroid injections, large volumes of saline with or without local anesthetics were injected through the caudal canal. It was believed that these treatments broke down adhesions that were the cause of pain.[25]

Steroid Use

Epidural steroids have been used to decrease low back pain and radiculopathy. The beneficial effects are believed to result from a reduction in the inflammation that was initiated by a mechanical or chemical insult to the nerve root.[26]

Experimental work on injured rat sciatic nerves demonstrates that steroids produce a rapid and prolonged suppression of on-going discharge in chronic neuromas that have already become active. The suppression of the neuroma discharge may be a direct membrane action rather than an anti-inflammatory action.[27]

Lindahl and Rexed noticed that posterior nerve roots examined and biopsied during laminectomy were inflamed and edematous with a proliferative response.[28]

A series of studies seems to indicate that epidural steroids are more effective in decreasing pain, which decreases analgesic requirements, and are more likely to result in patients returning to work than patients treated with placebo.[29–31]

Evaluation and Treatment

Before treatment with epidural steroid injections, patients should have a history, physical examination, and radiographic studies (CT, MRI, plain films, and electromyography when indicated).

It must be ascertained that the patients are suffering from lumbar radiculopathy. It is important to rule out neurologic conditions such as spinal cord tumors, subarachnoid cysts, arteriovenous malformations, and neurologic disorders such as multiple sclerosis, metastatic disease, and multiple myeloma.

Determine whether certain symptoms exist:

Complaint of low back pain or radicular pain over dermatomal distribution

Sensory deficits in the area supplied by the particular nerve root

Increase in the pain with coughing, sneezing, or straining

Certain conditions such as loss of bowel or bladder function or acute foot drop may require immediate surgical intervention.

A trial of conservative therapy with anti-inflammatory agents and bed rest should be carried out.

A course of epidural steroid injections may be instituted.

Disorders that are considered acceptable for epidural steroid injection are

Nerve root irritation

Acute herniated discs

Postlaminectomy syndrome

Postlaminectomy patients with scar tissue around nerve roots after laminectomy may show some relief after epidural injections.

Abnormal bony structures
This is a controversial indication; however, treatments are given because pain relief may be obtained, such as in cases of spinal stenosis or scoliosis.

Radicular pain from known metastatic cancer
Patients with cancer who have metastases with nerve root compression are candidates for epidural steroid injections, but it is necessary to know what is being treated.

Patients with arachnoiditis from surgery or dye from a myelogram may show little benefit and are usually not treated in these situations.

Epidural Steroid Use

The advantage of epidural injection over parenteral steroids is that the drug is deposited into the affected area and less systemic side effects are seen because of lower blood levels.

Winnie et al[29] have shown that the injection of epidural steroids close to the site of the affected nerve root is more effective than the injection of local anesthesia into the epidural space or bed rest.

Inflamed nerve roots can be seen myelographically and can be confirmed by histologic examination. Improvement in clinical symptoms coincides with diminution of nerve root edema even in the presence of a persistent herniated disc. Patients were evaluated for duration of pain relief and improvement in symptoms after injection of epidural steroids.

Duration	Improvement (%)
<3 mo	83–100
<6 mo	61–81
<1 yr	69
>1 yr	46

The response time to improvement appears to be highest 4 to 6 days after the injection. Relief is noted in 96 percent within 6 days of the injection.[26]

Medications, Dosage, and Number of Treatments
Medications most commonly used are triamcinolone diacetate (50 mg) or methylprednisolone acetate (80 mg).

The number of injections that patients are given varies.

Some clinicians administer only one injection. Others have found that there is a response to the second or third injections.

The addition of local anesthetic solution to epidural steroids (approximately 3 to 4 ml) in the patient with acute pain, will provide good pain relief for several hours. This will allow the patient to relax and stretch out, and it will also confirm the proper placement of the steroids.

Procedure

Place the patient in the lateral decubitus position or in the sitting position with the affected side down.

Prepare and drape the back in the usual manner.

Raise a skin wheal in the interspace that has been chosen for the injection.

Identify the epidural space by the loss of resistance technique.

Inject 80 mg (2 ml) methylprednisolone acetate or 50 mg (2 ml) triamcinolone diacetate added to 3 to 4 ml of 1 percent lidocaine or 0.25 percent bupivacaine into the epidural space.

Keep the patient on the side for 10 to 15 minutes for the mixture of drugs to gravitate toward the affected nerve root.

If pain relief is not complete, repeat injections can be performed. It is important that assessment be carried out after 2 to 3 days after the injection because the corticosteroids take time to exert an effect. Injections can be repeated until three have been administered.

Large volumes of epidural fluid injected rapidly may cause pain and should be avoided.

The injection of 6 ml of radiopaque dye at the L4-L5 interspace spreads up to L1 and down to S5.[32]

Intrathecal injection of steroids should be avoided because all the current preparations contain polyethylene glycol, benzyl alcohol, or phenol.[33]

Acute Discogenic Lumbar Radiculopathy

Acute discogenic radiculopathy should be treated with bed rest and analgesics.

A large midline disc will cause bowel and bladder problems, and prompt surgical intervention is indicated. Neurologic changes such as foot drop requires surgery.

Acute Herniated Disc

Epidural steroids can be used if conservative measures of bed rest and analgesics do not control the pain.

Drugs used most commonly are triamcinolone diacetate or methylprednisolone acetate in combination with local anesthetic agents.

Many patients obtain good pain relief when given this treatment in the acute state.

These patients may have severe spasm of the back muscles, making it very difficult to perform an epidural injection. Sedation with 2 mg midazolam and the administration of a narcotic for pain relief may be necessary to be able to position these patients properly. On occasion, injections into the tight paraspinal muscles with dilute local anesthetic solutions have relieved some of the muscle spasm and allowed the patient to be positioned for the injection.

Chronic Radicular Low Back Pain

Patients with chronic low back pain may not benefit as much from epidural steroid injections as those with acute signs and symptoms.[34]

Patients Who Have Undergone Surgery

Some patients who have undergone previous surgery may present with low back pain. If the patient has recently undergone surgery, pain may result from adhesions, which is considered postlaminectomy syndrome. Epidural steroid injections may be useful. Patients may present with a scar or multiple scars in the back and may not have any good landmarks. Patients with previous fusions will not have landmarks and only bone, making it impossible to enter the epidural space. With such patients, injections may have to be performed at a distance from the scar, and it may be difficult to determine whether the steroid preparation reaches the area of involvement.

In some patients, the only available area for the administration of the steroids into the epidural space is through the caudal canal.[35]

Postlaminectomy Pain

In patients with postlaminectomy pain, the injection should be made in the interspace as close to the surgical scar as possible. In some patients, there is an adherence of the dura to the ligamentum flavum, and a wet tap can occur even though strict adherence to technique has been carried out. In the older age group, such a wet tap on most occasions does not lead to any signs of headache; however, in a few patients, headache may result.

"Tight" Epidural Spaces

In some patients, the injection of 1 or 2 ml of air during the entrance of the needle into the epidural space may cause pain of a radicular nature, which mimics the pain from which the patient suffers. In such patients, the injection of the local anesthetic and steroid preparation should be performed very, very slowly to not increase the pressure in the epidural space. In one patient, after normal injection into the epidural space, there was complaint of severe pain in the thoracic area and a headache. The headache did not abate even though the patient was put into a flat position. The headache and backache were most likely caused by an increase in cerebrospinal fluid pressure as a result of the epidural injection. On subsequent injections, the medication was injected very slowly and the complaint of headache did not occur. Transitory headaches and fullness of the head, with mild exacerbation of the sciatic pain, were found to occur during rapid epidural injection.

Systemic Effects of Corticosteroids

Evidence of fluid retention, mental confusion, and adrenal suppression are possible and should be suspected, although these complications are not common.

Intrathecal Injection

The possibility of an inadvertent, unrecognized intrathecal injection could occur, although spinal fluid may not be detected in the needle before injection. A high spinal block with circulatory depression after accidental subarachnoid injection of steroid plus local anesthetic should always be considered, and equipment for treatment should be available and ready for use.

Epidural Hematoma

Epidural steroid injection should be avoided in any patient who has an abnormal coagulation profile, diseases associated with defective platelet function, or a history of bruising and easy bleeding. Spontaneous epidural hemorrhage with hematoma formation may develop in patients who do not receive anticoagulants as well as in those who do.[36]

Symptoms

An epidural hematoma should be suspected in patients who develop radiating back pain, sensory changes, and muscular weakness that progresses toward paraplegia. An immediate neuroradiologic examination should be obtained. If an epidural hematoma is found, immediate surgical decompression is indicated.

CERVICAL RADICULOPATHY

After careful evaluation, patients with cervical radiculopathy can be treated with a mixture of epidural steroids and a local anesthetic.

Procedure

Place the patient in the lateral decubitus position with the affected side down. Place a pillow under the patient's head to keep the cervical spine parallel to the table in line with the thoracic spine.

Flex the neck on the chest.

Palpate the spinous process of the C7 cervical vertebra. This is the most prominent spinous process in the cervical spine.

Give the injection in either the C6-C7 interspace or the C7-T1 interspace.

Cover the hair so it is not in the field.

Prepare and drape the neck in the usual manner.

Raise a skin wheal in the chosen interspace.

Make a hole in the center of the skin wheal with an 18-gauge needle to facilitate the passage of the epidural needle.

Insert the epidural needle through the previously prepared site.
   The ligamentum flavum is not as deep as in the lumbar area. Therefore, place the low-resistance glass syringe onto the hub of the needle as soon as the needle is passed through the skin.

Advance the needle carefully and look for loss of resistance.

Loss of resistance followed by slight "pop-back" indicates that the epidural space has been entered. *Do not be a hero and attempt to advance the needle farther—you are in the epidural space.* Inject 80 mg (2 ml) methylprednisolone or 50 mg (2 ml) triamcinolone diacetate with 2 ml of 0.25 percent bupivacaine. Keep the patient in a supine position with the affected side down for approximately 15 minutes.

Patients frequently feel some pain relief and should be told that this will be present as long as the local anesthetic is active but that the effect of the corticosteroid preparation will take several days to act.

Complications
   1. Dural puncture with post-dural puncture headache
   2. Cervical epidural abcess

Waldman[37] reported that approximately 72 hours after a third cervical epidural steroid injection for cervical radiculopathy, a patient had shaking chills and a stiff neck. He had a temperature of 39.3°C. Examination of the neck showed meningismus.

Myelography revealed a complete block of the subarachnoid space at the T1 level. This mass extended to the third cervical vertebral body.

At surgery, where a decompressive laminectomy was performed large amounts of material were drained, from which *Staphylococcus aureus* was cultured. After surgery, the patient became quadraparetic at the C6 level.

The diagnosis of epidural abcess should be considered in any patient who has undergone epidural nerve block and who has increased pain, spasm, new motor or sensory disturbances, and bowel and bladder dysfunction associated with fever. The offending organism is usually *S. aureus*.

Emergency radiographic studies and myelography should be performed to make the diagnosis of epidural abcess. Emergency laminectomy should be performed immediately.[37]

In a review of 790 consecutive cervical epidural steroid nerve blocks, Waldman[38] reported two patients who sustained unintentional dural punctures and three patients who experienced vasovagal syncope. One late complication of a superficial infection at the injection site was also reported.

Waldman reported that when removing the saline-filled syringe from the Hustead needle while using the loss of resistance technique to enter the epidural space, he noted spinal fluid coming from the needle. He first treated this with the installation of 10 ml of preservative-free normal saline and conservative therapy. This did not stop the headache. An epidural blood patch with 7 ml of autologous blood resulted in the relief of headache symptoms.

Three patients undergoing cervical epidural steroid injection had vasovagal reactions while in the sitting position.[38]

We believe that the procedure should be performed with the patient lying on one side, which would most likely prevent the occurrence of a vasovagal reaction.

Infection, both superficial as well as in the epidural space, is a dreaded complication.

Meticulous attention to preparing and draping, the use of masks by all involved in the treatment, and attention to handling of the medications are essential. All ampules and vials should be wiped with alcohol before entry with the needle. All vials and ampules should be single-use only, even though some unused medication may have to be discarded. These injections should be avoided in patients who are prone to infection such as immunocompromised individuals. When treating patients with diabetes, the anesthesiologist must be on the alert for the possibility of infection.

These precautions may not prevent infection from occurring. It is therefore important to follow the patients carefully and make certain that any infection is recognized early and treated vigorously.[38]

MYOFASCIAL PAIN

The myofascial syndrome is characterized by pain that is aggravated by movement and is associated with the development of "trigger points." Pressure applied over the trigger point area reproduces the pain, which is referred to an area some distance from the trigger point. The trigger points are associated with tight, rope-like bands of muscle.

There is no dermatomal or peripheral nerve distribution of the referred pain.

Biopsy of trigger points has demonstrated dystrophic and degenerative changes with the degree of change corresponding to the severity of symptoms.[39]

Pathophysiology

Travell and Simons[40] believe that disruption of sarcoplasmic reticulum with release of calcium after acute muscle strain causes sustained skeletal muscle contraction and fatigue. The increased metabolism and decreased circulation cause the affected muscle band to become taut. Adenosine triphosphate becomes depleted, preventing the release of myosin from actin, leading to rigid sarcomeres with tight muscles. Prostaglandins, kinins, serotonin, and histamine may be released from platelets and mast cells, leading to increased firing of muscle nociceptors.[40]

Common trigger point sites are

1. Scapulocostal
   The trigger point is just medial and superior to the upper portion of the scapula. Pain radiates to the occipital region, the shoulder, the medial aspect of the arm, or the anterior chest wall.
2. Gluteal muscle myofascial pain
   The pain is referred into the posterior thigh and calf, appearing as an S1 radiculopathy.
3. Piriform muscle myofascial pain
   This trigger point overlies the sciatic nerve and can produce sciatic irritation and hyperesthesia resembling radiculopathy.[41]

Several pain areas and trigger points may exist in the same patient.

Examination

The painful muscles are described as feeling like rope.

A positive "jump sign" occurs when the trigger area is palpated. The patient "jumps" away from the pain.

Treatment

Treatment for myofascial pain is directed toward stretching of muscles.

Reduce muscle pain before stretching exercises. Trigger point injections by infiltration of local anesthetics directly into the trigger point are carried out. Pain relief should result after the injection.

A series of several injections are performed before stretching of the muscles.

After the injections, repeated gentle stretching of the muscles is carried out daily or every other day.

At home, the patient can use vapocoolant sprays on the affected area, followed by gentle muscle stretching.

Transcutaneous electrical nerve stimulation (TENS) can be used on trigger point areas.[42,43]

LUMBAR FACET SYNDROME

Anatomy

The articular processes of the lumbar vertebrae form the facet joints. The intervertebral disc anteriorly combines with the facet joints to connect the adjacent vertebrae comprising a three-joint complex.

The facet joints are true joints, having a complete capsule and definite synovial membrane.

Pathology

Facet arthropathy may develop as a result of disc degeneration, torsion injury, or congenital malalignment of the joints.

Degeneration and inflammation of the lumbar facet joints can produce low back pain. The pain of facet joint origin may be felt in the low back or may radiate to the buttock mimicking sciatica.

Diagnosis

Physical Examination

Pain develops with

Lateral pressure on the adjacent spinous process

Pressure over the joint

Extension of the spine

Twisting or lateral bending or arching of the back in the sitting position

CT Scans

CT scans can demonstrate facet hypertrophy, narrowing of the joint space, cartilage, osteophyte formation, capsular calcification, subchondral erosions, or joint asymmetry.

Diagnostic Block

Diagnosis of the facet syndrome relies on the result of diagnostic blocks. Injection of 1 ml of local anesthetic into the joint capsule with relief of pain is a positive diagnostic test.

Marks[44] showed that referred pain from facet joint stimulation is not precise or diagnostic. The pain radiating to the buttock or trochanteric region may originate from L3 and L4 to L5–S1. The nerves supplying the facet joints give rise to distal referred pain significantly more commonly than the joints themselves.[44]

Procedure

Place the patient in a lateral oblique position, placing the facet joint perpendicular to the horizontal.

Under fluoroscopy, mark a point on skin overlying the facet.

Raise a skin wheal at the site of the mark. Use longer needle to anesthetize deep tissue.

Through this wheal, insert a 22-gauge 3.5-in. needle and point it directly downward toward the facet.

Under fluoroscopy, move the needle until it is inserted directly into the joint.

Passage into joint provides a feeling of "popping" through a ligament.

Inject local anesthetic and 40 mg (1 ml) methylprednisolone acetate or 25 mg (1 ml) triamcinolone diacetate.

Complications

Facet joint injections may lead to inadvertent spinal anesthesia. This may occur if the needle is inserted through or beside the facet joint into the intervertebral foramen to penetrate the dura.

The needle can enter the epidural space.

The needle may penetrate the dural cuff that protrudes through the intervertebral foramen.

The anesthetic may be injected into the lumbar nerve itself.

The volume of the facet joint is approximately 2 to 3 ml, so capsular rupture may occur when large volumes are injected. Contrast medium is noted to leak into the epidural space after capsular rupture when large volumes of solution are used.[45]

Before injection of the local anesthetic and steroids, injection of 0.5 to 1 ml of contrast material into the joint will outline the extent of the capsule. This injection may reproduce the patient's pain.

A study by Carrera[46] found that approximately one-third of patients who had injections of insoluble steroids into the joint had at least 6 months of pain relief. In those patients whose pain was initially relieved by local anesthetics, long-term success with steroid injections went up to 50 percent. If there was no facet pathology on CT, there was usually no relief from the injections.[46]

Bough et al[47] have found that the production of symptoms during facet arthrography is of little value as a screening procedure.

Lynch and Taylor[48] suggest that the injection for facet joint pain should be at the suspected level as well as the joint above the suspected level.

In a randomized study by Lilius et al,[49] cortisone and local anesthetic were injected into two facet joints, the same mixture around two facet joints, and physiologic saline into facet joints. A significant improvement was observed in work attendance, pain, and disability scores, but it was independent of the treatment given. Movement of the lumbar spine was not improved. The conclusion was that facet joint injection is a nonspecific method of treatment, and good results depend on the tendency to spontaneous regression and to the psychosocial aspects of pain.[49]

SACROILIAC JOINT ARTHROPATHY

Diagnosis

Present with low back pain

Have pain on palpation of the sacroiliac joint

Marked tenderness over the sacroiliac joint commonly found

Pain produced by lateral pressure to the iliac crest or by hyperextension of the hip joint

Pain relief obtained by the injection of local anesthetic and insoluble cortico-steroids

Position

The patient is placed on the operating table in the sitting position.

Procedure

Raise a skin wheal in the midline at the level of S2.

Through this wheal, pass a needle at a 45-degree angle laterally into the sacroiliac joint.

Inject 5 ml of local anesthetic to confirm the diagnosis with relief of pain.

Inject 80 mg (2 ml) methylprednisolone acetate.

Many patients may have improvement in their symptoms when corticosteroids are injected.

MERALGIA PARESTHETICA

Meralgia paresthetica (lateral femoral cutaneous neuralgia) is characterized by burning pain, numbness, and tingling in the anterolateral aspect of the thigh.

Paresthesias are confined to the trouser pocket area and may be aggravated when the skin is touched or rubbed.

The symptoms may disappear or may persist for years and may eventually give rise to numbness.

Associated Conditions

Obesity

Prolonged pressure from belts

Anatomic entrapment, with the nerve going through the inguinal ligament rather than deep to it

Pregnancy

Meralgia paresthetica has been reported during pregnancy. In one series, these patients were treated with TENS.[50]

After Coronary Bypass Surgery

Meralgia paresthetica after coronary bypass surgery has been reported in three patients. It was believed that the patients were laying on the operating table in a very relaxed position or that the frog position was used during vein harvest.[51]

Occupational Activity

Meralgia paresthetica was reported in four patients in whom the disease was a result of occupational activity. One individual was carrying large heavy trays supported on the anterior superior part of his right thigh. This patient had a right iliac crest triggered dysesthesia in the region. Another patient complained of a disagreeable "pin prick" numbness of the anterior lateral aspect of the right thigh. He had a history of loading and unloading heavy sacks, catching them on the anterior aspect of the right thigh. Another patient experienced dysesthesia of the anterior lateral aspect of the right thigh; palpation of the anterior superior iliac spine generated "pin pricks" in the area innervated by the right lateral femoral cutaneous nerve. He picked up 50-kg bags of cement from the floor to the anterior aspect of the right thigh. Another patient supported the edge of large sheets of plastic in the right groin. He complained of sharp electrical pains that extended to the lateral aspect of the right thigh. He had a positive Tinel sign elicited at the level of the anterior superior iliac spine. In all four cases, the pain disappeared when the patients changed their work habits. Percussion in the area of the nerve caused tingling in its distribution.[52]

Hypothyroidism

Meralgia paresthetica associated with hypothyroidism was thought to be caused by the deposition of water-attracting mucopolysaccharides in the perineurium and endoneurium, which would cause swelling of the nerve and reduce the space available for the lateral femoral cutaneous nerve as it passes between the inguinal ligament and the iliac spine.[53]

Surgical treatment may be necessary if conservative measures fail.[54,55]

Diagnosis

Tenderness to pressure immediately distal to the anterior superior iliac spine is a symptom of meralgia paresthetica.

The nerve may be palpable on the affected side.

In thin patients, symptoms may be aggravated by rolling or tapping the nerve.

Injection of local anesthetic into the area of the lateral femoral cutaneous nerve 1 in. medial and 1 in. inferior to the anterior superior iliac spine can aid in the diagnosis.

Lack of pain relief after injection does not exclude the diagnosis of meralgia paresthetica.

Pain from an intrapelvic lesion such as carcinoma of the uterus or prostate may cause the same syndrome. The lateral femoral cutaneous nerve has an intrapelvic course and may be involved by conditions in the pelvis because it lies under the parietal peritoneum adjacent to these organs. A block of the nerve at the anterior superior iliac spine would not relieve the pain from such involvement.

The idiopathic form of meralgia paresthetica is more common in muscular or obese individuals.

Women may suffer from meralgia paresthetica symptoms after pelvic osteotomies because women are more susceptible to hip dysplasia than men.

Meralgia paresthetica can also occur after the removal of an iliac crest bone graft.

Anatomic Considerations

The lateral femoral cutaneous nerve usually lies deep to the lateral end of the inguinal ligament but superficial to the sartorius muscle.

The nerve may lie in the following alternative positions:

1. It may overlie the anterior iliac wing.
2. It may pass between two slips of the inguinal ligament (entrapment is likely here).
3. It may pass deep to the sartorius muscle.
4. It may pass through the sartorius muscle.
5. It may be compressed distally where it passes through the deep fascia.

Conservative Treatment

Removal of constricting items about the waist (e.g., belts, tight clothes) may be all that is necessary.

Application of ice three times a day to the area of presumed constriction will alleviate the swelling of the nerve.

Nonsteroidal anti-inflammatory agents for 7 to days may be used.

Physical activities that lead to hip extension are avoided.

Nerve Block of the Lateral Femoral Cutaneous Nerves

Anatomy
The lateral femoral cutaneous nerve arises from L2 and L3. It lies on the iliacus muscle at the lateral border.

It runs on the medial side of the anterior superior iliac spine.

It pierces the fascia lata 1.5 to 2 in. below the inguinal ligament.

It innervates the lateral side of the skin of the thigh.

Equipment
  1 25-gauge 0.5-in. needle
  1 22-gauge 1.5-in. needle
  1 10-ml syringe

Drugs
  Short duration block: lidocaine 1 percent, 10 ml
  Long duration block: bupivacaine 0.25 percent, 10 ml
  Optional: corticosteroids: methylprednisolone acetate, 40 mg (1 ml)

Landmark
  Anterior superior iliac spine
  Inguinal ligament

Position
The patient is placed in the supine position.

Procedure
  Raise a skin wheal 2.5 cm inferior and 2.5 cm medial to the anterior superior iliac spine.
  Through this wheal, introduce a 22-gauge 1.5-in. needle attached to a 10-ml syringe with local anesthetic.
  Make injections upward and laterally through the skin wheal toward the iliac

crest behind the anterior superior iliac spine, with the needle touching the inner surface of the iliac crest. Inject 5 ml of local anesthetic.

Withdraw the needle to the skin wheal and make a fan-like injection lateral to the skin wheal; inject the remaining 5 ml of local anesthetic.

Subcutaneous infiltration as a field block in this area may also be useful.

After the injection of local anesthetic, inject 1 ml of corticosteroid.

GREATER OCCIPITAL NEURALGIA

Greater occipital neuralgia is frequently a cause of chronic unilateral or bilateral headaches. The greater occipital nerve originates in the second cervical nerve root and may become compressed, irritated, or inflamed.

Clinical Manifestations

Unilateral sharp, shooting, or continuous pain in the distribution of the greater occipital nerve in the back of the neck and scalp

Paresthesias, dysesthesias, or hypoesthesias

Tenderness to palpation over the greater occipital nerve trunk as it traverses over the superior nuchal line

Etiology

Cervical spine injuries

Cervical spine inflammatory diseases

Cervical spine degenerative diseases

Persistent posterior cervical muscle spasm

Diagnosis

Pain and tenderness on palpation of the greater occipital nerve as it passes over the nuchal ridge are signs of occipital neuralgia.

Landmark

The greater occipital nerve passes over the nuchal ridge in close proximity to the greater occipital artery, whose pulsations can be felt.

The greater occipital nerve lies on the superior nuchal line just lateral to the external occipital protuberance, which is a midline structure of the posterior aspect of the skull.

Treatment

Injection of local anesthetic into the area of the nerve at that superior nuchal line may provide relief.

Successful block of the nerve will lead to anesthesia on the posterior aspect of the scalp on the side of the block.

PHANTOM LIMB PAIN

Most patients who have an amputation of a limb experience the illusion that the limb is still present.

The phantom limb at first appears normal in size and shape, but it usually becomes smaller and in many cases gradually fades into the stump. In 5 to 30 percent of patients who have amputations, there can be persistent pain in the amputated limb.[56,57]

Tingling is the usual sensation, but the pain may be described as "cramping," "shooting," "burning," or "crushing."

Persistent phantom limb pain is associated with the following:

1. More common in the upper than in the lower limbs
2. Limbs usually seen as distorted or not whole
3. Movement of the limb felt
4. Sensation perceived (frequently occurs if the stump is stimulated)

Phantom limb pain has certain characteristics as outlined by Melzack.[58]

1. The pain remains for months or years after the tissues heal.
2. The pain develops more commonly in patients who have suffered pain in the limb before amputation.
3. Trigger areas, when stimulated, may bring on the pain.
4. The pain may be altered by increases or decreases in somatic input.

Phantom limb pain must be distinguished from stump pain. Stump pain develops after several days or weeks and may be caused by pressure on nerves.

Neuromas may form, which may cause abnormal impulses, leading to a locally painful stump. The painful stump may improve by repeatedly hitting the area directly with a firm object. Alternatively, the painful stump can be infiltrated with local anesthetics to provide pain relief.

Warning: Infiltration in a stump may cause infection if there is a problem with the blood supply or in diabetic patients.

Frequently, surgical resection of the neuroma may be necessary.

Phantom limb pain is more likely if the limb was painful before amputation and if the amputation was delayed for a long period of time after the injury.

Of those who develop phantom pain, it occurs in more than 50 to 85 percent of patients several years after limb loss.[59]

Phantom pain may be a reaction in which a painful imprint is established in the brain before amputation, leading to the concept of a central pain mechanism.[58,60]

Phantom limb pain noted immediately after amputation may be related to the preamputation pain that the patient was suffering.

The basis for the use of somatic nerve block such as lumbar epidural blocks in chronic pain is to interrupt the sensory input.

Increased sympathetic activity may sensitize peripheral sensory neurons in regions of damaged or ischemic tissues. Blocking of the sensory inputs may also block the sympathetic fibers and may eliminate sympathetic overactivity.

Prevention

The best method of managing the problem of phantom limb pain is to prevent its onset. The anesthesiologist can play an important role by pointing out the benefits of preoperative epidural block.

Lumber epidural blockade before amputation has been shown to decrease the incidence of phantom limb pain.[61]

When possible, patients with painful limbs who are to undergo amputation should have lumbar epidural blocks with anesthetic agents and narcotics for a few days before surgery to decrease the pain.

It is also suggested that placement of a prosthesis as soon as possible, even in the operating room, can decrease the incidence of phantom limb. Other treatment modalities include hypnosis, TENS, trigger point injections, having the patient move the limb in their mind, and medications for central pain such as phenytoin and carbamazepine[62] (H. Adelglass, M.D. personal communication).

HERPES ZOSTER

After an episode of childhood varicella infection has resolved, the varicella zoster virus may lay dormant in the dorsal root ganglia for up to 60 to 70 years. When the virus reactivates, it can result in a very painful disease process associated with skin eruptions and vesicle formation covering the dermatomal distribution of the infected dorsal root ganglia.[63–65]

The dermatomal distribution probably results from transport of virus by sensory axons to the skin.[66]

The dermatomal distribution is very striking in that the eruptions and rash do not cross the midline. Vesicles appear, pustulate, and finally scab over in 7 to 14 days. After a few weeks, the vesicles disappear.[64] However, the pain may remain.

Common sites of involvement are the thoracic and ophthalmic areas.

Although herpes zoster is usually found in the elderly population, it is commonly associated with

Cancer

Immunocompromised patients

Immunosuppressed patients

Patients with diabetes[63]

Treatment

Acute herpes zoster is a very painful condition. Treatment modalities are geared toward decreasing the duration of infection and decreasing the pain.

Acyclovir

Once the diagnosis of acute herpes zoster is made, the patient should receive high doses of oral acyclovir. This antiviral agent has helped decrease the duration of the acute phase.[63,66]

Acyclovir is effective in decreasing pain during the acute phase and in shortening the healing process.[65]

Topical acyclovir (Zovirax) can also be applied directly to the lesions.[66]

Steroids

Steroids have been advocated for use in acute herpes zoster. Loeser[65] believes there is some evidence that systemic steroids may decrease the severity and length of the acute herpetic infection, but topical or intradermal steroids are not effective. Post and Philbrick[67] also report that steroid use may decrease the early pain of herpes zoster but not the prolonged postherpetic neuralgia (PHN) pain.

Regional Nerve Blocks

Regional sympathetic blocks will provide pain relief during the acute stage of herpes zoster. Colding[68] reports beneficial effects of sympathetic blockade on acute herpes zoster and also reports that it may prevent PHN. Others have demonstrated relief during the acute state but no effect on the incidence of PHN.[69]

Analgesics

Pain medication is necessary to help alleviate the pain of an acute attack. Non-narcotic and narcotic analgesics are prescribed.

POSTHERPETIC NEURALGIA

Although acute herpes zoster infection is very painful and the pain may actually precede the development of the vesicles, in 10 percent of cases an even more painful condition known as PHN may occur.

Characteristics of PHN[63,65,70,71] include

  Pain that is continuously present and deep, burning, sharp, stabbing, and unbearable[63,70]

  Dysesthesia

  Paresthesia

  Decreased sensation

  Scarring

  Hyperpathia

  Hyperesthesia

  Hypoesthesia[63,65,70,71]

PHN appears to occur more frequently in the elderly with patients older than 60 years developing PHN more than 50 percent of the time.[63,70-72]

A very painful type of PHN can occur after ophthalmic herpes.[63,72]

The severe unremitting nature of the pain has led investigators to search for both a cause and cure for the pain, which is believed to result from nerve destruction.[65]

Noordenbos[73] has proposed that the pain associated with PHN is associated with destruction of large myelinated fibers, which have an inhibitory effect on pain, while small fibers continue to function.[63]

Treatment

Steroids

Steroids have been used to treat PHN.[63,67]

Post and Philbrick[67] evaluated the results of steroid use and were unable to conclude that steroids are efficacious in treating PHN.

Capsaicin Ointment

Topical capsaicin ointment (0.025 percent) is prescribed for PHN.[63,71]

The ointment should be applied three to four times daily. Capsaicin ointment works by decreasing pain by local depletion of substance P.[74]

EMLA Cream

Application of 5 percent EMLA cream has been shown to provide pain relief of short duration.[70]

Amitriptyline

A study by Watson et al[71] demonstrated a 60 percent rate of relief when amitriptyline was administered. Significant side effects include dry mouth, drowsiness, and constipation.

Carbamazepine and Dilantin

These anticonvulsants have been advocated for treating PHN.

Sympathetic Blocks

Sympathetic blocks have been advocated for relief of the pain associated with PHN, as well as for decreasing the incidence of PHN.[75] Although excellent pain relief is noted during the regional block, its effect on actually decreasing the duration of PHN is unclear.

A study by Milligan and Nash[75] demonstrated pain relief in patients who received stellate ganglion blocks for pain in the head, neck, and thorax within 1 year of the onset of symptoms. Stellate ganglion blocks were helpful in 75 percent of patients who had pain for less than 1 year, with 40 percent becoming pain-free. Results were not as good in patients treated after 1 year, with only 44 percent being helped and 22 percent becoming pain-free.[75]

The results of Watson et al[71] with blocks were not as successful as those of Milligan and Nash[75]:

Nine stellate blocks were used for ophthalmic PHN, none of which resulted in relief of pain.

Intercostal blocks were capable of relieving pain for the duration of the anesthetic and in some cases from 5 to 7 days.

Seven lumbar sympathetic blocks resulted in either no relief or relief for the duration of the action of the anesthetic.

Lidocaine plus methylprednisolone into the epidural space resulted in no effect.[71]

Paravertebral Thoracic Somatic Nerve Blocks

Paravertebral thoracic somatic nerve blocks may be useful in the treatment of herpes zoster in the thoracic area.

Procedure

Place the patient on the operating table in the prone position.

Prepare and drape the back in the usual manner.

Raise skin wheals 5 cm lateral to the spinous processes in the area of the nerve distribution of the herpetic involvement.

Through these wheals, direct a needle perpendicular to the skin until the transverse process is encountered.

Slide the needle off the transverse process and direct it inferiorly 1 to 2 mm deeper.

Inject 3 ml of local anesthetic at each level.

These blocks can be repeated on consecutive days for 3 to 5 days and then at longer and longer intervals as necessary (R. Alagesan, M. D. personal communication).

Summary

PHN is a very painful condition that is very difficult to treat. The anesthesiologist should coordinate with an internist and a neurologist and decide whether medication or blocks, or a combination, will be used on a given patient.

PAINFUL SHOULDER

Pain in the area of the shoulder can result from

Acute and chronic bursitis

Tears of the capsule

Glenohumeral arthritis

Chronic shoulder pain in rheumatoid arthritis

Pain from fractures of the scapula

Treatment

Painful conditions in the area of the shoulder can be relieved by blocking the suprascapular nerve.[76–78]

Anatomy

The suprascapular nerve is formed by branches from the fourth, fifth, and sixth cervical nerves. The suprascapular nerve enters the supraspinatus fossa through the suprascapular notch.

After the suprascapular nerve passes through the suprascapular notch, it branches to supply the supraspinatus muscle, the infraspinatus muscle, and the shoulder joint.

Equipment

1 2-ml syringe

1 25-gauge 0.5-in. needle

1 20-ml syringe

1 22-gauge 3.5-in. needle

Drugs

A dose of 15 ml of 1.5 percent lidocaine with 1:200,000 epinephrine or 10 ml of 0.5 percent bupivacaine is given.

Landmark

Spine of the scapula, which extends from the tip of the acromion on the lateral aspect to the scapular border on the medial aspect

Midpoint of the spine of the scapula on a vertical line parallel to the vertebral spine

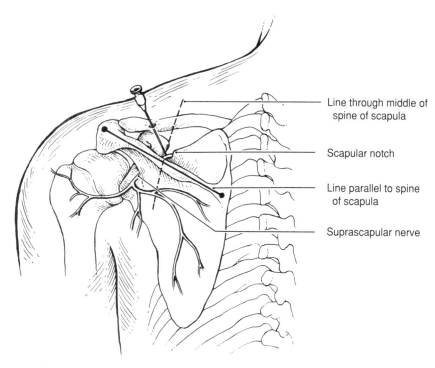

Line through middle of
spine of scapula

Scapular notch

Line parallel to spine
of scapula

Suprascapular nerve

Fig. 15-3. Suprascapular nerve block. Needle is inserted as shown until bone is contacted. The anesthesiologist walks needle along bone until it enters suprascapular notch.

In the upper outer quadrant, a line is drawn to bisect the angle of the upper outer quadrant. A mark is placed on this line 1 in. from the apex of the angle.

Position

The patient is placed in the sitting position, with the arms folded on the lap (Fig. 15-3).

Procedure

Raise a skin wheal on the line that bisects the upper outer quadrant of the line formed by the spine of the scapula and the line parallel to the vertebral bodies.

Through this wheal, pass a 3.5-in. 22-gauge needle 90 degrees perpendicular in all planes until bone is contacted. This will occur at a depth of 2 to 2.5 in., depending on the size of the patient.

The relationship of the needle to the skin must be 90 degrees in all planes to give the inward, downward, and forward direction toward the supra-scapular notch.

When bone is contacted, the needle should be on the bone surrounding the suprascapular notch.

Withdraw the needle and redirect either laterally, medially, or superiorly until it is felt to slide into the notch.

Inject 10 ml of local anesthetic solution.

Withdraw the needle slightly and check that the needle has been in the notch that is surrounded by bone. If the position of the needle is satisfactory, replace it into the notch and inject an additional 5 ml of local anesthetic solution.

If the needle is advanced and no bone has been contacted, it may be that the needle has been placed right into the suprascapular notch on the first pass. In that event, withdraw the needle and direct it medially, laterally, or inferiorly to contact bone. If this is not the case, the needle may have passed over the scapula.

Because there is no skin analgesia from this block, a successful block will be manifested by relief of pain.

Complications
Pneumothorax is a rare complication and may occur in less than 1 percent of cases. It is caused by advancing the needle deeper than recommended.

Indications

When administered for bursitis with a painful shoulder, it is advantageous if the block is given early to help relieve pain and allow the patient to exercise the shoulder and maintain a good range of motion.

The block can be repeated for further therapy as necessary.

If the block is not successful after the first injection, the block should be repeated.

Continuous Suprascapular Nerve Block

Use of the continuous suprascapular nerve block in the treatment of a fractured scapula involves the administration of the local anesthetic through an 18-gauge epidural catheter that was introduced through a 17-gauge Tuohy needle placed adjacent to the original 3-in. needle used to secure the block initially.

In one study the catheter was sutured to the skin and was used for 5 days with repeated injections of 10 ml of 0.25 percent bupivacaine with 1:200,000 epinephrine.[78]

NEUROPATHIC PAIN

Certain conditions can give rise to pain as a result of damage to peripheral nerves where A-δ and C-fibers are involved. These nociceptors are usually activated by injury. However, they can become damaged by pathologic conditions and produce impulses in reaction to acute, painful stimuli.

The pain can result from

Post-traumatic neuromas

Phantom limb pain

Diabetic neuropathy

PHN

Ischemic neuropathy

Nutritional neuropathy

Alcoholic neuropathy

Postradiation neuropathy[79]

Treatment

The treatment of conditions associated with neuropathic pain may be through the blocking of sodium channels by agents such as lidocaine, mexiletine, and carbamazepine.[80–82]

Intravenous Lidocaine

Patients who have conditions associated with neuropathic pain and appear to be resistant to other forms of therapy may respond to intravenous lidocaine administered in a dose of 70 mg/hr. While under treatment with intravenous lidocaine, the patients appear to have a decrease in the pain.

Mexiletine

Chabal et al[83] demonstrated a significant reduction in pain with oral mexiletine when compared with baseline or placebo. Patients were administered initial doses of 150 mg of mexiletine twice daily, which was gradually increased until a total daily dose of either 450 mg or 750 mg had been given. There were only mild side effects, and the patients reported improvement in symptoms.[83]

Others have started patients on intravenous lidocaine infusions and gradually instituted oral mexiletine, starting at 200 mg orally once per day to provide pain relief.

Carbamazepine

Carbamazepine can be administered for pain relief after the beneficial response to lidocaine infusion. A dose of 100 mg carbamazepine orally every hour is administered until pain control is achieved, with a maximum of 1,200 mg/day. The patient then can be maintained on a dose of carbamazepine orally, which results in a diminution in the pain.

FACTITIOUS PAIN

Factitious pain (*Münchausen syndrome*) involves feigning pain to gain special benefits. These benefits may be attention from the family, compensation, or other gains that would accrue as a result of having an illness.

Patients simulate fevers by heating thermometers; they may induce infection by injecting themselves with a contaminated substance.

Factitious disorders are divided into three types:

1. Factitious disorder with physical symptoms
2. Factitious disorder with psychological symptoms
3. Atypical factitious disorder[84]

The form of factitious disorder associated with physical symptoms is known as Münchausen syndrome.

Physicians involved in caring for patients with pain should be alert to the possibility that some patients may feign symptoms of pain and have a psychological need to be considered sick.

Patients with the Münchausen syndrome may wander from hospital to hospital for treatment; these patients may show medical sophistication, with anger and aggressive behavior toward the staff.

This syndrome is difficult to diagnose. The patient may present with problems that are very difficult to diagnose and may confound the physicians who are doing an evaluation.[85]

REFERENCES

1. IASP Subcommitte on Taxonomy: Pain terms a list with definitions and notes on usage. Pain 6:249, 1979
2. Mitchell SW, Morehouse OR, Keen WW: Gunshot Wounds and Other Injuries of Nerves. JB Lippincott, Philadelphia, 1864
3. Devor M: Nerve pathophysiology and mechanisms of pain in causalgia. J Auton Nerv Syst 7:371, 1983
4. Melzack R: Phantom limb pain: implications for treatment of pathologic pain. Anesthesiology 35:409, 1971
5. Roberts WJ: A hypothesis on the physiological bases for causalgia and related pains. Pain 24:297, 1986
6. Schwartzman RJ, McLellan TL: Reflex sympathetic dystrophy: a review. Arch Neurol 44:555, 1987
7. Smith DL, Campbell SM: Reflex sympathetic dystrophy syndrome diagnosis and management. Topics in primary care medicine. West J Med 147:342, 1987
8. Kozin F, Soin JS, Ryan LM et al: Bone scintigraphy in the reflex sympathetic dystrophy syndrome. Radiology 138:437, 1981
9. Ecker A: Contact thermography in diagnosis of reflex sympathetic dystrophy: a new look at pathogenesis. Thermology 1:106, 1985
10. Winnie AP, Collins VJ: The pain clinic: I. Differential neural blockade and pain syndromes of questionable etiology. Med Clin North Am 52:123, 1968
11. Homan J: Minor causalgia: a hyperesthetic neurovascular syndrome. N Engl J Med 222:870, 1940
12. Hannington-Kiff JG: Intravenous regional sympathetic blockade with guanethedine. Lancet 1:1019, 1974
13. Hannington-Kiff JG: Relief of Sudek's atrophy by regional intravenous guanethedine. Lancet 1:1132, 1977
14. Hannington-Kiff JG: Relief of causalgia in limbs by regional intravenous guanethedine. Br Med J 2:367, 1979
15. Hannington-Kiff JG: Hyperadrenergic-effected limb causalgia: relief by IV pharmacologic norepinephrine blockade. Am Heart J 103:152, 1982
16. Benzon HT, Chomka CM, Brunner EA: Treatment of reflex sympathetic dystrophy with regional intravenous reserpine. Anesth Analg 59:500, 1980
17. Ford SR, Forrest WH, Eltherington L: The treatment of reflex sympathetic dystrophy with intravenous regional bretylium. Anesthesiology 68:137, 1988
18. Cooper DE, DeLee JC, Ramamurthy S et al: Reflex sympathetic dystrophy of the knee. J Bone Joint Surg 71(A):365, 1989
19. Dietz FR, Mathews KD, Montgomery WJ: Reflex sympathetic dystrophy in children. Clin Orthop 258:225, 1990
20. Sherry DD, Weisman R: Psychologic aspects of childhood reflex neurovascular dystrophy. Pediatrics 81:572, 1988
21. Marshall LL, Trethwie ER, Curtain CC: Chemical radiculitis. Clin Orthop 29:61, 1977
22. McCarron RF, Wimpee MW, Hudkins PG et al: The inflammatory effect of nucleus pulposus, a possible element in the pathogenesis of low back pain. Spine 12:760, 1987
23. Finneson BE: Low Back Pain. JB Lippincott, Philadelphia, 1973

24. Mixter WJ, Barr JS: Rupture of intervertebral discs with involvement of the spinal cord. N Engl J Med 211:210, 1934
25. Davidson JT, Robin GC: Epidural injections in the lumbosciatic syndrome. Br J Anaesth 33:595, 1961
26. Benzon HT: Epidural steroid injections for low back pain and lumbosacral radiculopathy. Pain 24:277, 1986
27. Devor M, Govrin-Lippmann R, Raber P: Corticosteroid suppress ectopic neural discharge originating in experimental neuromas. Pain 22:127, 1985
28. Lindahl O, Rexed B: Histologic changes in spinal nerve roots of operated cases of sciatica. Acta Orthop Scand 20:215, 1950
29. Winnie AP, Hartman JT, Myers HL et al: Pain clinic II: intradural and extradural corticosteroids for sciatica. Anesth Analg 51:990, 1972
30. Dilke TFW, Burry HC, Graham ER: Extradural corticosteroid injection in management of lumbar root compression. Br Med J 2:635, 1973
31. Breivik H, Hesla PE, Molnar I et al: Treatment of chronic low back pain and sciatica: comparison of caudal epidural steroid injections of bupivacaine and methylprednisolone with bupivacaine followed by saline. p. 927. In Bonica JJ, Albe-Fessard D (eds): Advances in Pain Research and Therapy. Vol. 1. Raven Press, New York, 1976
32. Harley C: Extradural corticosteroid infiltration. A follow-up study of 50 cases. Ann Phys Med 9:22, 1967
33. Bernat JL: Intraspinal steroid therapy. Neurology 31:168, 1981
34. Abram SE, Anderson RA: Using a pain questionnaire to predict response to steroid epidurals. Reg Anaesth 5:11, 1980
35. Warr AC, Wilkinson JA, Burn JMB et al: Chronic lumbosciatic syndrome treated by epidural injection and manipulation. Practitioner 209:53, 1972
36. Costabile G, Husag L, Probst C: Spinal epidural hematoma. Surg Neurol 21:489, 1984
37. Waldman SD: Cervical epidural abcess after cervical epidural nerve block with steroids. Anesth Analg 72:713, 1991
38. Waldman SD: Complications of cervical epidural nerve blocks with steroids: a prospective study of 790 consecutive blocks. Reg Anaesth 14:149, 1989
39. Miehlke K, Schulze G, Eger W: Klinsche Und Experimentelle Untersuchungen Zum Fibrositis-Syndrom. Z Rheumaforsch 19:310, 1960
40. Travell JG, Simons DG: Myofascial Pain and Dysfunction. Williams & Wilkins, Baltimore, 1983
41. Berges PV: Myofascial pain syndromes. Postgrad Med 53:161, 1953
42. Garvey TA, Marks MR, Wiesel SW: A prospective randomized double-blind evaluation of trigger-point injection therapy for low-back pain. Spine 14:962, 1991
43. Graff-Radford SB, Reeves JL, Baker RL et al: Effects of transcutaneous electrical nerve stimulation on myofascial pain and trigger point sensitivity. Pain 37:1, 1989
44. Marks R: Distribution of pain provoked from lumbar facet joints and related structures during diagnostic spinal infiltration. Pain 39:37, 1989
45. Goldstone JC, Pennant JH: Spinal anaesthesia following facet joint injection—a report of two cases. Anaesthesia 42:754, 1987
46. Carrera GF: Lumbar facet joint injection in low back pain and sciatica. Radiology 137:665, 1980
47. Bough B, Thakore J, Davies M et al: Degeneration of the lumbar facet joints, arthrography and pathology. J Bone Joint Surg 72(B):275, 1990

48. Lynch MC, Taylor JF: Facet joint injection for low back pain. J Bone Joint Surg 68(B):138, 1986
49. Lilius G, Laasone EM, Myllynen P et al: Lumbar facet joint syndrome: a randomized clinical trial. J Bone Joint Surg 71(B):681, 1989
50. Fisher AP, Hanna M: Transcutaneous electrical nerve stimulation in meralgia paraesthetica of pregnancy. Br J Obstet Gynaecol 94:603, 1987
51. Parsonnet V, Karasakalides A, Gielchinsky I et al: Meralgia paresthetica after coronary bypass surgery. J Thorac Cardiovasc Surg 101:219, 1991
52. Garcia-Alba E, Plomo F, Tejeiro J et al: Occupational meralgia paraesthetica. J Neurol Neurosurg Psychiatry 53:708, 1990
53. Suarez G, Sabin TD: Meralgia paresthetica and hypothyroidism. Ann Intern Med 112:149, 1990
54. Williams PH, Trzil KP: Management of meralgia paresthetica. J Neurosurg 74:76, 1991
55. MacNicol MF, Thompson WJ: Idiopathic meralgia paresthetica. Clin Orthop 254:270, 1990
56. Sunderland S: Nerves and Nerve Injuries. Churchill Livingstone, Edinburgh, 1978
57. Krebs B, Jensen TS, Kroner J et al: Phantom limb phenomena in amputees seven years after limb amputation. Pain (suppl 2):S85, 1948
58. Melzack R: Phantom limb pain. Anesthesiology 35:409, 1971
59. Sherman RA, Sherman CJ: Prevalence and characteristics of chronic phantom limb pain among American veterans. Am J Phys Med 62:227, 1983
60. Melzack R, Loeser JD: Phantom body pain in paraplegics: evidence for central pattern generating mechanism for pain. Pain 4:195, 1978
61. Bach S, Norang MF, Tjellden NU: Phantom limb pain in amputees during the first twelve months following limb amputation, after preoperative lumbar epidural blockade. Pain 33:297, 1988
62. Murphy TM: Chronic pain. p. 1931. In Miller R (ed): Anesthesia. 3rd Ed. Churchill Livingstone, New York, 1990
63. Schmidt SI, Moorthy SS, Dierdorf SF et al: Current therapy for herpes zoster and postherpetic neuralgia. Anesthesiol Rev 18:35, 1991
64. Burgoon CF Jr, Burgoon JS, Baldridge GA: The natural history of herpes zoster. JAMA 164:265, 1957
65. Loeser JD: Herpes zoster and postherpetic neuralgia. Pain 25:149, 1986
66. Petershund NA, Apsen J, Schonheyden H et al: Acyclovir in herpes zoster. Lancet 2:827, 1981
67. Post BT, Philbrick J: Do corticosteroids prevent postherpetic neuralgia? J Am Acad Dermatol 18:605, 1988
68. Colding A: The effect of regional sympathetic blocks in the treatment of herpes zoster. Acta Anaesth Scand 13:133, 1969
69. Jollup J: Treatment of shingles and post herpetic neuralgia. Br J Med 299:740, 1989
70. Stone PJ, Glynn CJ, Minor B: EMLA cream in the treatment of post-herpetic neuralgia. Efficacy and pharmacokenetic profile. Pain 39:301, 1989
71. Watson CPN, Evans RJ, Watt VR et al: Post-herpetic neuralgia: 208 cases. Pain 35:289, 1988
72. Demoragas JM, Kierland RR: The outcome of patients with herpes zoster. Arch Dermatol 75:193, 1957
73. Noordenbos W: Pain problems pertaining to transmission of nerve impulses which give rise to pain: preliminary statement. Elsevier Science Publications, Amsterdam, 1959

74. Physicians' Desk Reference. 46th Ed. Medical Economics Data, Medical Economics, Montvale, NJ, 1992
75. Milligan WS, Nash TP: Treatment of postherpetic neuralgia. A review of 77 consecutive cases. Pain 23:381, 1985
76. Brown DE, James DC, Roy S: Pain relief by suprascapular nerve block in glenohumeral arthritis. Scand J Rheumatol 17:411, 1988
77. Emery P, Bowman S, Wedderburn L et al: Suprascapular nerve block for chronic shoulder pain in rheumatoid arthritis. Br Med J 299:1079, 1989
78. Breen TW, Haigh JD: Continuous suprascapular nerve block for analgaesia of scapular fracture. Can J Anaesth 37:786, 1990
79. Tanelian DL, Brose WG: Neuropathic pain can be relieved by drugs that are use-dependent sodium channel blockers: lidocaine, carbamazepine and mexiletine. Anesthesiology 74:949, 1991
80. Tanelian DL, Cousin MJ: Combined neurogenic and nociceptive pain in a patient with Pancoast tumor managed by epidural hydromorphone and oral carbamazepine. Pain 36:85, 1989
81. Kastrup J, Petersen P, Dejgard A et al: Intravenous lidocaine infusion: a new treatment of chronic painful diabetic neuropathy? Pain 28:69, 1987
82. Bejgard A, Petersen P, Kastrup J: Mexiletine for treatment of chronic painful diabetic neuropathy. Lancet 2:9, 1988
83. Chabal C, Jacobson L, Mariano A et al: The use of oral mexiletine for the treatment of pain after peripheral nerve injury. Anesthesiology 76:513, 1992
84. American Psychiatric Association: Diagnostic and Statistical Manual of Mental Disorders: Revised (DSM-III-R). 3rd Ed. American Psychiatric Association, Washington, DC, 1987
85. Fishbain DA, Goldberg M, Rosomoff RS et al: Munchausen syndrome presenting with chronic pain: case report. Pain 35:91, 1988

Index

Page numbers followed by *f* represent figures; those followed by *t* represent tables.

A

Abdomen
  examination, in juvenile rheumatoid arthritis, 328
  postoperative considerations with, in trauma patient, 85
Abscess, epidural, after epidural steroid injection, 479–480
Acetabular fracture, 79
  repair, intrathecal/epidural narcotics for, 433–434
Acetaminophen, for postoperative pain relief, in children, 443
Acetylsalicylic acid therapy, 12, 15
Achondroplasia
  anesthetic considerations in, 312
  cervical spine in, 298
  clinical features of, 311
  spinal involvement in, 312
Acquired immune deficiency syndrome, transmission, prevention, 40
Acrocephalosyndactyly, 306
Acromegaly
  anesthetic considerations in, 23
  manifestations of, 22–23
  pathophysiology of, 22
Acyclovir, for herpes zoster, 492–493
Adriamycin. *See* Doxorubicin
Adult respiratory distress syndrome
  incidence of, with early fracture repair, 74, 74*f*
  pulmonary artery catheterization in, 58
  after reinfusion of shed blood, 129
Air embolism
  with general anesthesia in sitting position, 147

with lumbar disc surgery, 398
  in spinal surgery, 372–373
  in total hip replacement, 137
Airway
  assessment of
    in neurofibromatosis, 30
    preanesthetic, 270–271
    in rheumatoid arthritis patient, 12
  management. *See also* Cricothyrotomy
    in acromegaly, 22, 23
    in ankylosing spondylitis, 18
    in cerebral palsy, 323
    in cervical spine surgery, with transoral retropharyngeal approach, 390, 392
    in hemophilia A, 39
    in juvenile rheumatoid arthritis, 327–328
    in mucopolysaccharidoses, 325–327
    in osteogenesis imperfecta, 314
    in Parkinson's disease, 100
    in rheumatoid arthritis, 4–7
    in scleroderma, 26
    in systemic lupus erythematosus, 21
    in trauma patient, 46–51
  obstruction, postoperative, 85
  pressures, elevated, 51–52
Alcoholism, 28
Aldomet. *See* Methyldopa
Alfentanil
  administration, for ambulatory surgery, 281
  for tourniquet pain, 248
Algodystrophy, 451
Allodynia, definition of, 448
Ambulatory surgery, 269–292
  anesthesia for, induction and maintenance of, 281–282
  candidates

Ambulatory surgery *(Continued)*
  discussion of anesthetic management
    with, 272–273
  ECG, preanesthetic review of, 271
  laboratory tests for, 272
  medical evaluation of, 269
  physical examination of, 270–271
  preoperative anesthesia assessment for,
    269–273
  discharge criteria, 291
  hospital admission after, 289
  management of, 282–287. *See also specific*
    procedure
  medications for, 276–278
  nausea and vomiting after, prevention of,
    287–288
  patient
    assessment of, on day of surgery, 280
    characteristics of, 273
    diabetic, management of, 274
    discharge, 289–292
    discharge instruction for, 290–291
    early release of, 290
    elderly, 275
    information for, 275–276
    interventions by anesthesiologist for,
      275
    with multi-organ system disease, 275
    postoperative care of, 273–274
    postrelease assistance for, 291–292
    preoperative call to, by nurse, 278
    problems with, 274–275
    transfer from recovery bed to chair,
      288–289
    who has not undergone preoperative
      testing, 280
  postanesthesia recovery scoring system for,
    290
  premedication for, 276–278
  preoperative preparation for, 269–278
    surgeon's role in, 276
  procedures not suited to, 280
  procedures suited to, 278–280
  recovery room care after, 288–289
  recovery room stay after, reducing,
    287–288
American Society of Anesthesiologists, risk
    classification

and anesthetic technique for hip fracture
    repair, 104, 104*t*
  and hip fracture outcome, 92–93, 93*t*
Amitriptyline, for postherpetic neuralgia,
    494
Amputation
  lower extremity
    for bone tumors, 414
    for sarcoma, 412
  upper extremity
    for bone tumors, 414
    for sarcoma, 412
Amyloidosis, renal problems with, 4
Analgesia. *See also* Patient-controlled
    analgesia
  definition of, 448
  intermittent intravenous doses, 422–423
  therapeutic effectiveness, paradigm for,
    422, 422*f*
Analgesics. *See also specific agent*
  administration, in trauma patient, 55–56
  for herpes zoster, 493
  precautions with, in trauma patient, 56
Anaphylactoid/anaphylactic reactions, with
    dextran, 154–155
Anemia
  hypochromic microcytic
    in ankylosing spondylitis, 18
    in rheumatoid arthritis, 3
  in juvenile rheumatoid arthritis, 328
  secondary to gastrointestinal bleeding,
    evaluation for, 120
  in sickle cell disease, 31
  in systemic lupus erythematosus, 21
Ankle
  arthroscopy of, 287
  surgery
    in ankylosing spondylitis, 20
    special considerations with, 265
Ankle block, 15, 265
  for ambulatory surgery, transfer from
    recovery bed to chair after, 289
  anatomy for, 223–224, 224*f*
  cutaneous innervation, 202*f*
  indications for, 222–223
  landmarks for, 225, 225*f*, 226*f*
Ankylosing spondylitis, 16–20
  airway management in, 18

anesthetic considerations in, 17
cardiovascular involvement in, 17
cervical osteotomy in, 401–402
cervical spine in, 17
conduct of anesthesia in, 18–19
endotracheal intubation in, 18
epidemiology of, 16
intraoperative considerations with, 19–20
juvenile, 329–330
pathology of, 16–17
preoperative considerations in, 271
respiratory involvement in, 17–18
spinal surgery for, 399–400
and thoracic kyphosis
  flexible deformity, 400
  rigid deformity, 400
  thoracic osteotomy for, 400–401
  Zielke's technique for, 401
ventilation in, intraoperative, 19
Antacid(s), preoperative administration of, 277–278
Anterior cord syndrome, 67
Anterior femoral cutaneous nerve, dermatomal distribution of, 202f
Antibiotic(s), prophylactic, for total knee replacement, 143
Anticholinergics, preoperative administration of, 276–277
Anticoagulant(s)/anticoagulation
  and regional anesthesia, 156
  and reinfusion of shed blood, 129
Anticonvulsant therapy/antiepileptic medication
  lupus-like syndromes caused by, 22
  perioperative management of, 346
Antihypertensives
  contraindications to, 100
  perioperative management of, 118
Aortic insufficiency, in children, 330
Aortic valve calcification, in osteitis deformans, 24
Apert syndrome, 306
  clinical features of, 315
  treatment of, 316
Arachnodactyly. See Marfan syndrome
Arm(s). See also Upper extremity
  reimplantation of, 261

Arterial blood gases
  monitoring. See also Pulse oximetry
    postoperative, 85
    with neuromuscular scoliosis, preoperative determination of, 345
Arterial line(s)
  contraindications to, 122
  in total hip replacement, 122
Arterial puncture(s), contraindications to, in scleroderma, 27
Arteriography, with pelvic fracture, 77
Arteritis, in rheumatoid arthritis, 4
Arthritis. See also Rheumatoid arthritis
  cricoarytenoid, 5, 6–7, 17
Arthrogryposis, 309–311
  associated conditions, 310
  clinical features of, 310
  special considerations with, 348
  types of, 310
Arthropathy, hemophilic, 37
Arthroplasty, total hip. See Hip(s), total replacement
Arthroscopy
  anesthesia for, 276
  of ankle, 287
  of elbow, 283
  of hip, 284
  indications for, 279
  of knee, 284–287
  of shoulder, 282–283
l-Asparaginase, side effects of, 407t
Aspiration
  prevention of, 277–278
  risk of
    factors increasing, 277–278
    and hand surgery, 259
    in Parkinson's disease, 100–101
    in scleroderma, 27
    in trauma patient, 46, 47
Aspirin therapy. See also Acetylsalicylic acid therapy
  contraindications to, in children, 443
  perioperative management of, 119–120, 156
Asthma, versus cricoarytenoid arthritis, 7
Asthmatic patient
  SSEP monitoring in, 368, 369f–370f
  tourniquet release in, 253

Atlantoaxial dislocation, in neurofibromatosis, 30
Atlantoaxial instability, in osteogenesis
imperfecta, 313
Atlantoaxial subluxation
in juvenile rheumatoid arthritis, 327
in rheumatoid arthritis, 7–9, 8f, 10f
traumatic, 298–299
Atlas dens interval, 8–9, 10f, 298
in children, 298
Atracurium, administration, in trauma
patient, 63
Atropine
administration, during intubation of spinal
cord-injured patient, 69
cardiac effects, in spinal shock, 70, 70t
in local anesthetic toxicity, 165
Autologous predonation
contraindications to, 411
erythropoietin and, 127, 351
iron and, 127
for scoliosis surgery, 350–351
for total hip replacement, 127–128
Autonomic hyperreflexia
prevention of, 72
signs and symptoms of, 71
Autotransfusion
contraindications to, 53
in sickle cell disease, 35
for total hip replacement, 127–128
in trauma, 53
Axillary artery, injury, 79
Axillary nerve block. See Brachial plexus
block, axillary approach; Brachial
plexus block, infraclavicular
approach
Azathioprine, side effects of, 5t, 12, 407t
Azulfidine, side effects, 5t

B

Bamboo spine, 16
Barbiturate(s), administration, in trauma
patient, 61
Beach chair position, for shoulder
arthroscopy, 282–283
Becker's dystrophy, 318

Benzodiazepines, contraindications to, 353
β-Blocker therapy, in Marfan syndrome, 29–30
Bier block(s)
in lower extremity, 466–467
mini-dose, 238–239
monitoring for, 464
for reflex sympathetic dystrophy, 463–467
in upper extremity, 229f, 229–232,
464–466
Bilateral simultaneous procedures, approach
to, 259–260
Biopsy, in orthopedic oncology, 405
of bone tumor, 413
Bleeding. See also Blood loss; Hemorrhage
with epidural catheter, 438
in hemophilia B, treatment of, 39–40
Bleeding time, in juvenile rheumatoid arthritis, 329
Bleomycin, pulmonary toxicity of, 407t,
408–409
Blood. See also Transfusion therapy
autologous predonation. See Autologous
predonation
cross-matching, 53–54
in systemic lupus erythematosus, 22
intraoperative scavenging of, 352, 357
reinfusion, protocol for, 353
salvaged from wound drainage
contraindications to, 411
reinfusion, problems with, 129
in scoliosis surgery, 353
washed versus unwashed, 129
warming, 54
Blood glucose, preoperative testing of, 272
Blood loss
with biopsy and curettage of bone tumor,
413
control of, in spinal surgery, 357–358
during limb-sparing surgery, 416
monitoring
in bilateral total knee replacement, 146
after spinal surgery, 374
operative, in neuromuscular disease, 349
in total hip replacement, 126
estimation of, 130
and fluid replacement, 130
Blood pressure
arterial, monitoring, in trauma patient, 58

arterial, monitoring, in trauma patient, 58
elevation, with tourniquet use, 247–248
   in head-injured patient, 249, 249*f*
monitoring
   during hip fracture repair, 102
   with tourniquet use, 247–248
Blood salvage devices. *See also* Cell Saver
   contraindications to, in sickle cell disease,
      35
Blood urea nitrogen, preoperative testing of,
   272
Body temperature. *See also* Hypothermia
   effects of tourniquet use on, 250*f*, 250–251
   monitoring
      intraoperative, in children, 302
      in trauma patient, 59
   postoperative
      maintenance of, 141
      monitoring, after spinal surgery, 374
Bone(s)
   metastatic disease involving, management
      of, 418
   in osteitis deformans, 24
   in rheumatoid arthritis, 1
Bone graft(s)
   iliac, 263
      anesthesia for, 260
      postoperative analgesia at harvest site,
         440
   sources of, 262
Bone marrow embolization, with methyl-
      methacrylate cement, 133
Bone scan(s), in reflex sympathetic dystro-
      phy, 455
Bone tumor(s)
   definitive surgical procedures for, 413–414
   surgery for, 413–414
Brachial artery, injury, 79
Brachial plexus
   anatomy of, 174–177, 175*f*, 176*f*
   injury, with general anesthesia in sitting
      position, 146
Brachial plexus block
   anesthetic agent for, 179
      choice, 179
      dosage, 179
   approaches for, 63
   assessment of, 174

axillary approach, 14, 176*f*, 178, 189–192
   anatomy for, 189–190
   in children, 236
   drug for, 191
   equipment, 190–191
   indications for, 177*t*, 178*t*, 178, 189–190
   landmark for, 191, 192*f*
   patient positioning for, 191
   procedure, 191–193
   single versus multiple injections for,
      190
   stimulating current used for, 174*t*
continuous, 193–194
   equipment for, 193
   indications for, 193
   kits for, 193–194
   procedure, 193–194
for elbow arthroscopy, 283
and exercise, 179–180
factors affecting, 179–180
infraclavicular approach, 15, 176*f*,
      184–186
   anatomy for, 184
   drug for, 184
   equipment, 184
   indications for, 177*t*, 178*t*, 179, 189
   landmarks for, 184–185, 185*f*
   patient positioning for, 184
   procedure, 185–186
interscalene approach, 14–15, 176*f*,
      177–178, 180–183
   in children, 236
   drugs for, 181
   equipment, 181
   indications for, 63, 177*t*, 177, 178*t*, 189
   landmarks for, 181–182, 182*f*
   patient positioning for, 181
   in preparation for Bier block in upper
      extremity, 465
   procedure for, 182–183
   for shoulder arthroscopy, 283
   stimulating current used for, 174*t*
onset of
   factors affecting, 179–180
   patient management until, 174
   and pain, 179–180
for reimplantation of digits, 260
for reimplantation of forearm/arm, 261

Brachial plexus block *(Continued)*
  sensory only, 179
  subclavian perivascular approach, 176*f*,
      186–188
    anatomy for, 186
    drug for, 187
    equipment, 187
    indications for, 177*t*, 178*t*, 189
    landmarks for, 187, 188*f*
    patient positioning for, 187
    problems with, 188
    procedure, 187–188
  supraclavicular approach, 179
  for upper extremity surgery, in short
      (1-hour) procedures, 284
Bradycardia, with spinal cord injury, 70
Bretylium, regional sympathetic blockade
    using, 463–464, 466
Brown-Sequard syndrome, 67
Bupivacaine
  for brachial plexus block, 179
  continuous epidural blockade with, for
      reflex sympathetic dystrophy,
      467–468
  dosage and administration, 166*t*
  epidural, for postoperative pain manage-
      ment, 435–436
  hyperbaric, for tourniquet pain, 248
  indications for, 167
  intra-articular, after knee surgery, 439
  isobaric, for spinal anesthesia, 105, 106, 125
  pharmacology of, 166*t*
  toxicity, management of, 165
  wound infiltration with, for postoperative
      analgesia, 440
Buprenorphine, epidural
  characteristics of, 433
  dosage and administration, 433
Busulfan, side effects of, 407*t*
Butterfly rash, in systemic lupus erythema-
    tosus, 20
Butyrophenone derivative(s), contraindica-
    tions to, 100

C

Café au lait spots, 30

Caplan syndrome, 3
Capsaicin ointment, for postherpetic neural-
    gia, 494
Captopril, administration, in preparation for
    hypotensive anesthesia, 354
Carbamazepine
  for neuropathic pain, 500
  for postherpetic neuralgia, 494
Carbon dioxide, end-tidal
  monitoring, in total hip replacement, 122
  after tourniquet release, 251–252, 252*t*
Cardiac risk, assessment of, 98–99, 99*t*
Cardiomyopathy
  in acromegaly, 22, 23
  in muscular dystrophy, 320
Cardiovascular system. *See also* Heart
  in acromegaly, 22, 23
  in juvenile rheumatoid arthritis, 328
  in Marfan syndrome, 29
  in neuromuscular disease, 345
  preoperative management, in hip fracture
      patient, 98–99
Carmustine, side effects of, 407*t*
Carpenter syndrome, 306, 316
Cast syndrome, after spinal surgery, 375
Catheter(s)
  epidural
    bleeding with, 438
    infection with, 438
    migration of, 438
  in nerve sheath, for postoperative pain
      relief, 440
  in wound, infiltration with local anesthetics,
      for postoperative analgesia, 440
Cauda equina syndrome, in ankylosing
    spondylitis, 18
Caudal anesthesia, in infants and children,
    238
Causalgia, 449, 451–452
  case report of, 469
Cell Saver, 16
  contraindications to, 411
    in sickle cell disease, 35
  use of
    in bilateral total knee replacement, 146
    problems with, 128
    in scoliosis surgery, 352
    in spinal surgery, 357

in total hip replacement, 128
Central cord syndrome, 67
Central nervous system, in systemic lupus
    erythematosus, 21
Central pain, 491
    definition of, 448
Central venous lines, indications for, 122
Central venous pressure, monitoring
    during hip fracture repair, 102–103
    in trauma patient, 58
Cerebral blood pressure measurement, dur-
    ing general anesthesia in sitting
    position, 147
Cerebral palsy
    anesthetic considerations in, 323
    clinical features of, 322
    scoliosis in, 347
    selective posterior rhizotomy in, 323–324
    spasticity in, 323–324
    surgical procedures in, 323
Cerebral thrombosis, in sickle cell disease, 31
Cervical plexus, 180
Cervical plexus block. *See also* Brachial
    plexus block, interscalene approach
    for shoulder arthroscopy, 283
Cervical spine. *See also under* Atlantoaxial
    in achondroplasia, 298, 312
    in ankylosing spondylitis, 17, 401–402
    disc herniation, operative repair of,
    383–384
    evaluation of, 9–10
    flexion deformity, in ankylosing spondylitis,
        surgical correction of, 20
    fracture. *See also* Cervical spine, injury
    in osteogenesis imperfecta, 314
    fusion, posterior, in pediatric patient, 300
    in Hurler syndrome, 325
    injury. *See also* Spinal cord, injury
        associated injuries and problems, 67
        in children, 298–299
        intubation with, 46, 69
        pulmonary edema after, 65, 70
        respiratory problems with, 68
    in juvenile rheumatoid arthritis, 300, 327
    myelopathy, decompressive surgery for,
        389
    in neurofibromatosis, 30
    normal anatomy of, 66*f*

osteotomy
    in ankylosing spondylitis, 401–402
    awake technique, 401–402
    general anesthesia for, 402
    problems, in children, 296–300
    protection/precautions with, in trauma
        patient, 46–48, 64–65, 68
    radiculopathy, treatment of, 478–480
    radiography
        in rheumatoid arthritis, 12
        in trauma patient, 65, 66*f*
    in rheumatoid arthritis, 5, 7–11
        surgery for, 16
    surgery
        anterior approach, 382
        for cervical spondylosis, 384–388
        for decompression of myelopathy, 389
        for herniated cervical disc, 383–384
        retropharyngeal approach, 392–393
        transoral retropharyngeal approach,
            390–392
    in trisomy 21, 299
Cervical spondylosis (chronic disc degenera-
        tion)
    associated conditions with, 384–385
    clinical features of, 385
    operative repair of, 384–388
        anterior approach for, 386–387
        patient positioning for, 386–388
        posterior approach for, 387–388
        surgical procedures for, 386
Champion Trauma Score, 44, 45*t*
Charcot-Marie-Tooth disease, special consid-
        erations in, 347
Chemonucleolysis, with chymopapain,
        402–403
Chemotherapy, 405–411
    cardiotoxicity of, 406–408, 407*t*
    hematologic effects of, 410
    hepatotoxicity of, 407*f*, 410
    nephrotoxicity of, 407*t*, 409–410
    neurotoxicity of, 407*t*, 410
    pulmonary toxicity of, 407*t*, 408–409
    side effects of, 406, 407*t*
        relevant to anesthesiology, 406–410
Chest
    assessment of, preanesthetic, 271
    postoperative considerations with, in

trauma patient, 85
Chest radiograph(s)
in juvenile rheumatoid arthritis, 328
postoperative, in trauma patient, 85
preoperative, 272
Chest tube(s), removal, pneumothorax developing after, 60–61
Chest wall, in rheumatoid arthritis, 3
Chewing gum, effect on gastric volume, 278
Child(ren)
achondroplasia in, 311–312
ambulatory surgery patients, postoperative care of, 274
anesthetic induction and maintenance in, 301–302
aortic insufficiency in, 330
arthrogryposis in, 309–311
atlantoaxial subluxation in
in juvenile rheumatoid arthritis, 327
traumatic, 298–299
body temperature
effects of tourniquet use on, 250f, 250–251
intraoperative monitoring of, 302
caudal anesthesia in, 238
with cerebral palsy, 322–324
cervical spine problems in, 296–300
radiographic evaluation of, anesthetic management during, 299
club foot in, 300–303
surgery for, 300–303
congenital constrictive bands in, 307
congenital high scapula in, 295–296
congenital pseudarthrosis of tibia in, 305–306
coxa vara in, 304
craniofacial abnormalities in, 306–307, 315–318
cricoarytenoid arthritis in, 327–329
developmental dislocation of hip in, 303–304
doxorubicin cardiotoxicity in, 408
intravenous access in, securing, 301
intravenous lines for, starting, 301–302
intravenous regional anesthesia for, 239
juvenile ankylosing spondylitis in, 329–330

juvenile rheumatoid arthritis in, 327–329
limb abnormalities in, associated problems with, 307–308
lower extremity problems in, 300–306
malignant hyperthermia in. See Malignant hyperthermia
mucopolysaccharidoses in, 324–327
muscular dystrophy in, 318–322
myelodysplasia in, and allergy and anaphylactic reactions to latex, 308–309
neck problems in, 293–295
osteogenesis imperfecta in, 312–315
patient-controlled analgesia in, 444
posterior cervical spine fusion in, anesthetic management for, 300
postoperative pain relief for, 302, 442–445
preparation for surgery, 442–443
reflex sympathetic dystrophy in, 468–469
regional anesthesia for, 234–239
scoliosis in. See Scoliosis
slipped capital femoral epiphysis in, 305
supracondylar humeral fracture in, 261, 307
surgical patient
monitoring for, 301
parents accompanying, 301–302
with runny nose, 301
syndactyly in, 306
upper extremity problems in, 306–308
Chlorambucil, side effects of, 407t
Chloroprocaine
dosage and administration, 166t, 167
pharmacology of, 166t, 167
Christmas disease, 39–40
Chymopapain, chemonucleolysis with, 402–403
Cimetidine, preoperative administration of, 276, 278
Circulation, in trauma patient, 52–53
Circulatory hemodynamics, in scleroderma, 27
Cis-platinum, nephrotoxicity of, 407t, 409–410
Club foot
acquired, 300
congenital, 300–303
Coagulopathy
dilutional, 55
with limb-sparing surgery, 417

in systemic lupus erythematosus, 21–22

Coma, with fat embolism, 83

Common peroneal nerve
anatomy of, 220
dermatomal distribution of, 202*f*

Common peroneal nerve block, at knee,
220–221, 222*f*
drug for, 221
equipment, 221
patient positioning for, 221
procedure, 221, 222*f*

Comorbidity, and postoperative mortality in
surgical patient, 93–94

Compartment pressure, measurement of, 81

Compartment syndrome, 80–81

Complement activation, with reinfusion of
shed blood, 129–130

Compression boots, intermittent pneumatic,
152
with spinal surgery, 158

Compression stockings, graduated, 152
with spinal surgery, 158

Congestive heart failure, and spinal anesthesia, in hip fracture patient, 102–103
postanesthesia care for, 110

Constrictive bands, congenital, 307

Continuous passive motion machine, intra-
thecal/epidural narcotics with, 434

Contrast agent(s), for myelography, adverse
reactions to, 379–380

Convulsions, in local anesthetic toxicity, 163,
165

Corticosteroids. *See also* Steroids
for reflex sympathetic dystrophy, 468
for spinal cord injury, 65–66

Coxa vara, 304

Craniofacial abnormalities, in children,
306–307, 315–318
airway management with, 317
anesthetic considerations with, 317
intraoperative monitoring with, 317

Craniosynostosis, 315–316

Creatine kinase, in malignant hyperthermia,
331, 335

Creatinine, preoperative testing of, 272

Cricoarytenoid arthritis, 5–7, 17
in children, 327–329

Cricoid pressure, in trauma patient, 47

Cricothyrotomy, 48–49, 50*f*

Crouzon syndrome, 306, 316

Cryoprecipitate administration, in hemophilia
A, 38

Crystalloid infusion, in trauma, 53

Cyclophosphamide, side effects of, 5*t*, 407*t*

Cytosine arabinoside, side effects of, 407*t*

D

Dantrolene administration, in malignant
hyperthermia, 333*t*, 333–334

Daunorubicin, cardiotoxicity of, 406, 407*t*

Deafness, in osteitis deformans, 25

Deep peroneal nerve
anatomy of, 223–224, 224*f*
block, 225, 225*f*
dermatomal distribution of, 202*f*

Deep vein thrombosis
incidence of, 151
prevention of, 151–156
risk factors for, 151–152
signs and symptoms of, 156–157

Degenerative joint disease, total hip replacement for, 117–118

Dehydration, in hip fracture patient, 101, 102

Dementia, in hip fracture patient, preoperative
evaluation of, 100

Demerol. *See* Meperidine

Dens, ligamentous anatomy of, 7, 9*f*

Desflurane, administration, for ambulatory
surgery, 282

Desmopressin acetate, administration, in
hemophilia A, 38

Dextran
anaphylactoid/anaphylactic reactions with,
154–155
for prevention of venous thromboembolism,
153–155
renal toxicity of, 155

Diabetes mellitus
and hip fracture outcome, 93
perioperative management of, 97–98, 118,
120

Diaphragmatic breathing, in ankylosing spondylitis, 17–18

Diazepam, for convulsions, in local anesthetic

toxicity, 165
Digit(s), reimplantation of, 260
Digital nerve block, 199–201, 200f
Dilantin, for postherpetic neuralgia, 494
Dislocation(s), management of, 75–76
Diuresis, in trauma patient, 55, 59
Doxorubicin, cardiotoxicity of, 406–408, 407t
    in children, 408
Droperidol
    antiemetic effects of, 287–288
    contraindications to, 100
    side effects, 288
Drug(s), lupus-like syndromes caused by, 22
Duchenne's muscular dystrophy, 319
    cardiovascular abnormalities in, 345–346
    and malignant hyperthermia, 319, 321, 322
    postanesthetic considerations in, 322
    special considerations in, 348
    succinylcholine contraindicated in, 321
    vital capacity in, preoperative determina-
        tion of, 345–346
Dysesthesia, definition of, 448

E

Edema, postoperative, with tourniquet use, 245
Elbow
    arthroscopy of, 283
    fracture, nerve injury with, 261
    innervation of, 183
    nerve blocks at, 194–197
        anatomy for, 194
        drug for, 194
        landmarks for, 194–195
        regional anesthesia for, 178t, 183–188
    surgery, ambulatory procedures, 280
Elderly patient
    ambulatory surgery for, 275
    autologous predonation, for total hip
        replacement, 128
    cardiac status of
        in PACU, 112
        preoperative evaluation of, 119
    comorbidity in, 117–118
    extubation of, 108–109
    general anesthesia for, 107–108
    hematologic status of, preoperative evalua-

tion of, 119
    hip fracture in. See Hip fracture
    hypothermia in, in PACU, 111
    intravascular volume status, in PACU, 112
    metabolic status of, in PACU, 110
    neurologic status of, preoperative evalua-
        tion of, 119
    neurovascular status of, in PACU, 111
    with organic mental syndrome, manage-
        ment of, 109–110
    orientation (mental status), in PACU, 113
    perioperative problems in, 117
    postoperative pain management for,
        112–113
    preoperative management, 97–101
    pulmonary status of
        in PACU, 111
        preoperative evaluation of, 119
    renal status of, preoperative evaluation of,
        119
    respiratory therapy for, in PACU, 111
    shivering in, in PACU, 111
    special considerations with, 91, 117–118
        in postanesthesia care, 110–113
Electrocardiography
    intraoperative, during hip fracture repair,
        102
    in muscular dystrophy, 320
    preoperative, 272
        preanesthetic review of, 271
    in total hip replacement, 122
Electrolytes, in hip fracture patient, 101
Embolization, in pelvic trauma, 78
EMLA cream, for postherpetic neuralgia,
    494
Endocarditis, in systemic lupus erythematosus,
    20, 21
Endotracheal intubation
    in acromegaly, 23
    in ankylosing spondylitis, 18
    fiberoptic
        in rheumatoid arthritis, 13–14
        in scleroderma, 26
        in trauma patient, 48
    and halo traction, 298–300
    in Hurler syndrome, 325
    in Marfan syndrome, 29
    with pelvic trauma, 77

retrograde wire technique, 51
  in rheumatoid arthritis, 13–14
Ephedrine, in local anesthetic toxicity, 165
Epidural anesthesia
  in acromegaly, 23
  for ambulatory surgery, transfer from
    recovery bed to chair after, 289
  contraindications to, 63
  patient information about, 275–276
  total joint replacement, 125
Epidural blockade, continuous, for reflex
    sympathetic dystrophy, 467–468
Epinephrine
  added to local anesthetic, 167–168
    contraindications to, 168
    method for adding, 167–168
    optimal dose, 167
  contraindications to, in scleroderma, 28
  in local anesthetic toxicity, 165
Epsilon-aminocaproic acid, administration, in
    hemophilia A, 39
Erythropoietin, and autologous predonation,
    127, 351
Esmarch's bandage, for upper extremity
    exsanguination, 228–229
Esophagus, in scleroderma, 26–27
Ethylene oxide, allergy to, 309
Etidocaine
  for brachial plexus block, 179
  dosage and administration, 166t
  indications for, 167
  pharmacology of, 166t
Evoked potentials. See Neurogenic motor
    evoked potentials; Somatosensory
    evoked potentials
Exchange transfusion, in sickle cell disease,
    32, 32t, 35
Extremity(ies). See also Lower extremity;
    Upper extremity
  disarticulation, anesthetic management for,
    414–418
  nerve blocks in, in children, 235–237
  trauma
    compartment syndrome with, 80–81
    nerve injury in, 81
Extubation
  of elderly patient, 108–109
  renarcotization after, 108–109
  in rheumatoid arthritis, 14
  in sickle cell disease, 36
  after spinal surgery, 374

F

Facioscapulohumeral dystrophy, 318
Factitious pain, 500
Factor VIII
  antibody to, 39
  deficiency. See Hemophilia A
  therapy with, 38
Factor IX deficiency, 39–40
Factor XI deficiency, 40
Fanconi syndrome, 308
Fasciotomy, for compartment syndrome, 81
Fat embolism syndrome, 81–84
  in general circulation, 82
  with methylmethacrylate cement, 133
  pathophysiology of, 82
  prevention of, 83–84
  signs and symptoms of, 82–83
  in total hip replacement, 137
  treatment of, 83–84
Felty syndrome, risk of infection in, 4
Femoral cutaneous nerve(s). See Anterior
    femoral cutaneous nerve; Lateral
    femoral cutaneous nerve; Posterior
    femoral cutaneous nerve
Femoral head, aseptic necrosis, causes of, 116
Femoral neck fracture(s), 94f, 94–95
Femoral nerve, anatomy of, 202
Femoral nerve block, 64, 203–205. See also
    Inguinal paravascular block
  in children, 236–237
  drug for, 203
  equipment, 203
  indications for, 201
  landmarks for, 203
  for postoperative analgesia, after knee
    surgery, 439–440
  procedure, 204f, 204–205
Femoral-sciatic nerve block, 64
Femoral shaft fracture(s)
  regional anesthesia for, 64
  special considerations with, 266

Femur *(Continued)*
    derotational osteotomy of, with develop-
        mental dislocation of hip, 304
Fentanyl
    administration
        for spinal surgery, 354–355
        in trauma patient, 62
    in continuous epidural blockade, for reflex
        sympathetic dystrophy, 468
    epidural
        characteristics of, 432
        dosage and administration, 432
        infusions, 434–436
        for tourniquet pain, 248, 434
    in patient-controlled analgesia, total hourly
        dose for, 425
    transdermal administration, for post-
        operative pain relief, 440–441
Fever, in malignant hyperthermia, 331
Fibula, fracture, 265
Fluid overload, postoperative, 106, 140–141
Fluid resuscitation
    rapid infusion systems for, 52
    in spinal shock, 70
    in trauma, 52–53
5-Fluorouracil, side effects of, 407t
Foley catheter(s), use of, 122–123
Folic acid, therapy, in sickle cell disease, 33
Foot, surgery
    ambulatory procedures, 280
    in rheumatoid arthritis, 15
    special considerations with, 265, 287
Foot drop, postoperative, causes of, 136
Forearm
    innervation of, 189
    regional anesthesia for, 178t, 189
    reimplantation of, 261
Fracture(s)
    acetabular, 79
        repair, intrathecal/epidural narcotics for,
        433–434
    associated conditions, 261
    closed, management of, 75
    closed reduction, special considerations
        with, 262
    combined tibial and femoral, 266
    compartment syndrome with, 80–81
    elbow, nerve injury with, 81

fat embolism with, 82–84
femoral neck, 94f, 94–95
femoral shaft
    regional anesthesia for, 64
    special considerations with, 266
fibular, 265
in hemophilia A, 37
hip. *See* Hip fracture
humeral
    midshaft, nerve injury with, 261
    nerve injury with, 81
    supracondylar, in children, 261, 307
long bone, management of, 75
open
    management of, 75
    surgery for, special considerations with,
        262
open book, 77–78
open reduction and internal fixation,
        special considerations with, 262
pelvic. *See* Pelvic fracture(s)
pubic rami, 78
repair, early, 73–74
sacroiliac complex, 78
straddle, 78
subtrochanteric, 94f, 94–95
surgery for
    anesthetic considerations, 263
    general anesthesia for, 263
    regional anesthesia for, 263
    types of, 262
tibial, repair, special considerations with,
        265–266
vascular injury with, 79
Fresh frozen plasma, administration, in hemo-
        philia A, 38
Friedreich's ataxia
    cardiovascular abnormalities in, 346
    special considerations in, 347
    vital capacity in, preoperative determina-
        tion of, 345

G

Gastric volume
    effect of chewing gum on, 278
    preoperative reduction of, 276

Gastrointestinal system
  in muscular dystrophy, 320
  in neuromuscular disease, 346
  in systemic lupus erythematosus, 21
General anesthesia
  in acromegaly, 23
  administration, in geriatric patient, 107–108
  for ambulatory surgery, transfer from
      recovery bed to chair after, 288
  with induced hypotension, 16
  patient information about, 275
  positioning with, 108
  for shoulder arthroscopy, 283
  total joint replacement, 125–126
Glucose solution(s), contraindications to, 66
Glycopyrrolate, premedication, for spinal
    surgery, 353
Gold therapy, side effects, 5t
Gowers sign, 319
Greater occipital nerve, anatomy of, 489
Greater occipital nerve block, 490
Greater occipital neuralgia, 489–490
Grisel syndrome, 297
Guanethidine, regional sympathetic blockade
    using, 463

H

Haloperidol, contraindications to, 100
Halo traction, and endotracheal intubation,
    298–300
Hand
  regional anesthesia for, 178t, 189–199
    and infection, 257
    special considerations in, 257–258
    and tumor, 258
  surgery
    ambulatory procedures, 279
    patient positioning for, 258
    quick cases, 259
    in rheumatoid arthritis, 14–15
    special considerations in, 257–260
    table for, 258
    tourniquet use for, 259
H$_2$ antagonists, preoperative administration
    of, 277–278
Headache

after cervical epidural steroid injection, 480
  with epidural steroid injection, 478
  history of, in surgical candidate, 270
  after myelography, 379–381
  postdural puncture, patient information
      about, 276
  post-dural puncture, 380–381
Head injury
  and airway management, 46–47
  and tourniquet use, 249, 249f
  and ventilation, 51–52
Heart
  in acromegaly, 22, 23
  in ankylosing spondylitis, 17
  assessment of, preanesthetic, 271
  in Carpenter syndrome, 316
  and chemotherapy, 406–408, 407t
  function, with scoliosis, 343
  in Hurler syndrome, 325
  in Marfan syndrome, 29
  in myotonic dystrophy, 346
  postoperative considerations with, in
      trauma patient, 85
  in rheumatoid arthritis, 2
  in scleroderma, 26
  in sickle cell disease, 31
  in systemic lupus erythematosus, 20–21
Heart failure
  high-output, in osteitis deformans, 24
  intraoperative, in Duchenne's dystrophy, 322
Hematocrit
  in hip fracture patient, 101
  preoperative testing of, 272
Hematologic disease
  in rheumatoid arthritis, 3
  in systemic lupus erythematosus, 21
Hematoma(s), epidural, with epidural steroid
    injection, 478
Hemidiaphragmatic paralysis, with inter-
    scalene brachial plexus block, 183
Hemipelvectomy
  anesthetic management for, 414–418
  extended, for sarcoma, 412
  for sarcoma, 412
Hemodilution, intraoperative isovolemic,
    351–352
Hemodynamic instability, with fat embolism,
    82–84

Hemoglobin, in hip fracture patient, 101
Hemoglobin C, 31, 33
Hemoglobin S, 31, 36
  levels, lowering, 32–33
Hemoglobinuria, in trauma patient, 59
Hemolytic transfusion reaction(s), 54
Hemophilia
  classification of, 36–37
  universal precautions in, 40
Hemophilia A, 36–39
  airway management in, 39
  factor VIII therapy in, 38
  surgical management, 37–38
Hemophilia B, 39–40
  bleeding in, treatment of, 39–40
Hemophilia C, 40
Hemorrhage
  occult, in total hip replacement, 137, 142
  with pelvic fracture
    initial management of, 76–77
    management of, 77–78
Heparin, low-molecular-weight, for preven-
    tion of venous thromboembolism,
    153, 155
Heparinization
  during fracture repair, 80
  for prevention of venous thromboem-
    bolism, 152
Hepatitis, transmission, prevention, 40
Herpes zoster, 492–493
  associated conditions, 492
  distribution of, 492
  treatment of, 492–493
Hip(s)
  arthroscopy of, 284
  congenital dislocation, repair, sciatic nerve
    injury in, 135–136
  developmental dislocation of, 303–304
  dislocation, nerve injury with, 81
  in osteitis deformans, 25
  revision surgery, 138–140
    anesthetic management for, 139–140
    general anesthesia for, 139–140
    monitoring in, 140
    positioning for, 140
    sciatic nerve injury in, 136
    spinal anesthesia for, 139
    after total joint replacement, 138–139

surgery. *See also* Hip(s), revision surgery;
    Hip(s), total replacement; Hip frac-
    ture, surgical repair
  ambulatory procedures, 280
  deep vein thrombosis after, 151
  postoperative pain control with, 142
  postoperative problems with, 140–142
  prevention of venous thromboembolism
    in, 152–156
  pulmonary complications after, 142
  regional anesthesia for, 201
  sciatic nerve injury in, 135–136, 141
  vascular complications of, 141–142
total replacement, 115–137
  anesthetic management for, 119–120
  autologous predonation for, 127–128
  bilateral, 137–138
  blood loss during, 126, 130
  Cell Saver in, 128
  choice of anesthesia for, 124–126
  conditions leading to, 115–116
  conduct of anesthesia in 15, 18–19, 34
  epidural anesthesia for, 125
  epidural fentanyl infusions after, 435
  equipment for, 122–123
  fluid replacement in, 130
  general anesthesia for, 125–126
  homologous transfusion in, avoiding,
    127, 130
  with induced hypotension, 126
  induction of anesthesia for, 124–126
  intraoperative blood pressure control in,
    126–130
  intrathecal/epidural narcotics for,
    433–434
  medication history for, 119–120
  monitoring during, 122–123
  operating room for, 120–121
  operation for, 123–124
  for osteoarthritis, 117–118
  patient evaluation for, 117–119
  perioperative problems with, 118
  positioning for, 123
  postoperative blood salvage with, from
    wound drains, 129–130
  prevention of venous thromboembolism
    in, 152–156
  regional anesthesia for, 124–125

revision surgery after, 138–139
spinal anesthesia for, 125
sudden hypotension during, 136–137
Hip fracture, 91–114
American Society of Anesthesiologists risk status with
and anesthetic technique for repair, 104, 104*t*
and outcome, 92–93, 93*t*
anatomy of, 94*f*, 94–95
comorbidity with, 92–94, 93*t*
and anesthetic technique for repair, 104
as emergency, 95–96
epidemiology of, 91
extracapsular, 94*f*, 94–95
geriatric
preoperative management, 97–101
special considerations with, 91
intertrochanteric, 94*f*, 94–95
repair, 108
intracapsular, 94*f*, 94–95
repair, 108
mortality with, 92–94, 93*t*
and anesthetic technique, 104*t*, 104–105
outcome
and age, 93*t*
and diabetes, 93
effect of comorbidity, 92–94, 93*t*
risk factors for, 91–92
surgical repair
anesthetic technique for, 103–108, 105*t*
blood loss during, 109
evaluation of patient for, 97–101
fatal pulmonary embolism with, 151
fracture table for, 108
general anesthesia for, 104, 104*t*, 105*t*, 107–108
intrathecal/epidural narcotics for, 433–434
methylmethacrylate cement in, 109
monitoring during, 102–103
oxygen administration during, 109
positioning for, 108
postanesthesia care, 110–113
preoperative considerations with, 95–101
preoperative laboratory determinations for, 101
regional anesthesia for, 104, 104*t*, 105*t*, 105–107

special considerations with, 264–265
spinal anesthesia for, 105–107
Hip spica, application of, with developmental dislocation of hip, 303
HLA B-27, and ankylosing spondylitis, 16
Holt-Oram syndrome, 307
Horner syndrome, 63
with stellate ganglion block, 459, 460
Humerus, fracture
midshaft, nerve injury with, 261
supracondylar, in children, 261, 307
Hydralazine, lupus-like syndromes caused by, 22
Hydration
in sickle cell disease, 33–34
of trauma patient, 55
Hydromorphone, in patient-controlled analgesia, total hourly dose for, 425
Hydroxyzine, premedication, for spinal surgery, 353
Hyperalgesia, definition of, 448
Hypercarbia, and sickle cell disease, 34
Hyperesthesia, definition of, 449
Hyperkalemia
in Duchenne's dystrophy, 319
intraoperative, in Duchenne's dystrophy, 322
Hyperpathia, definition of, 449
Hypertension
in neurofibromatosis, 30
perioperative management of, 118
and postoperative mortality in surgical patient, 93
preoperative management, in hip fracture patient, 97
in scleroderma, 27
Hyperviscosity syndrome, in rheumatoid arthritis, 3
Hypnotics, preoperative administration of, 277
Hypokalemia, in hip fracture patient, 101
Hyponatremia, in hip fracture patient, 101
Hypotension. *See also* Vasodilators
with general anesthesia in sitting position, 147
induced. *See also* Hypotensive anesthesia
general anesthesia with, 16
in spinal surgery, 357–358
for total hip replacement, 126

Hypotension *(Continued)*
  intraoperative, with methylmethacrylate
    cement, 132
  and sickle cell disease, 34
  sudden, in total hip replacement, 136–137
Hypotensive anesthesia. *See also* Vasodilators
  management of, 382
  in spinal surgery, 354–355, 358–359
Hypothermia
  in elderly patient, in PACU, 111
  prevention of
    in spinal surgery, 354
    in trauma patient, 59
  and sickle cell disease, 34
Hypovolemia, and sickle cell disease, 34
Hypoxemia, intraoperative, with methyl-
    methacrylate cement, 132
Hypoxia
  with fat embolism, 82–84
  and sickle cell disease, 34

I

Ileus, after spinal surgery, 375
Iliac crest bone graft(s), 263
  anesthesia for, 260
  postoperative analgesia at harvest site, 440
Ilioinguinal nerve, dermatomal distribution
    of, 202*f*
Immunologic alterations, in rheumatoid
    arthritis, 3
Indomethacin, for postoperative pain relief,
    442
Induction of anesthesia
  for ambulatory surgery, 281–282
  in children, 301–302
  for spinal surgery, 354–355
  for total hip replacement, 124–126
  in trauma patient, 61–62
Infant(s)
  caudal anesthesia in, 238
  postoperative pain relief for, 443
  spinal anesthesia in, 237–238
Infection(s)
  after cervical epidural steroid injection, 480
  as contraindication to tourniquet use, 254
  of epidural catheter, 438

  risk of
    in rheumatoid arthritis, 3–4
    in sickle cell disease, 31, 33
Infection control
  anesthesiologist's role in, 120
  in operating room, 120–121
  ultraviolet light in, 121
Inguinal paravascular block, 209–210
  landmarks for, 209
  procedure, 209*f*, 209–210
Inhalation agent(s)
  administration, in geriatric patient, 107
  in Marfan syndrome, 29
Intercostal nerve block, for postherpetic
    neuralgia, 495
Intercostobrachial nerve block, 193. *See also*
    Brachial plexus block, infraclavicular
    approach
Intervertebral disc(s), herniation, 472–474
  acute, management of, 477
  cervical spine surgery for, 383–384
  nerve root compression by, physiology of,
    473
  nonsurgical approaches to, 473–474
  saline injections for, 473
  site of involvement, 473
  steroid therapy for, 473–476
  surgery for, 473
Intracranial pressure, effects of tourniquet use
    on, 249, 249*f*
Intravenous access
  in arthrogryposis, 311
  preanesthetic assessment of, 271
  in trauma patient, 52
Intubation. *See also* Endotracheal intubation;
    Nasotracheal intubation
  in arthrogryposis, 311
  and cervical spine injury, 46, 69
  in trauma, 46
    with awake patient, 46
    and full stomach, 47
    with unconscious patient, 47
Iridocyclitis, in juvenile rheumatoid arthritis,
    327
Iron, and autologous predonation, 127
Isoflurane, administration, in geriatric patient,
    107–108
Itching. *See* Pruritus

J

Joint(s). *See also specific joint*
    in osteitis deformans, 25
    surgery, in ankylosing spondylitis, intraoperative considerations, 19
    in systemic lupus erythematosus, 20
    total replacement, 115–149
        operating room for, 120–121
        patient evaluation for, 117–119

K

Ketamine
    contraindications to, 62
    for pediatric patient, during radiographic evaluation of cervical spine injury, 299
    for trauma patient, 62
Ketorolac
    for analgesia, 441–442
    side effects of, 441
Kidney(s). *See* Renal failure; Renal function
Klippel-Feil syndrome, 294–295, 343
Knee(s)
    arthroscopy of, 284–287
        choice of anesthesia for, 285
        infusion pump for, 286
        lateral releases, special observation after, 286
        local anesthesia with sedation for, 285
        patient positioning for, 284–285
        sensory block only for, 285
        tourniquet use in, 285
    floating, 266
    injury, special considerations with, 266
    ligament repair, 279
        arthroscopic, 286–287
    in osteitis deformans, 25
    surgery
        postoperative pain relief techniques for, 439–440
        regional anesthesia for, 201–203
    total replacement, 142–146
        anesthetic management for, 143
        antibiotic prophylaxis for, 143
        bilateral, 145–146
        conditions leading to, 142

epidural anesthesia for, 143
epidural fentanyl infusions after, 435
general anesthesia for, 143
indications for, 142
intrathecal/epidural narcotics for, 433–434
operation for, 142–143
peroneal nerve palsy after, 145
positioning for, 142
postoperative management in PACU, 145
in rheumatoid arthritis, 15
spinal anesthesia for, 143
tourniquets used in, 144
vascular injury in, intraoperative management of, 144
Kyphoscoliosis
    in Marfan syndrome, 29
    in neurofibromatosis, 30

L

Labetalol administration, in preparation for hypotensive anesthesia, 354
Laminar flow system(s), 120–121
Laryngoscopy, fiberoptic, in rheumatoid arthritis, 13–14
Larynx, in rheumatoid arthritis, 11
Lateral decubitus position
    precautions with, 123
    for shoulder arthroscopy, 282
Lateral femoral cutaneous nerve
    anatomy of, 202, 487–488
    dermatomal distribution of, 202f
Lateral femoral cutaneous nerve block. *See also* Inguinal paravascular block
    anatomy for, 205
    drug for, 205
    equipment, 205
    indications for, 201, 205
    for meralgia paresthetica, 488–489
        drugs for, 488
        equipment, 488
        landmarks for, 488
        patient positioning for, 488
        procedure, 488–489
    patient positioning for, 205
    procedure, 205–206, 206f

Lateral femoral cutaneous neuralgia. *See* Meralgia paresthetica
Latex, allergy and anaphylactic reactions to, 308–309
Left ventricular end-diastolic pressure, in chronic CHF, anesthetic considerations with, 103, 103*f*
Leg(s). *See* Lower extremity
Lidocaine
  administration, in geriatric patient, 107
  for brachial plexus block, 179
  dosage and administration, 166*t*
  indications for, 167
  intravenous, for neuropathic pain, 499–500
  pharmacology of, 166*t*
Limb-girdle dystrophy, 318
Limb-sparing surgery, 414–418
  anesthetic management for, 414–417
  blood loss during, 416
  coagulopathy with, 417
  for lower extremity, 416
  major resections and, 415–417
  postoperative care with, 417
  postoperative pain management with, 417–418
  preoperative preparation for, 414–415
  procedures for, 414
  psychological preparation of patient/family for, 415
  sedation before, 415
  for upper extremity, 416
Liver function test(s), preoperative, 272
Local anesthetics/anesthesia. *See also specific agent*
  for ambulatory surgery, 284
  bolus, for postoperative pain relief, 438
  choice of, 165–167, 166*t*
  with epidural steroids, 476
  epinephrine-containing, 167–168
  hematologic effects of, 156
  intra-arterial injection, prevention of, 162
  intravenous injection
    management of, 163, 166*t*
    toxicity with, 162–163, 166*t*
  oropharyngeal, for fiberoptic intubation, 13–14
  sodium bicarbonate added to, 168–169

solution alkalinization, for intravenous regional anesthesia, 228
solution temperature, for intravenous regional anesthesia, 228
with steroid injection
  for lumbar facet syndrome, 483–484
  for sacroiliac joint arthropathy, 484–485
toxicity, 162–165
  factors affecting, 163
  management of, 164, 164*t*, 165, 166*t*
  prevention of, 164–165
  signs and symptoms of, 162–163, 166*t*
vasoconstrictor added to, 167–168
warming, and onset of brachial plexus block, 180
wound infiltration with, for postoperative analgesia, 440
Lomustine, side effects of, 407*t*
Low back pain, 471–480
  chronic radicular, management of, 477
  differential diagnosis, 471–472
  postlaminectomy, treatment of, 474–475, 477
  in previous surgical patient, treatment of, 477
  and radiculopathy, 471–474
    from metastatic cancer, 475
    steroid therapy for, 473–476
  with sacroiliac joint arthropathy, 484–485
Lower extremity. *See also* Extremity(ies)
  amputation, 412, 414
  anesthesia for, 64
  blood flow, with regional anesthesia, 156
  differential neural blockade, in diagnosis of reflex sympathetic dystrophy, 455
  intravenous regional anesthesia in, 232–234
  limb-sparing surgery for, 416
  nerve blocks in, 201–227
    in children, 236–237
  nerves of, dermatomal distributions of, 202*f*
  prevention of venous thromboembolism in, 152–156
  problems, in children, 300–306
  regional sympathetic blockade using Bier blocks in, 466–467

resection, for tumor, intrathecal/epidural narcotics for, 433
surgery
  epidural fentanyl infusions after, 434–436
  intrathecal/epidural narcotics for, 433–434
  neurovascular evaluation with, 267
  patient positioning for, 264–265
  regional anesthesia for, 203, 236–237
  special considerations with, 264–267
Lumbar epidural blockade, in prevention of phantom limb pain, 491
Lumbar facet joints, anatomy of, 482
Lumbar facet syndrome, 482–484
  diagnosis of, 483
  diagnostic block in, 483
  pathology of, 482
  treatment of, 483
    complications of, 484
Lumbar plexus block. *See also* Inguinal paravascular block
  anatomy for, 215, 217*f*
  drug for, 216
  equipment, 216
  indications for, 201
  landmark for, 217
  patient positioning for, 216
  for postoperative analgesia, after knee surgery, 439–440
  procedure, 217–218, 218*f*
  of Winnie, 219
Lumbar spine
  injury
    associated injuries and problems, 68
    intraoperative considerations with, 73
  laminectomy, for disc removal, 395–398
    air embolism with, 398
    anesthetic management of, 396, 398
    in lateral position, 398
    patient positioning for, 396–397
    spinal anesthesia for, 398
    surgical procedure for, 397–398
  osteotomy, 399–400
  radiculopathy, 472–474
    acute discogenic, management of, 476
    evaluation and treatment of, 472–478
  surgery

for percutaneous discectomy, 395
for spinal stenosis, 398–399
Lumbar sympathetic block
  paravertebral
    anatomy for, 460
    drugs for, 461
    effects of, 463
    equipment for, 460–461
    landmarks for, 461
    patient positioning for, 461
    procedure, 461–462, 462*f*
    for reflex sympathetic dystrophy in lower extremity, 460–463
  for postherpetic neuralgia, 495
Lumboinguinal nerve, dermatomal distribution of, 202*f*
Lung(s). *See also under* Pulmonary
  apical fibrosis, in ankylosing spondylitis, 18
Lupus-like syndrome(s), drug-related, 22

M

Magnetic resonance imaging, of cervical spine, in rheumatoid arthritis, 10–11, 11*f*
Malignancy. *See also* Orthopedic oncology
  biopsy of, 405
  hemostatic alterations in, 410–411
  metastatic
    bleeding from, 411
    involving bone, management of, 418
    low back pain and radiculopathy from, 475
  thoracic spine surgery in, 394–395
Malignant hyperthermia
  cart, 333, 333*t*
  clinical manifestations of, 332–333
  creatine kinase in, 331, 335
  dantrolene pretreatment for, 335
  dantrolene treatment in, 333*t*, 333–334
  diagnosis, in operating room, 332
  genetic studies of, 331
  Hotline, 336
  keeping current with, 336
  masseter muscle rigidity and, 331
  in muscular dystrophy, 319, 321–322

Malignant hyperthermia *(Continued)*
in osteogenesis imperfecta, 313
patient management, 331–332
postoperative management, 334
susceptible patients, anesthetic management of, 334–335
treatment of, 333–334
triggering events, 330, 330*t*
Malignant Hyperthermia Association of the
United States, 336
Mandible
in acromegaly, 22–23
in arthrogryposis, 310–311
in rheumatoid arthritis, 4, 7
Mannitol, 55
Marfan syndrome, 28–30
anesthetic considerations in, 29–30
cardiac defects in, 343
clinical features of, 28–29
pulmonary involvement in, 29
Masseter muscle rigidity, and malignant
hyperthermia, 331
Mechanical ventilation, with pelvic
trauma, 77
Median nerve
causalgia, 451
distribution, at wrist, 197*f*
injury, with elbow fracture, 261
Median nerve block. *See also* Brachial plexus
block, axillary approach
at elbow
anatomy for, 194, 195*f*
procedure, 195
indications for, 189
at wrist, 197–198, 198*f*
Medication history
with hip fracture, 97
of rheumatoid arthritis patient, 12
for total hip replacement, 119–120
Melphalan, side effects of, 407*t*
Meningitis, pneumococcal, risk of, in sickle
cell disease, 31
Mental status
of elderly patient, in PACU, 113
postoperative, in trauma patient, 84–85
preoperative evaluation of, in hip fracture
patient, 100
Meperidine

for acute post-traumatic pain, 86
in continuous epidural blockade, for reflex
sympathetic dystrophy, 468
in patient-controlled analgesia, total hourly
dose for, 425
premedication, for spinal surgery, 353
to treat shivering, in elderly patient, in
PACU, 111
Mepivacaine
for brachial plexus block, 179
dosage and administration, 166*t*
pharmacology of, 166*t*
Meralgia paresthetica, 485–489
anatomic considerations in, 487
associated conditions, 485–486
conservative treatment of, 487–488
after coronary artery bypass surgery, 486
diagnosis of, 486–487
features of, 485
and hypothyroidism, 486
nerve block for, 488–489
and occupational activity, 486
in pregnancy, 486
6-Mercaptopurine, side effects of, 407*t*
Methotrexate, side effects of, 5*t*, 407*t*
Methyldopa, contraindications to, 100
Methylmethacrylate cement
adverse effects of, 131–135
cardiovascular effects of, 131–135
in hip fracture repair, 108–109
mode of action, 131–132
precautions with, 132
pulmonary effects of, 133–135
in total hip replacement, 131–135
vascular involvement, 139
Methylprednisolone, dosage and administration, with spinal cord injury, 65
Methylprednisolone acetate, epidural, dosage
and administration, 475–476
Metoclopramide, preoperative administration
of, 276, 278
in hip fracture patient, 98
Mexiletine, for neuropathic pain, 499–500
Midazolam administration
preoperative, 277
in trauma patient, 62
Migraine, history of, in surgical candidate, 270
Military antishock trousers, application of, 76

Mithramycin, side effects of, 407*t*
Mitomycin, side effects of, 407*t*
Mitral valve prolapse, and scoliosis, 343
Monitoring, intraoperative, 122–123. *See also*
    Neurogenic motor evoked potentials;
    Somatosensory evoked potentials
  for children with craniofacial abnormalities,
    317
  in hip fracture repair, 102–103
  in hip revision surgery, 140
  for pediatric surgical patient, 301
  in spinal surgery, 381–382
  in total hip replacement, 122–123
  for trauma patient, 57–61
Morphine
  for acute post-traumatic pain, 86
  in continuous epidural blockade, for reflex
    sympathetic dystrophy, 468
  epidural
    characteristics of, 431
    for children, 444–445
    side effects of, 431
    with total knee replacement, 143
  intra-articular, after arthroscopic knee
    surgery, 439
  intramuscular administration, in children,
    443
  intrathecal
    characteristics of, 431
    side effects of, 431
    with total hip replacement, 125
    with total knee replacement, 143
    for tourniquet pain, 248
  intravenous administration, in children, 443
  in patient-controlled analgesia
    basal infusion for, 425
    bolus (loading) dose, 424
    demand dose, 424
    lockout interval for, 424
    total hourly dose for, 425
  premedication, for spinal surgery, 353
  preservative-free, intrathecal/epidural
    administration of, 431
Morquio syndrome, 325–327
  with odontoid hypoplasia, 298
Mouth. *See also* Mandible
  assessment of, preanesthetic, 271
  opening, in scleroderma, 26

Mucopolysaccharidosis, 324–327
  type I (Hurler syndrome), 324–325
  type II (Hunter syndrome), 325
  type IV. *See* Morquio syndrome
Münchausen syndrome, 500
Muscle(s), in rheumatoid arthritis, 1
Muscle relaxant(s), administration
  for ambulatory surgery, 282
  in trauma patient, 62–63
Muscular dystrophy
  anesthetic considerations in, 320–321
  cardiac changes in, 343
  in children, 318–322
  malignant hyperthermia in, 319, 321–322
  postanesthetic considerations in, 322
  succinylcholine contraindicated in, 321
  surgical procedures in, 320
Musculocutaneous nerve block. *See also*
    Brachial plexus block, axillary
    approach; Brachial plexus block,
    infraclavicular approach
  at elbow
    anatomy for, 194, 195*f*
    procedure, 196
  indications for, 189
Musculoskeletal injury, in trauma patient,
    73–75
Myelodysplasia, and allergy and anaphylactic
    reactions to latex, 308–309
Myelography
  contrast agents for, adverse reactions to,
    379–380
  headache after, 379–381
  and renal function, 380
  before spinal surgery, 379–381
  surgery immediately after, special consid-
    erations with, 380
Myelomeningocele, 308
Myocardial infarction, recent, in hip fracture
    patient, 100
Myocarditis, in systemic lupus erythematosus,
    20
Myofascial pain, 481–482
Myoglobinuria
  after spinal surgery, 375
  in trauma patient, 59
Myotonic dystrophy, cardiovascular abnor-
    malities in, 346

N

Naloxone
dosage and administration, in children, 444
after scolosis surgery, 374
for wake-up test, 361
Narcotics. *See also specific agent*
combined with NSAIDs, 442
in continuous epidural blockade, for reflex sympathetic dystrophy, 467–468
epidural, for children, 444–445
intra-articular, after arthroscopic knee surgery, 439
intramuscular administration, 421
intrathecal/epidural
complications of, 436–438
intraoperative use of, 433–434
order sheet for, 429–430, 430*f*
with and without local anesthetics, 429–438
lipid solubility of, effect on therapeutic effectiveness, 430–431
lipophilic, characteristics of, 432
transdermal administration, for postoperative pain relief, 440–441
for trauma patient, 62
Nasotracheal intubation, precautions with, in trauma patient, 47
Nausea and vomiting
after ambulatory surgery, prevention of, 287–288
with intrathecal/epidural narcotics, 431, 437
in children, 444
Neck. *See also* Airway; Cervical spine
postoperative considerations with, in trauma patient, 85
Neck problems, in children, 293–295
Nerve block. *See also specific nerve block*
assessment of, 174
for children
with general anesthesia, 235
with sedation, 235
differential, in diagnosis of reflex sympathetic dystrophy, 455–457
digital, 199–201, 200*f*
at elbow, 194–197
failed, 163–164
lower extremity, 201–227

regional
for herpes zoster, 493
for postherpetic neuralgia, 494
successful
as function of decreasing stimulating current with nerve stimulator, 173, 174*t*
techniques for, 169
technique, 172–173
toxicity from. *See* Local anesthetics, toxicity
upper extremity, 174–201
at wrist, 197–199
Nerve compression, in osteitis deformans, 25
Nerve injury
caused by mechanical trauma, 162
in extremity trauma, 81
Nerve palsy, in hemophilia A, 37
Nerve stimulator
characteristics of, 170
insulated needles for, 171, 171*f*
use of, 162, 170–173
advantages of, 170
in axillary brachial plexus block, 191–193
in continuous brachial plexus block, 193–194
equipment for, 171–172
in femoral nerve block, 204–205
in infraclavicular brachial plexus block, 185–186
in inguinal paravascular block, 209–210
in interscalene brachial plexus block, 182–183
in pediatric extremity block, 235
in sciatic nerve block, 210–215
set-up for, 173*f*
in subclavian perivascular brachial plexus block, 187–188
technique, 172–173
Nesacaine, methylparaben-free, for regional anesthesia in short (1-hour) procedures, 284
Neuralgia. *See* Greater occipital neuralgia; Meralgia paresthetica; Postherpetic neuralgia
Neural tube defect(s), 308
Neurofibromatosis, 30
Neurogenic motor evoked potentials monitoring

interpretation of results, 370–372, 372*f*,
  373*f*
during spinal surgery, 360, 368–372
response characteristics of, 370, 371*f*
Neurologic changes
  in ankylosing spondylitis, 18
  in osteitis deformans, 25
  in systemic lupus erythematosus, 21
Neurologic evaluation
  preoperative, in hip fracture patient, 100
  in rheumatoid arthritis, 12
  after spinal surgery, 373
Neuromuscular disease. *See also specific
    disease*
  gastrointestinal system in, 346
  scoliosis with. *See* Scoliosis, neuromus-
    cular
  surgery-related problems in, 349
Neuropathic pain, 499–500
Nitrogen mustards, side effects of, 407*t*
Nitrous oxide
  administration, in geriatric patient, 107
  contraindications to, 61
Nonsteroidal anti-inflammatory drugs
  adverse effects of, 441
  for analgesia, 441
  side effects of, 5*t*
  therapy with, perioperative management of,
    119–120, 156
NPO status
  for ambulatory surgery patient, 274, 278
  for children, 317
Nucleus pulposus, material from, inflammato-
    ry effect of, 472

O

Obtunded patient
  missed injury in, 76
  radiologic evaluation of, 76
Obturator nerve
  anatomy of, 202–203
  dermatomal distribution of, 202*f*
Obturator nerve block, 206–208. *See also
    Inguinal paravascular block*
  anatomy for, 206
  drug for, 207

equipment, 207
indications for, 201, 206
landmark for, 207
patient positioning for, 207
procedure, 207–208, 208*f*
Ocular involvement, in juvenile rheumatoid
    arthritis, 327
Odontoid process
  abnormalities, 297–298
    in osteogenesis imperfecta, 313
  anatomy of, 296–297
  congenital separation of, 297
  hypoplasia of, 297–298
  ligamentous anatomy of, 7, 9*f*
  superior migration of, in rheumatoid
    arthritis, 8*f*, 10–11, 11*f*
  trauma to, 297
Operating room
  equipment for, 122–123
  infection control in, 120–121
  laminar flow, 120–121
  monitoring in, 122–123
Operative site, postoperative considerations
    with, in trauma patient, 86
Opioids
  high lipid solubility, 430–431
  lipid solubility of, effect on therapeutic
    effectiveness, 430–431
  low lipid solubility, 431
  preoperative administration of, 277
Organic mental syndrome, uncooperative
    patient with, management of, 109–110
Orthopedic oncology, 405–420. *See also
    Malignancy; Tumor(s)*
  biopsy in, 405
  chemotherapy in, 405–411
  definitive surgical procedures in,
    413–414
  limb-sparing surgery in, 414–418
  patient, preoperative evaluation of, 405
  surgery in, 411–418
Os odontoideum, 297
Osteitis deformans, 23–25
  anesthetic considerations in, 25
  epidemiology of, 23
  manifestations of, 24–25
  pathology of, 24
  sites of involvement, 24

Osteoarthritis, total hip replacement for,
117–118
Osteogenesis imperfecta, 312–315
    airway management in, 314
    anesthetic considerations with, 314
    cardiovascular abnormalities in, 313, 315
    clinical features of, 312
    intraoperative considerations with,
        314–315
    metabolic abnormalities in, 313–314
    postoperative care with, 315
    surgical procedures in, 314
    types of, 312
Osteomyelitis, in sickle cell disease, 31
Oxygen
    administration
        during hip fracture repair, 109
        in sickle cell disease, 34
    concentrations, during anesthesia, in
        bleomycin chemotherapy patient, 409
Oxygenation, arterial, decreases, with methyl-
    methacrylate cement, 133–135, 134*f*,
    135*f*

P

Paget's disease of bone, 23–25
Pain/pain syndrome(s), 447. *See also*
        Causalgia; Low back pain; Myofascial
        pain; Phantom limb pain; Reflex sym-
        pathetic dystrophy; Tourniquet pain
    approach to patient with, 447–448
    comprehensive management of, 448
    definition of, 448
    factitious, 500
    neuropathic, 499–500
    sympathetic mediated, 449
Pain management. *See also* Patient-controlled
        analgesia
    acute post-traumatic, 86
    emergency, in trauma patient, 55–56
    epidural narcotics for, 429–438
    intramuscular narcotic administration for,
        421
    intrathecal narcotics for, 429–438
    postoperative, 421–446
        in children, 302, 442–445

for elderly patient, 112–113
with hip surgery, 142
intrathecal/epidural narcotics for,
    429–438
with limb-sparing surgery, 417–418
local anesthetic bolus for, 438
with pelvic fracture, 79
planning for, 421
techniques for, 421
with total hip replacement, 124
with total knee replacement, 143
for trauma patient, 86
Pancuronium, administration, in trauma
    patient, 63
Paralysis, post-tourniquet, 245
Paraplegia, in neurofibromatosis, 30
Parkinson's disease, and hip fracture, preop-
    erative management of, 100–101
Partial thromboplastin time
    in hemophilia A, 37
    preoperative testing of, 272
Patient-controlled analgesia, 422–429
    basal infusion, 425, 427
    bolus (loading) dose, 424, 426–427
    in children, 444
    demand dose, 424, 427
    development of, 422–423
    disadvantages of, 429
    with epidural fentanyl infusions, 434–436
    flow sheet for, 427, 428*f*
    lockout interval, 424
    method for, 423–424
    order sheet, 425–426, 426*f*
    pain with, 429
    paradigm for, 422, 422*f*
    for postoperative pain, 86
    starting, 426–427
    terminology for, 424–425
    total hourly dose, 425
    with total knee replacement, 143
Pediatric orthopedics, 293–338. *See also*
        Child(ren); Infant(s)
Pediatric patient(s). *See* Child(ren); Infant(s)
Pelvic fracture(s), 76–79
    anesthetic technique with, 79
    associated problems, 78
    exsanguinating, protocols for, 78
    external fixation, 77

hemorrhage with
  embolization for, 78
  initial management of, 76
  management of, 77–78
  management of, 76–77
  mechanism of injury in, 78
  mortality with, 77
  open book, 77–78
  postoperative pain relief with, 79
  repair, intrathecal/epidural narcotics for,
    433
  respiratory problems with, 78
Penicillamine, side effects, 5t
Pericardial effusion, in rheumatoid arthritis, 2
Pericarditis, in rheumatoid arthritis, 2
Peritoneal lavage, diagnostic, 76
Peroneal nerve, palsy, after total knee
  replacement, 145
Pertrach Tracheotomy Set, 49, 50f
Pfeiffer syndrome, 306, 316
Phantom limb pain, 490–492
  prevention of, 491–492
Physical therapy, for reflex sympathetic
  dystrophy, 468
Piroxicam, combined with morphine, 442
Plantar nerve
  lateral, dermatomal distribution of, 202f
  middle, dermatomal distribution of, 202f
Plaquenil, side effects, 5t
Pleural effusion, in rheumatoid arthritis, 3
Pneumatic antishock garment, application of,
  76–77
Pneumatic compression boots, intermittent,
  152
Pneumococcal infection, risk of, in sickle cell
  disease, 31
Pneumoconiosis, in rheumatoid lung disease, 3
Pneumonia, and hip fracture, 98
Pneumothorax, 85
  intraoperative development of
    after chest tube removal, 60–61
    in trauma patient, 60–61
  after spinal surgery, 375
  in trauma patient, 60
Popliteal artery, injury, 79
Positioning
  in Marfan syndrome, 29
  of trauma patient, 55

Posterior femoral cutaneous nerve, dermatomal
  distribution of, 202f
Posterior tibial nerve
  anatomy of, 224, 224f
Posterior tibial nerve block, 226f, 226–227
Postherpetic neuralgia, 493–495
  characteristics of, 493–494
  treatment of, 494–495
Premedication
  for ambulatory surgery, 276–278
  for Bier block, 464
  for lumbar sympathetic block, 460
  for spinal surgery, 353
  for total hip replacement, 120
Procainamide, lupus-like syndromes caused
  by, 22
Procarbazine, side effects of, 407t
Progressive systemic sclerosis. See
  Scleroderma
Promit, for prevention of anaphylactoid-/
  anaphylactic reactions with dextran,
  154–155
Propofol
  administration, for ambulatory surgery, 281
  for tourniquet pain, 248
Propranolol, administration, in preparation for
  hypotensive anesthesia, 354
Prostaglandin inhibitors, for postoperative
  pain relief, 441–442
Prothrombin time, preoperative testing of,
  272
Pruritus, with intrathecal/epidural narcotics,
  431, 436–437
  in children, 444
Psoas compartment block of Chayen,
  218–219
Pulmonary artery catheterization
  during hip fracture repair, 102–103
  in trauma patient, 58
Pulmonary artery lines, indications for, 122
Pulmonary edema, after cervical spine injury,
  65, 70
Pulmonary embolism
  fatal
    incidence of, 151
    prevention of, 151–156
  occult (subclinical), 156, 158
  prevention of, 151–156

Pulmonary embolism *(Continued)*
  signs and symptoms of, 156–158
  in total hip replacement, 137
  with tourniquet use, 246, 252–253
  workup for, 157
Pulmonary evaluation, after spinal surgery,
    373–374
Pulmonary function
  with arthrogryposis, 348
  in scoliosis, 341–342
Pulmonary function test(s)
  in ankylosing spondylitis, 18
  in chemotherapy patient, 409
  with neuromuscular scoliosis, 345
  in scleroderma, 27
Pulmonary hypertension, in scoliosis,
    342–343
Pulmonary involvement
  in Marfan syndrome, 29
  in mucopolysaccharidoses, 325–326
  in rheumatoid arthritis, 3
  in scleroderma, 26
  in sickle cell disease, 31
  in systemic lupus erythematosus, 21
Pulmonary system, preoperative management,
    in hip fracture patient, 98
Pulse oximetry
  intraoperative, during hip fracture repair,
    102
  in total hip replacement, 122
  in trauma patient, 57–58

R

Radial nerve
  distribution, at wrist, 197*f*
  injury
    with elbow fracture, 261
    with humeral shaft fracture, 261
    traumatic, 81
Radial nerve block. *See also* Brachial plexus
    block, axillary approach
  at elbow
    anatomy for, 194, 195*f*
    procedure, 195–196
  indications for, 189
  at wrist, 199, 199*f*

Ranitidine, preoperative administration of,
    276, 278
Rash, in systemic lupus erythematosus, 20
Raynaud's phenomenon, in scleroderma, 26
Referred pain, from facet joint stimulation, 483
Reflex sympathetic dystrophy, 449–471
  cardinal features of, 449
  case reports, 469–470
  in children, 468–469
  clinical features of, 454
  diagnosis of, 453–456
    differential neural blockade in, 455–457
  differential diagnosis, 456
  in lower extremity
    diagnosis of, 455
    lumbar sympathetic block for, 460–463
  pathophysiology of, 452
  physical therapy for, 468
  precipitating factors, 449–451
  radiographic findings in, 454
  scintigraphy in, 455
  stages of, 452–453
  thermography in, 455
  treatment of, 456–468
    by Bier blocks, 463–467
    with continuous epidural blockade,
      467–468
    with corticosteroids, 468
    by sympathetic ganglion blockade,
      456–463
  with underlying surgically correctable
    disease, 470–471
  in upper extremity
    diagnosis of, 455
    stellate ganglion block for, 457–460
  variants, 451
Regional anesthesia, 161–242. *See also* Nerve
    block
  in ankylosing spondylitis, 19
  and anticoagulation, 156
  antithrombotic effect of, 155–156
  Bernstein's rules of, 161
  in children, 234–239
    drugs for, 235–237
  choice of anesthetic for, 165–167, 166*t*
  intravenous, 227–234
    in children, 239
    complications of, 234

continuous, in upper extremity, 232
contraindications to, 227
equipment, 227–228
exsanguination technique for, 228–229
in lower extremity, 232–234
solution alkalinization for, 228
solution temperature for, 228
in upper extremity, 229–232
needle for, 162
patient information about, 275–276
preoperative patient preparation for,
        161–162
preparation for, 169
for reimplantation of digits, 260
in scleroderma, 28
sedation with, 161–162, 169, 174
in sickle cell disease, 34
total joint replacement, 124–125
in trauma patient, 63–64
for upper extremity, in rheumatoid arthritis,
        14
Regurgitation, in scleroderma, 26–27
Reimplantation
of arm, 261
of digits, 260
of forearm, 261
Relton-Hall frame, 355, 356f
Renal failure, in trauma patient, prevention,
        55, 60
Renal function
in ankylosing spondylitis, 18
and chemotherapy, 407t, 409–410
in juvenile rheumatoid arthritis, 327
and postoperative mortality in surgical
        patient, 93
in rheumatoid disease, 4
in scleroderma, 26
in sickle cell disease, 32
in systemic lupus erythematosus, 21–22
Renarcotization, after extubation, 108–109
Reserpine, regional sympathetic blockade
        using, 463
Respiratory depression, with intrathecal/-
        epidural narcotics, 431, 436–437
in children, 444
Respiratory function
intraoperative monitoring, in trauma patient,
        57–58

and spinal cord injury, 68–69
Respiratory involvement
in ankylosing spondylitis, 17–18
with pelvic fracture, 78
Respiratory muscle weakness, in muscular
        dystrophy, 319–320
Respiratory physiology, with scoliosis, 341
Respiratory therapy, for geriatric patient, in
        PACU, 111
Rhabdomyolysis, in Duchenne's dystrophy,
        319
Rheumatoid arthritis, 1–16
airway management in, 4–7
cervical spine in, 5, 7–11
cricoarytenoid involvement in, 5–7
endotracheal intubation in, 13–14
juvenile, 327–329
    airway management in, 327–328
    cervical spine in, 300
    patient positioning in, 329
mandibular involvement in, 4, 7
pharmacotherapy, side effects of, 4, 5t
preoperative considerations in, 12–13,
        271
surgical procedures in, 14–16
systemic effects of, 1–4, 2f
treatment of, 4, 5t
Rheumatoid nodules, 1
Rhizotomy, selective posterior, 323–324
Ropivacaine
dosage and administration, 166t
pharmacology of, 166t

S

Sacroiliac joint, arthropathy, 484–485
Salicylates, side effects, 5t
Saline injections, for low back pain and
        radiculopathy, 473
Saphenous nerve
anatomy of, 202, 221, 224, 224f
dermatomal distribution of, 202f
Saphenous nerve block, 225f, 226
at knee
    drug for, 222
    equipment for, 222
    procedure, 222, 223f

Sarcoma(s), surgery for, 411–413
    muscle compartment excision, 413
    wide excision, 412
Scapula, congenital high, 295–296
Sciatic nerve
    anatomy of, 203
    causalgia, 451
    injury
        in hip surgery, 135–136, 141
        traumatic, 81
Sciatic nerve block, 64, 210–215
    anatomy for, 210
    anterior approach of Beck
        indications for, 213
        landmark for, 213
        patient positioning for, 213
        procedure, 214f, 214–215
    in children, 236
    equipment, 210
    indications for, 201
    lateral approach of Ischiyanaga, 215, 216f
    posterior approach of Labat
        drug for, 211
        landmark for, 211
        patient positioning for, 211, 211f
        procedure, 211–212
    supine approach of Raj
        patient positioning for, 212
        procedure, 212–213, 213f
Scintigraphy, in reflex sympathetic dystrophy, 455
Sclerae, blue, 312
Scleroderma, 25–28
    airway management in, 26
    arterial puncture in, 27
    endotracheal intubation in, 26
    epidemiology of, 25
    manifestations of, 25–26
    postoperative care in, in postanesthesia care unit, 28
    regurgitation in, 26, 27
    ventilatory support in, postoperative, 28
Scleromalacia perforans, 4
Scoliosis, 339–377
    with arthrogryposis, 310–311, 348
    cardiac changes with, 343
    in cerebral palsy, 347
    in Charcot-Marie-Tooth disease, 347

classification of, 339
congenital deformities with, 343
in Duchenne's muscular dystrophy, 348
in Friedreich's ataxia, 347
idiopathic, 343
mitral valve prolapse with, 343
neuromuscular, 341
    arterial blood gas determination in, 345
    cardiovascular evaluation in, 345
    characteristics of, 344
    classification of, 344
    gastrointestinal problems with, 346
    preoperative considerations with, 344–349
    pulmonary function in, 349
    pulmonary function tests with, 345
    respiratory considerations with, 344–345
    seizure disorders with, 346
    surgery-related problems in, 349
    vital capacity in, 345
operative correction of
    anesthetic equipment for, 353–354
    blood loss after, monitoring, 374
    blood loss in, control of, 357–358
    blood salvage in, 357
    body temperature monitoring after, 374
    cast syndrome after, 375
    combined anterior and posterior approaches, 356–357
    extubation after, 374
    homologous blood transfusion in, methods to decrease, 350–353
    hypotensive anesthesia in, 354–355, 358–359
    ileus after, 375
    induced hypotension in, 357–358
    myoglobinuria after, 375
    neurogenic motor evoked potential monitoring during, 360, 368–372
    neurologic evaluation after, 373
    patient positioning for, 355, 356f
    pneumothorax after, 375
    postoperative care, 373–375
    premedication for, 353
    preoperative preparation and evaluation for, 349–350
    prevention of hypothermia in, 354
    pulmonary evaluation after, 373–374

spinal cord function during, 359–372
spinal cord injury in, steroid use for, 372
SSEP monitoring during, 360, 362–368
urine output after, monitoring, 375
venous air embolism in, 372–373
volume status after, 374
wake-up test in, 350, 360–362
in osteogenesis imperfecta, 315
pulmonary function with, 341–342,
    344–345, 349
pulmonary hypertension in, 342–343
respiratory physiology with, 341
spinal curvature in, determination of, 339,
    340f
with spinal muscle atrophy, 348
in syringomyelia, 347–348
treatment of, historical advances in, 339,
    340t
vital capacity with, 345
    and postoperative ventilatory manage-
    ment, 342
Sedation
for fiberoptic intubation, 14
with intrathecal/epidural narcotics, 438
for knee arthroscopy, 285
before limb-sparing surgery, 415
precautions with, in scleroderma, 28
with regional anesthesia, 161–162, 169, 174
with spinal anesthesia, for hip fracture
    repair, 107
Sedatives, preoperative administration of,
    277
Seizure disorders, with neuromuscular scol-
    iosis, 346
Seizure threshold, drugs affecting, 379
Septicemia, pneumococcal, risk of, in sickle
    cell disease, 31
Shivering, in elderly patient, in PACU, 111
Shock. *See also* Spinal shock
hemorrhagic, 52
Shoulder
arthroscopy of, 282–283
    anesthesia for, 283
    patient positioning for, 282–283
innervation of, 180
painful, 496–499
    causes of, 496
regional anesthesia for, 178t, 180–183

surgery
    neutral head position for, 264
    special considerations with, 263–264
total replacement
    anesthetic management for, 147
    general anesthesia for, 147
    indications for, 146
    operation for, 146
    positioning for, 146–147
    postoperative care with, 147
    regional anesthesia for, 147
Shoulder-hand syndrome, 451
Sickle cell disease, 31–36
anesthetic management in, 33–34
and blood salvage devices, 35
as contraindication to tourniquet use, 33,
    254
extubation in, 36
factors that induce sickling in, 34
hydration in, 33–34
manifestations of, 31–32
pathophysiology of, 31
postoperative care in, 36
preoperative considerations in, 32–33
surgical procedures in, 34–36
transfusion therapy in, 32t, 32–33
Sickle cell trait, 33
anesthetic management with, 36
as contraindication to tourniquet use, 254
Sitting position
for cervical spine surgery, 388
general anesthesia in, problems associated
    with, 147
Skin
in rheumatoid arthritis, 1
in scleroderma, 25
in systemic lupus erythematosus, 20
trophic changes
    in causalgia, 452
    in reflex sympathetic dystrophy, 449, 453
Skull, cloverleaf-shaped, 316
Slipped capital femoral epiphysis, 305
Sodium bicarbonate, added to local anesthet-
    ics, 168–169
Sodium nitroprusside, 358
Somatosensory evoked potentials
alterations in, 366–367, 367f
    anesthesiologist's response to, 367–368

Somatosensory evoked potentials *(Continued)*
  deteriorated, and wake-up test, 368
  factors affecting, 364–365
  and inhalation agents, 365–366, 366*f*
  monitoring
    in asthmatic patient, 368, 369*f*–370*f*
    during cervical spine fusion, 383, 384, 385*f*
    with epidural electrodes, 368, 369*f*–370*f*
    in hip surgery, 136
    in pelvic fracture repair, 79
    principles of, 362–363, 363*f*
    procedure, 363–364, 364*f*–365*f*
    during shoulder arthroscopy, 282
    with spinal cord injury, 72
    during spinal surgery, 360, 362–368
    during thoracic spine surgery, 393–394
  and neurogenic motor evoked potentials,
    simultaneous monitoring of, during
    spinal surgery, 371–372
Spasticity, in cerebral palsy, 323–324
Spina bifida, 308
Spinal anesthesia
  in acromegaly, 23
  for ambulatory surgery, transfer from
    recovery bed to chair after, 289
  contraindications to, 63
  fluid balance with, 106, 141
  for hip fracture repair, 105–107
    contraindications to, with valvular heart
      disease, 107
    and hypotension, 106
    nausea and vomiting with, 107
    sedation during, 107
  in infants, 237–238
  for lumbar disc surgery, 398
  patient information about, 275–276
  total joint replacement, 125
Spinal cord
  blood supply to, 359–360, 360*f*
  function, during operative correction of
    scoliosis, 359–372
  injury. *See also* Cervical spine, injury
    acute, management of, 64–75
    associated cord syndromes, 67
    associated injuries and problems, 67–68
    bradycardia with, 70
    corticosteroid treatment with, 65–66
  distribution of, 64
  epidemiology of, 64
  hemodynamic responses to, 69
  intraoperative considerations with, 72–75
  intubation with, 69
  perioperative considerations with, 72
  and respiratory function, 68–69
  perfusion pressure, after spinal cord injury,
    66
  sensory pathways of, 362–363, 363*f*
Spinal deformities, conditions associated
  with, 296
Spinal muscle atrophy, special considerations
  with, 348
Spinal nerve roots
  C3-C6, block. *See* Brachial plexus block,
    interscalene approach
  C5-C8, block, 183–184
  C5-T1, block, 189
  L2-S2, block, 201
  L5-S1, irritation, in disc disease, 473–475
  T10-S2, block, 201
  T1-T2, block, 181, 183–184
Spinal shock, 64
  and autonomic hyperreflexia, 71
  duration of, 71
  etiology of, 70–71
  fluid therapy in, 70
Spinal surgery, 379–403. *See also* Scoliosis,
    operative correction of
  anesthetic considerations with, 381
  anesthetic management of, 381–382
  for ankylosing spondylitis, 399–400
  blood pressure control during, 382
  for fixed flexion deformity, 399
  hypotensive anesthesia for
    β-blockade before, 354
    induction and maintenance of, 354–355
    preparation for, 354
  monitoring during, 381–382
  myelography before, 379–381
  patient positioning for, 382
  positioning for, 355, 356*f*
  prevention of thromboembolism in, 158,
    382
  venous access for, 382
Sprengel's deformity, 295–296, 343
Steel's rule of thirds, 8

Stellate ganglion, anatomy of, 457
Stellate ganglion block
    complications of, 460
    drugs for, 458
    effects of, 459
    equipment for, 457
    Horner syndrome with, 459–460
    landmarks for, 458
    patient positioning for, 458
    for postherpetic neuralgia, 495
    procedure, 458–459, 459f
    in reflex sympathetic dystrophy
        diagnostic, 455
        therapeutic, 457–460
    side effects of, 460
Steroids
    epidural
        for cervical radiculopathy, 478–480
        dosage and administration, 475–476
        drugs for, 475
        epidural hematoma with, 478
        indications for, 474–475
        local anesthetics with, 476
        for low back pain and radiculopathy,
            473–476
        systemic effects of, 478
        and tight epidural space, 478
    injection
        for lumbar facet syndrome, 483–484
        for sacroiliac joint arthropathy, 484–485
    intrathecal injection, 478
    prophylactic, for fat embolism, 83–84
    for spinal cord injury, 65–66
        in spinal surgery, 372
    systemic, for herpes zoster, 493
Steroid therapy, for rheumatoid arthritis,
    complications of, 3
Streeter's dysplasia, 307
Streptozocin, side effects of, 407t
Stroke, and hip fracture, management of, 101
Stump pain, 490–491
Subaxial subluxation, in rheumatoid arthritis,
    8f, 10, 11f
Subclavian artery, injury, 79
Succinylcholine
    administration, in trauma patient, 62–63
    contraindications to, in Duchenne's
        dystrophy, 321

Sudeck's atrophy of bone, 451
Sufentanil
    administration
        for spinal surgery, 354–355
        in trauma patient, 62
    epidural
        characteristics of, 432
        dosage and administration, 432
Superficial peroneal nerve
    anatomy of, 224
    dermatomal distribution of, 202f
Superficial peroneal nerve block, 225f, 226
Supine position, precautions with, 123
Suprascapular nerve, anatomy of, 496
Suprascapular nerve block
    complications of, 498
    continuous, 498–499
    drugs for, 496
    equipment for, 496
    indications for, 498
    landmarks for, 496–497
    for painful shoulder, 496–498
    patient positioning for, 497
    procedure, 497f, 497–498
Sural nerve
    anatomy of, 224, 224f
    dermatomal distribution of, 202f
Sural nerve block, 226, 226f
Sympathetic ganglion blockade, in reflex
        sympathetic dystrophy, 456–463
Syndactyly, 306, 315–316
    surgery for, 317–318
Syndrome of inappropriate antidiuretic
        hormone secretion, with vincristine,
        410
Syringomyelia, special considerations in,
        347–348
Systemic lupus erythematosus, 20–22
    airway management in, 21
    anesthetic considerations in, 21–22
    manifestations of, 20–21

T

Tache cérébrale, 468
Talipes equinovarus. See Club foot,
        congenital

T-cell abnormalities, in rheumatoid arthritis, 3–4
Temporomandibular joint, abnormalities, 4, 17
Tension pneumothorax, 60–61
β-Thalassemia, 31, 33
Thermography, in reflex sympathetic dystrophy, 455
Thiopental
  administration
    in geriatric patient, 107
    in trauma patient, 61
  for convulsions, in local anesthetic toxicity, 165
Thoracic somatic nerve block, paravertebral, for postherpetic neuralgia, 495
Thoracic spine
  injury
    associated injuries and problems, 67
    intraoperative considerations with, 72–73
    respiratory problems with, 68
  osteotomy, for thoracic kyphosis, 400–401
  surgery
    indications for, 393
    with malignancy, 394–395
    in trauma, 393–394
Three-in-one block. See Inguinal paravascular block
Thromboembolism, 151–160
  incidence of, 151
    and anesthetic technique, 155–156
  prevention of, 151–156, 382
    during spinal surgery, 158
  risk factors for, 151–152
  signs and symptoms of, 156–158
Thromboplastic elements, with methyl-methacrylate cement, 133
Thumb, base of, surgery at, anesthesia for, 189
Tibia
  congenital pseudarthrosis of, 305–306
  fracture, repair, special considerations with, 265
  saber sword appearance, in osteitis deformans, 25
Tibial nerve

anatomy of, 219
dermatomal distribution of, 202f
Tibial nerve block, at knee, 219–220, 220f
  equipment for, 218
  patient positioning for, 218
  procedure, 220, 220f
Tibial plateau, fracture, repair, special considerations with, 265–266
Torticollis, congenital muscular, 293–294
Tourniquet(s), 243–255
  in Bier block
    in lower extremity, 466–467
    in upper extremity, 464–465
  bilateral simultaneous
    contraindications to, 253, 267
    effects on body temperature, 250, 250f
  on calf, complications of, 253–254
  contraindications to, 144, 254
    in head-injured patient, 75, 249, 249f
    in sickle cell disease, 33, 254
  creeping deflation of, 244
  duration of inflation (tourniquet time), 244–245
    maximizing, 246
    two-hour limit on, 244–245
  effect on body temperature, 250f, 250–251
  equipment, 243
  forearm
    complications of, 253–254
    intravenous regional anesthesia with, 231–232
  hemodynamic effects of, 247–248
  inflation pressure, 244
  postoperative edema with, 245
  preparation solution, skin damage from, 246
  and pulmonary embolism, 246, 252–253
  puncture, 246
  release, 246
    in asthmatic patient, 253
    effect on body temperature, 250–251, 251f
    hemorrhage after, in total knee replacement, 144
    metabolic changes with, 251–252, 252t
    systemic effects, 144, 251–253
  removal, 246, 288

size of, 244
tissue damage with, 245–246
use of
   and atherosclerotic disease, 245–246
   with intravenous regional anesthesia,
     227–234
   in knee arthroscopy, 285
   paralysis after, 245
   procedure, 243
   in total knee replacement, 144
Tourniquet pain, 247–248, 259
  blocking, 143, 184, 193
  epidural fentanyl for, 434
Trachea. *See also* Airway
  in rheumatoid arthritis, 11
Tranquilizers, preoperative administration of,
   277
Transcutaneous electrical nerve stimulation,
   for trigger points, 482
Transfusion reaction(s), 54
Transfusion therapy. *See also* Autotransfusion; Blood, reinfusion
  in hip fracture patient, 109
  homologous
   in scoliosis surgery, methods to
    decrease, 350–353
   in total hip replacement, avoiding, 127,
    130
   in tumor surgery, 411
  in sickle cell disease, 32*t*, 32–33, 35
  in trauma patient, 53–54
  in tumor surgery, 411
Transverse axial ligament, 7, 9*f*
  disruption of, 8, 9*f*
Trauma (patient), 43–89
  airway management in, 46–51
  anesthetic management in, 61–64
  autotransfusion in, 53
  cervical spine protection/precautions in,
   46–48
  circulation in, 52–53
  cricothyrotomy in, 48–49, 50*f*
  crystalloid infusion in, 53
  fluid resuscitation in, 52–53
  induction in, 61–62
  intraoperative monitoring of, 57–61
  intravenous access in, 52
  intubation, 46

  with awake patient, 46
  and full stomach, 47
  retrograde wire technique, 51
  with unconscious patient, 47
jet ventilation with intravenous catheter in,
   49–51
mortality, 43
muscle relaxants for, 62–63
musculoskeletal injury in, 73–75
pain management in, 55–56
pneumothorax in, 60–61
positioning, 55
postoperative considerations, 84–86
regional anesthesia in, 63–64
transfusion therapy in, 53–54
transport to operating room, 56
treatment of
  anesthesiologist's role in, 46–61
  essential components of, 43–44
urinary output, 55
  intraoperative monitoring of, 59
ventilation in, 51–52
Trauma operating room, 56
  equipment, 56–57
Trauma score, 44, 45*t*
Triamcinolone acetate, epidural, dosage and
   administration, 475–476
Trigger points, 481–482
Trisomy 21, cervical spine in, 299
Tuberculosis, and rheumatoid arthritis
   therapy, 3
Tumor(s). *See also* Bone tumor(s); Malignancy; Orthopedic oncology;
   Sarcoma(s)
  as contraindication to axillary block, 258
  as contraindication to tourniquet use, 254
  metastatic, bleeding from, 411
Tumor surgery, transfusion in, 411

U

Ulnar nerve
  distribution, at wrist, 197*f*
  injury
   with elbow fracture, 261
   intraoperative, 258
   traumatic, 81

Ulnar nerve *(Continued)*
  neuropathy, postoperative, 258–259
Ulnar nerve block. *See also* Brachial plexus
    block, axillary approach
  at elbow
    anatomy for, 194, 196*f*
    procedure, 196*f*, 196–197
  at wrist, 198*f*, 198–199
Ultraviolet light, in infection control, 121
Unconscious patient
  intubation, 47
  missed injury in, 76
  radiologic evaluation of, 76
Uncooperative patient, with organic mental
    syndrome, management of,
    109–110
Universal precautions, 40
Upper extremity. *See also* Arm(s); Extrem-
    ity(ies); Hand; Wrist
  amputation
    for bone tumors, 414
    for sarcoma, 412
  anesthesia for, 63
  differential neural blockade, in diagnosis
    of reflex sympathetic dystrophy,
    455
  intravenous regional anesthesia for, 229*f*,
    229–232
  large, intravenous regional anesthesia for,
    231
  limb-sparing surgery for, 416
  nerve blocks in, 174–201
    in children, 235–236
  peripheral nerves of, 175*f*, 176*f*, 177
  problems, in children, 306–308
  regional sympathetic blockade using Bier
    blocks in, 464–466
  surgery
    regional anesthesia for, in children, 235
    in rheumatoid arthritis, 14–15
Urinary output
  monitoring
    in hip fracture patient, 103
    postoperative, 86, 123
    after spinal surgery, 375
    in total hip replacement, 122–123
  of trauma patient, 55
    intraoperative monitoring of, 59

Urinary retention, with intrathecal/epidural
    narcotics, 431, 438
  in children, 444

V

Vascular injury
  with fracture dislocations, 79
    of knee, 266
  presenting signs (five P's), 80
  in total knee replacement, intraoperative
    management of, 144
Vasoconstrictor, added to local anesthetics,
    167–168
Vasodilator(s). *See also* Hypotension,
    induced; Hypotensive anesthesia
  precautions with, in Marfan syndrome, 29
  use of, with tourniquet, 248
Vasovagal reaction, with cervical epidural
    steroid injection, 480
Vater syndrome, 307–308
Vecuronium, administration, in trauma
    patient, 63
Venous access, for spinal surgery, 382
Ventilation
  during anesthesia, in ankylosing spondylitis,
    19
  jet, with intravenous catheter, in trauma
    patient, 49–51
  in trauma patient, 51–52
Ventilatory problems, in arthrogryposis, 311
Ventilatory support, in scleroderma, post-
    operative, 28
Vertebral artery involvement, in rheumatoid
    arthritis, 13
Vertebrobasilar artery insufficiency, 13
Vinblastine, neurotoxicity of, 407*t*, 410
Vincristine, neurotoxicity of, 407*t*, 410
Vindesine, neurotoxicity of, 410
Vital capacity, with scoliosis
  and postoperative ventilatory management,
    342
  preoperative determination of, 345
Volume status, monitoring, after spinal
    surgery, 374
von Recklinghausen's disease. *See* Neuro-
    fibromatosis

W

Wake-up test
  and deteriorated somatosensory evoked
    potentials, 368
  in scoliosis surgery, 350, 360–362
Warfarin, for prevention of venous thrombo-
    embolism, 155
Whistling face syndrome, 317
Wrist
  anatomic distribution of nerves at, 197, 197*f*

fracture, complications of, 261
nerve blocks at, 197–199
regional anesthesia for, 178*t*, 189–193
surgery, in rheumatoid arthritis, 14–15

Z

Zielke's technique, for correction of kyphosis
  in ankylosing spondylitis, 401
Zovirax. *See* Acyclovir